Practical Pediatric Gastrointestinal Endoscopy

Practical Pediatric Gastrointestinal Endoscopy

Third Edition

Edited by

George Gershman
Professor of Pediatrics, David Geffen School of Medicine
Chief, Division of Pediatrics Gastroenterology, Hepatology and Nutrition
Harbor-UCLA Medical Center
Torrance, California, USA

Mike Thomson
Professor of Paediatric Gastroenterology and Interventional Endoscopy
Director of the International Academy for Paediatric Endoscopy Training
Centre for Paediatric Gastroenterology, Nutrition and Haepatology
Sheffield Children's Hospital NHS Foundation Trust
Sheffield, UK;
Portland Hospital for Women and Children
London, UK

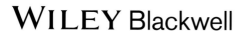

Edition history
Blackwell Publishing Ltd. (2e, 2011)

Registered Offices
John Wiley & Sons, Inc., 111 River Street, Hoboken, NJ 07030, USA
John Wiley & Sons Ltd, The Atrium, Southern Gate, Chichester, West Sussex, PO19 8SQ, UK

Editorial Office
9600 Garsington Road, Oxford, OX4 2DQ, UK

For details of our global editorial offices, customer services, and more information about Wiley products visit us at www.wiley.com.

Wiley also publishes its books in a variety of electronic formats and by print-on-demand. Some content that appears in standard print versions of this book may not be available in other formats.

Library of Congress Cataloging-in-Publication Data
Names: Gershman, George, editor. | Thomson, Mike (Mike Andrew), editor.
Title: Practical pediatric gastrointestinal endoscopy / edited by George
   Gershman, Mike Thomson.
Description: Third edition. | Hoboken, NJ : Wiley-Blackwell, 2021. |
   Includes bibliographical references and index.
Identifiers: LCCN 2020022834 (print) | LCCN 2020022835 (ebook) | ISBN
   9781119423454 (hardback) | ISBN 9781119423416 (adobe pdf) | ISBN
   9781119423485 (epub)
Subjects: MESH: Endoscopy, Gastrointestinal | Pediatrics–methods | Child |
   Infant
Classification: LCC RJ446 (print) | LCC RJ446 (ebook) | NLM WI 190 | DDC
   618.92/3307545–dc23
LC record available at https://lccn.loc.gov/2020022834
LC ebook record available at https://lccn.loc.gov/2020022835

Cover Design: Wiley
Cover Image: © FatCamera/Getty Images

Set in 9.5/12.5pt STIXTwoText by SPi Global, Pondicherry, India

Printed and bound in Singapore by Markono Print Media Pte Ltd
10 9 8 7 6 5 4 3 2 1

Contents

Personal statements

George Gershman
To the new generations of pediatric gastroenter-ologists and endoscopy enthusiasts: a letter to the future.

Once upon a time, there was a young fellow in Moscow, Russia, who was a resident working in one of the oldest hospitals in Moscow, named after Yevgeny Botkin, court physician to Tsar Nicholas II (who was murdered along with the entire Tsarust family by Bolsheviks in 1918).

The training was all about patient care. The diagnostic tools were limited to a stethoscope, basic laboratory support, and X-rays. The time felt almost frozen.

One day, I heard a rumor that one of the attending physician named Eduard Rokhlin was performing unique procedures, and out of curiosity I asked for permission to watch.

To my surprise, I was allowed not only to observe the study but look inside the endo-scope. I still remember that moment of excite-ment and disbelieve that I was looking inside the stomach of a live person in real time. It was the moment which changed my life. I was fortunate to witness the fast progression of flexible endoscopy from a primitive stage of large-caliber fiberscopes with an eyepiece resembling that of old microscopes to modern high-definition, slim and ultra-slim video endoscopes, single- and double-balloon enter-oscopes, endoscopic capsules, and many other innovations which have opened unlimited diagnostic and therapeutic possibilities in the field of pediatric gastroenterology.

You, my young colleague, who have opened a new page of your life, step into a fascinating journey of new discoveries in pediatric gastroenterology.

I express my deep gratitude to Dr Eduard Rokhlin, who was my endoscopy mentor and dear friend; Professor Samy Cadranel and Jean-François Mougenot: two remarkable phy-sicians and endoscopists who opened the door for me to enter the world of European commu-nity of pediatric gastroenterology; Professor Jon A. Vanderhoof, who gave me the opportu-nity to share my endoscopy skills and scientific data with my American colleagues at the Annual Meeting of North American Society of Pediatric Gastroenterology and Hepatology in 1989; and Professor Marvin E. Ament, one of the pioneers of pediatric GI endoscopy, who invited me to work with him at UCLA in Los Angeles. Finally, this book would not be pos-sible without love abd support of Irina, my amazing wife and healer and my daughter Zhenya, a talanted artist, educated and art historian and my grandauphter Nikka, a truly gifted musician and composer.

Mike Thomson

Why Pediatric Endoscopy?

Please forgive this indulgence, but as you may divine from this, I am clearly a little too focussed, and some may say 'sad and obsessed', with this area of medicine!

Like most things in life, and particularly in the serendipitous, chaotic and mal-designed world of medical careers, I 'fell' in to endoscopy in children. Which does sound a little 'messy'!

I am very grateful to George my co-Editor and massive contributor for the opportunity to join him in this venture - we did it together for the Second Edition 10 years ago, and this version has massively surpassed that one. Marvin Ament should not be forgotten as an integral part of the first and second Editions - a real progenitor of paediatric endoscopy. We hope that this Third Edition has kept pace with this fast-changing field.

I was first exposed to endoscopy in children in 1986 in a large teaching hospital in the North of England where it was 'hold them down, minimally sedate, and get on with it.' Things have changed a bit since then! However, to be fair, at that point, I did not 'get the bug' for pediatric endoscopy. It was really still in its infancy, having been championed in the late 1970s and early 1980s by such giants of the field as Sami Cadranel (so sadly, recently left us), Marvin Ament and Jean-Francois-Mougenot. Sami, Jean-Francois and I were (much) later get to know each other and become friends. They and many others set the scene for the undertaking of children's endoscopy by children's specialists in GI – a cause I have always believed in and tried to implement. Who wants an adult surgeon doing a quick sigmoidoscopy on your child with suspected Crohn's and taking no biopsies? Never mind not getting to the ileum! Hobby horse time – I always call the lower GI procedure an ileo-colonoscopy not simply a colonoscopy. Why, for instance, would you be happy with having a bronchoscopy where the bronchoscopist only examined the trachea and main left and right bronchi without going further? Or even just the left lung and not the right?!

My first inspirational moment came when I took up the position of GI/Hepatology Fellow in the Royal Brisbane Children's Hospital in Australia in 1989 - a perfect equation of work hard/play hard. My mentor Prof Ross Shepherd was, and is, one of the most astute clinicians I have had the good fortune to learn from - and luckily he was a great teacher of endoscopy as well. Prof Geoff Cleghorn and Dr Mark Patrick deserve mention here as well and imparted knowledge and skill tips that I have not forgotten. Australia at this point were streets ahead of Europe in this area and in the 5 years I was there I had an accelerated endoscopy training, which, like many things in medicine, was down to good luck rather than good management. Also undertook my MD Doctorate on CF here.

Quick story - on our research staff we had a vet called Ristan Greer and I had a patient who had recurrent H pylori type bug called then Gastrospirillum hominis (now Helicobacter heilmanii) only usually previously seen in cats and dogs – we agreed to scope the cats and dogs at their farm with Ristan anesthetising them and using an old scope that was to be thrown out we identified the micro-organism in the cats, gave eradication to the girl and the cats simultaneously, and she was 'cured'. Cue a paper in The Lancet.

Watersheds occur in life, and I chose, for family reasons, to return to the UK in 1994. Birmingham and Dame Professor Deirdre Kelly CBE and her world-leading liver unit awaited. Gulp. Without doubt one of the most inspirational women and doctors in the UK, to this day. When I first arrived, I met Sue the amazing PA to Deirdre, and after she had shown me my office – in a Portacabin! – I asked her 'Are you doing that accent for a joke?' It took a while for me to get back in to her good books! It was easy transferring skills but not so easy adapting back to a West Midlands climate. I loved my time there but the only things that the two cities have in common is the letter 'B'.

No beach or surf in Brummie. Made some great life-long friends there though. I clearly remember getting a phone call, possibly 'tongue in cheek', from the head histopathologist in Birmingham Children's Hospital two weeks after I had started. I had performed a scope on a post-transplant girl and sent the biopsies off. He said I had mislabelled the samples because I had put 'terminal ileum' on one, and they hadn't seen that label for years, so was I sure! And so to another mentor, the extraordinary Deirdre Kelly, from whom I learnt many things - but not much endoscopy. But another good friend which the journey of medicine has allowed me to make. She was instrumental in my application to then become a Consultant with the incomparable Prof John Walker-Smith, one of the fathers of our discipline, at the Royal Free Hospital in London. Got lost, nearly missed the interview, swore I would never work and live in London - got the job and moved to London.

The next ten years were eye-opening. The 'dream-team' of JAWS (which acronym I know he dislikes), Simon Murch, Alan Phillips, me and latterly Rob Heuschkel were as close to a medical family as is possible. We should remember here our friend Dave Casson who sadly passed away from gastric cancer. Importantly I was privileged to learn at John's feet but almost, if not more, significant for me, I was able to hone my apprentice-type ileo-colonoscopy skills with the greatest of them all, Prof Christopher Williams. A unique character is a fair way to describe him, but he is acknowledged as having been the best of the best when it came to ileo-colonoscopy training. Simon Murch, John Fell and I learnt a great deal. We were in the mid-nineties, however, still iv drug users! Eric Hassall, the famous North American paediatric gastroenterologist and a good and wise friend, once wrote a paper 'Why pediatric endoscopists should not be iv drug users.' Referring to the dual role of performing a procedure and also administering the iv sedation. Holding down a child should never be part of an endoscopy, nor should respiratory rescue. 'Let the anaesthetists do what they want to keep the child still, unknowing and amnesic and don't get involved' has always been my mantra. Cost and availability of anaesthetists is the only reason why it still happens in the bad old way.

So I had a vision - please forgive me for sounding like a prima donna! The John Walker-Smith Unit had been running a brilliant Paeds Gastro Course in December in London for at least 12 years. As the young guy and the endoscopy enthusiast I thought 'why not add on a live endoscopy day?' John was very receptive and the first one was a real experiment but it worked. I still owe Simon an apology for training the room camera on him as he was scoping and videoing his 'gurnying' (facial movements as if in pain), during a live ileo-colonoscopy, to 150 people in the main auditorium! Fortunately, he has a great and forgiving sense of humour. It was probably the first ever successful live paediatric endoscopy meeting. The close interaction with scientists such as Alan Phillips also came out in this Course with biopsy orientation and handling adding another dimension. The Meeting seemed, apparently, to work smoothly - but a bit like a swan gliding serenely over the lake's surface, meanwhile its legs swimming frenetically beneath, we were frantically trying to get all the pieces of the jigsaw to fit together and at the appropriate time. It was amazing and a real privilege to be able to invite the great and good from the world of paediatric endoscopy over to London to teach over the next 10 years - Victor Fox, Luigi Dall'Oglio, Jean-Francois Mougenot, Jean-Pierre Olives, Sami Cadranel, Yvan Vandenplas, Ernie Seidman, Harland Winter, Athos Bousvaros, Raoul Furlano and of course Eric Hassall. Other giants of the field I was to meet later.

Over the next ten years we worked closely with the adult GI Unit and Prof Owen Epstein and I produced a DVD with over 400 endoscopy videos and stills, which is still available and remains for me a great resource for Powerpoint presentations etc. This textbook has many other videos on the accompanying webpage if you are interested. The Paediatric Endoscopy Unit evolved and we started pioneering therapeutic techniques with close clinical governance, and always learning from meetings such as the BSG, ESGE, UEGW, and DDW which showcased new and exciting techniques in endotherapy. The Unit did however produce a non-endoscopy virtue - a wife and our first daughter - Kay was a part of our team at middle grade level for a while which is how we met (Mills and Boon or not!) and I remain so grateful that she threw her towel in with me!

Eventually the 'pull to the North' became overwhelming for me - back to where I grew up - and in 2004 I took the difficult and painful decision to leave John, Alan, Simon and Rob and move to the relative peds GI virgin territory of Sheffield Children's Hospital. Back to 'God's Own County', Yorkshire. Thanks to Kay, my incredible and long-suffering partner for agreeing and sacrificing her promising career in 'Pharma' to which she had made a transfer and a name for herself in a short time. I appreciate it more than you can know.

So, now a blank canvas - almost. Prof Chris Taylor was the only paeds GI there when I arrived on, fittingly, April the 1st 2005. I remember that in the very first list I broke their only colonoscope! Oops! Time to get some more then.......

Chris was a very generous host and indulged my ambitions. He was even kind enough as we became friends to ask me to be his best man and I was delighted - only embarrassing him slightly.

In 2005 we carried on with the Royal Free Course but then transferred it to Sheffield the year after and converted it to a Hands-On small group ileo-colonoscopy Course over 2–3 days. This was to be the template for the nest 15 years and has increased in frequency driven by demand to about 6–8 a year.

Meanwhile we began to build the Unit and with my colleagues and friends we have now over 50 staff. Prof Chris Taylor and Prof Stuart Tanner (hepatology) retired (Chris only recently) and I was joined by consultant colleagues Sally Connolly (now also retired), David Campbell, Prithviraj Rao, Priya Narula, (temporarily Dalia Belsha, Franco Torrente and Camilla Salvestrini), Arun Urs, Natalia Nedelkopoulou, Shishu Sharma, Zuzana Londt, Intan Yeop and Akshay Kapoor. Amazing team who all bring something different to the table. The Gastro Nurses are so important to us led very ably by Valda Forbes. Dietitians also brilliant led by Lynn Hagin, SALT by Jane Shaw, and psychology by Charlotte Merriman are also hugely important and fantastic. Prof Marta Cohen, head of histopathology and I have collaborated on research over the years and she is always energetic and a great colleague to have.

The people of Sheffield and the region are, contrary to popular belief of a Yorkshireman being a 'Scotsman robbed of his generosity', incredibly generous. The Sheffield Children's Hospital Charity (led by my friend David Vernon-Edwards) were, and have been, pivotal in financial help to make the Unit the most fantastic place to work - the Endoscopy Unit of the Future, the double balloon enteroscopy set up, the wireless capsule endoscopy service and the new magnetic-controlled capsule technology, and most recently the Symbionix virtual endoscopy training simulator, are amongst a few of the things that they have kindly and generously funded for us, allowing us to stay at the cutting edge of training and diagnostic and endo-therapeutic capability.

An area that I am particularly happy with is the ESPGHAN Council's open-minded approach to the Endoscopy Special Interest Group initiatives in terms of Training. Hands-On Courses are spreading, the Endoscopy Learning Zone at the Annual Meeting has been fantastic and is going from strength to strength under the guidance now of Prof Raoul Furlano, and the first ever live endoscopy session occurred in 2019 in Glasgow at the Annual ESPGHAN Meeting and was very well received. There is nothing like performing live endoscopy to 500 people to get the cardiovascular system energised! Thank you to the recent Presidents of ESPGHAN Raanan Shamir and the ever-enthusiastic Sanja Kolacek. Sanja has pushed for, and obtained funding for, the ESPGHAN Pediatric Endoscopy Fellowships which are starting in early 2021, which will be amazing - thank you!

My endoscopic 'raison d'être' is to attempt to put the paediatric surgeons out of work! Hence pushing the boundaries in such areas as are covered in this Textbook. Nevertheless, I think it is critical that we work hand in hand with our surgical colleagues, many of who perform endoscopy, in order to blur the interface between our approaches. I am extremely fortunate to work with some fantastic and enlightened individuals in the surgical team and we are almost a joint Unit nowadays – as can be seen by our innovations with laparoscopic assisted endoscopic percutaneous jejunostomy and duodenal web division, amongst many others. Maybe I am a frustrated surgeon after all! Hopefully the web page is educational to those that access it with many videos etc. I am particularly indebted to the open-minded attitude and team-spirited nature of Mr Sean Marven, Mr Richard Lindley, Prof Ross Fisher, Mr Suresh Murthi, Prof Prasad Godbole, Ms Emma Parkinson, and more recently Ms Liz Gavens and Ms Caroline McDonald. Sparring with Jenny Walker was always fun and we are now good friends. Rang Shawis and Julian Roberts should not be missed out here.

Endoscopy in the modern world in children could not occur - especially endo-therapeutic - without the excellence of our anaesthetists - my stars are Dr David Turnbull, Dr Liz Allison, Dr Kate Wilson, Dr Rob Hearn, Dr George Colley at the Royal Free, and most importantly of all, the best paediatric anesthetist of them all, Dr Adrian Lloyd-Thomas (AL-T). A quick story - the modern practice of topical application of Mitomycin C after esophageal dilation came from a chance conversation with AL-T, who told me that the ENT guys used Mitomycin C post-laryngeal reconstruction to prevent circumferential stenosis - we tried it and it worked in the esophagus of a girl requiring multiple frequent esophageal dilation. Cue a paper in

The Lancet. Perhaps we should have more cross-specialty conversations?

We should remember that this is the only truly 'procedure-specific' paediatric specialty and stick to our guns with respect of the importance of endoscopy in our training. The Guidelines and Position Papers, some joint with ESGE and NASPGHN have been extremely well received and, in addition, have helped in raising the JPGN Impact Factor to its new dizzying height of nearly 3.

Medicine is a vocation amongst us of course, and training the next generation has been one of my major aims. In this I am particularly grateful to Prof Sanja Kolacek in her unswerving support and application of her considerable energy in moving forward the recent amazing ESPGHAN Endoscopy Fellowship Program - worth mentioning again!

We should, in my view, never compromise on the quality of training or care delivery afforded by paediatric endoscopy by those of us fortunate enough to have benefitted by it in our careers. Adult GI endoscopists should be involved only if we cannot avoid it - that comes down to our learning the correct skills and techniques and making their involvement redundant. We still have plenty to learn from them though, I will acknowledge.

Recently we have created a global community for Pediatric Endoscopy - adult GI, European, North American, South American, Asian, Australasian Peds GI - and Joint Endoscopy Guidelines have emerged – this is fantastic and I am sure that this fruitful collaboration will continue. Special mention should go to the drivers of these collaborative efforts and the contributors - Catharine Walsh, Doug Fishman, Jenifer Lightdale, Jorge Amil-Dias, Andrea Tringali, Mario Vieira, Raoul Furlano, Victor Fox, Looi Ee, Patrick Bontems, Matjaz Homan, Rok Orel, Frederick Gottrand, Alexandra Papadopoulou, Salvatore Oliva, Erasmo Miele, Claudio Romano, Luigi Dall'Oglio, Rob Kramer, Mike Manfredi, Diana Lerner, Marsha Kay, Tom Attard, Warren Hyer, Joel Freidlander, 'The Richards' Hansen and

Russell, David Wilson, Dan Turner, Pete Gillett, Pat McKiernan, Stephen Murphy, Christos Tzivinikos, Ari Silbermintz, Rupert Hinds, Marta Tavares, Bruno Hauser, Yvan Vandenplas, Ron Bremner, Pete Lewindon, Petar Mamula, Orin Ledder, Merit Tabbers, Ilse Broekaert, Cesare Hassan, Marc Benninga, Alessandro Zambelli, Nikhil Thapar, Iva Hojsak, Stefan Husby, Ilektra Athiana, Andreia Nita, Sara Isoldi, Paola DeAngelis, Lissy De Ridder, the incomparable Samy Cadranel, all in the Sheffield Team and many many more - apologies if I have missed you out!

Thank you to the numerous members of the endoscopy Companies that have been so helpful over the years with Courses etc etc. You will know who you are but to numerous to mention here.

Kevin and Kat in ESPGHAN Head Office have always been very receptive to any Qs needed and I am grateful to them.

There is no ceiling to what we can achieve in pediatric endoscopy. Attending 'adult' GI and endoscopy meetings is illuminating e.g. 'ESGE Days'. We are no longer the Cinderella part of pediatric GI but we still need to achieve parity with the adult Societies - a place at the 'top table' i.e. Societal Councils – as occurs in all adult GI Societies.

I would like to thank all the trainees from so many countries and backgrounds for their personal commitment and sacrifice over the last 25 years in coming to train with us - it never ceases to amaze me how mothers and fathers and spouses can leave their loved ones for months, on occasions a year or more, in order to train in this fantastic compelling area. Their ability to do so has been facilitated by my amazing Endoscopy Fellow and Course Coordinator, without whom it would have been truly impossible to run such a successful training program - Sam Goult. Thankyou Sam.

And then, if you have got this far then 'well done'. It is so important to me to hold up my hand and say that, in all honesty, I could have not done all that I have done (admittedly a microcosm in the great scheme of things)

without the forbearance and tolerance of my wife Kay and my exceptional and talented and kind daughters Ella, Jess and Flo. Incredible people and my driving force. I am sorry to you all for being away so much giving lectures and all that stuff when you were growing up and when you, Kay, were managing them so amazingly, almost single-handedly. I would have done things differently if I had had the time again and know what I know now. Medicine as a job is not necessarily life, although some times it is difficult to see beyond the vocation.

Lastly, I want to say a special thankyou to all the families and children that it has been my pleasure and privilege to help over the last 35 years.

As a small post-script it would be remiss of me to not thank all the authors who have been extremely patient over the last 4 years and I hope that you will be happy with the labour of love that has produced this book with your extraordinary help. Nearly all of you are good friends – some are friends yet to make – some are friends during this process that have sadly passed. Gábor (Veres) was a great and a good man and I never saw him be anything but kind and intelligent and helpful and energetic. A particularly sad event occurred recently – Prof Samy Cadranel lost his battle against cancer. He trained and touched so many in our discipline from the late 1970s to the modern day. He was a real giant in the field of pediatric endoscopy – he produced the first bespoke pediatric endoscope in 1978, led the field in diagnostics and then in therapeutic endoscopy. He trained a generation across the world leaders in the field such as Carlo di Lorenzo, Luigi Dall'Oglio and many many others. I was asked by him to lecture on advances in endoscopy at his Festschrift in Brussels some 15 years ago – he may have retired but he maintained a phenomenally active role in ESGPHAN. Most recently he taught on our Endoscopy Learning Zone at the Annual ESPGHAN Meeting and was always there for me if I needed a bit of guidance or advice. What he did not know about pediatric endoscopy is not worth knowing.

A polymath and a multi-linguist, but above all a really nice man and a wise and good doctor. We will miss both of these guys greatly in the future.

Please enjoy this text if you can, and believe me when I say that this is the distillation of a life's work, but not just mine - it is a distillation of all that I have been taught and that George has been taught - it is therefore the 'handing down of knowledge' which is key to keeping a discipline moving forwards.

YOU! – the next generation – continue to push paediatric endoscopy forwards – training, research, Courses, expansion of the ELZ, further collaboration with our friends all over the world and push for live endoscopy at all the annual meetings – but please remember that, like our counterparts in adult GI endoscopy, we should be recognized and have a say on the Councils of our respective Societies.

Can I just mention some amazing people that deserve it who have been mentioned and some who have not? Andrei Nita; Jorge Amil-Dias; Alexandra Papadopoulos; Marc Benninga; Nikhil Thapar; Pete Lewindon; Tom Attard; Warren Hyer; Muftah Eltumi; Paul Hurlstone; Mark Donnelly; Mark McAlindon; Stuart Riley; Deb Salvin (of the world-famous 'Salvin procedure'); Dom Hughes; Helen Wigmore; Ben Roebuck, Jamie Shepherd; Dave Turnbull; Liz Allison; and of course all the extremely patient authors of all the Chapters.

Our work would not have been possible without the trust and cooperation of all the children and families, so much heartfelt gratitude goes to these – tens of thousands!

My working life has been orchestrated by two amazing PAs without whom I would never have found the time to do all of this. Sam – thank you! Kate – thank you! You are both incredible.

Thank you to the amazing team at the publishing house – Anupama Sreekanth and editing team all along the gestation and birth i.e. April 2021, including lastly Holly Regan-Jones, who was amazing during 'labour'. Lastly the production to completion expertly orchestrated by Hari Sridharan – thanks for your patience!

Undoubtedly there will be mistakes somewhere in all these pages, and if there are then, we'll get it right next time (please let us know) - but it has been a labour of love and thank you to everyone – absolutely everyone – that has contributed, in even the smallest way.

The FatBoys Fell Running Club of Hathersage deserve a special mention for keeping me sane and balancing my life – to whom I lost my virginity (in fell racing terms!) – 'a drinking club with a running problem'!

Lastly a big hug and love to my dear long-suffering wife Kay – thank you for putting up with me. And my fab daughters Ella, Jess and Flo, of whom I am immensely proud – sorry for the holiday time taken up with writing etc!!!

And as Sir Steve Redgrave, the most famous Olympic rower, said, on winning his last gold medal 'If you ever see me in a boat again, shoot me!' - and that goes for textbooks for me as well.

Contributors

Jorge Amil-Dias
Department of Pediatric Gastroenterology,
Centro Hospitalar de São João, Porto, Portugal

Paul Arnold
Histopathology Department, Sheffield
Children's Hospital NHS Foundation Trust,
Sheffield, UK

Thomas Attard
Department of Gastroenterology, Children's
Mercy Hospital, Kansas, MO, USA

Vasile Daniel Balaban
"Dr. Carol Davila" Central Military
Emergency University Hospital and "Carol
Davila" University of Medicine and Pharmacy,
Bucharest, Romania

Valerio Balassone
UOC di Chirurgia ed Endoscopia Digestiva,
Ospedale de Bambino Gesù, Rome, Italy

Dalia Belsha
Centre for Paediatric Gastroenterology
and International Academy of Paediatric
Endoscopy Training, Sheffield Children's
Hospital NHS Foundation Trust, Sheffield,
UK

Natalie Bhesania
Department of Pediatric Gastroenterology,
Hepatology and Nutrition, The Cleveland
Clinic, Cleveland, OH, USA

Jernej Brecelj
Department of Gastroenterology, Hepatology
and Nutrition, University Children's Hospital,
University Medical Centre Ljubljana,
and Department of Pediatrics, Faculty of
Medicine, University of Ljubljana, Ljubljana,
Slovenia

Samy Cadranel
Queen Fabiola Children's Hospital, Free
University of Brussels, Brussels. Belgium

Marta C. Cohen
Department of Paediatric Histopathology,
Sheffield Children's Hospital NHS Foundation
Trust; Honorary Senior Lecturer, University of
Sheffield, Sheffield, UK

Luigi Dall'Oglio
UOC di Chirurgia ed Endoscopia Digestiva,
Bambino Gesù, Rome, Italy

Paola de Angelis
UOC di Chirurgia ed Endoscopia Digestiva,
Bambino Gesù, Rome, Italy

Looi Ee
Department of Gastroenterology, Hepatology
and Liver Transplant, Lady Cilento Children's
Hospital, Brisbane, Australia

Simona Faraci
Department of Surgery, Ospedale de Bambino
Gesù, Rome, Italy

Victor Fox
Department of Gastroenterology, Boston
Children's Hospital, Boston, MA, USA

Douglas S. Fishman
Department of Gastrointestinal Endoscopy
and Therapeutic Endoscopy, Texas Children's
Hospital, Houston, TX, USA

Chris Fraser
Department of Gastroenterology, Edinburgh
Royal Infirmary, Edinburgh, Scotland, UK

Joel A. Friedlander
Childrens's Hospital Colorado/Digestive
Health Institute,
University of Colorado School of Medicine,
Aurora, CO, USA

Raoul Furlano
Departement of Pediatric Gastroenterology
and Nutrition, University Children's Hospital,
Basel, Switzerland

Glenn T. Furuta
Digestive Health Institute, Section of Pediatric
Gastroenterology, Hepatology and Nutrition,
Children's Hospital Colorado, Gastrointestinal
Eosinophilic Diseases Program, Department
of Pediatrics, Mucosal Inflammation Program,
University of Colorado School of Medicine,
Aurora, CO, USA

George Gershman
Harbor-UCLA Nedical Center, David Geffen
School of Medicine, UCLA, Torrance, CA
USA

Jonathan Goring
Paediatric Surgical Unit, Sheffield Children's
Hospital NHS Foundation Trust, Sheffield,
UK

Frederick Gottrand
Pediatric Gastroenterology, Hepatology and
Nutrition Department, CHU Lille, University
of Lille, Lille, France

Matjaz Homan
Department of Gastroenterology, Hepatology
and Nutrition, University Children's Hospital,
University of Ljubljana, Ljubljana, Slovenia

Paul Hurlstone
Department of Endoscopy, Doncaster and
Bassetlaw Hospitals NHS Foundation Trust,
Doncaster, UK

Warren Hyer
Department of Gastroenterology, St Mark's
Hospital, London, UK

Sara Isoldi
Department of Digestive Endoscopy,
"Sapienza" University, Sant'Andrea Hospital,
Rome, Italy

Lauren Johanson
Pittsburgh Liver Research Center, Children's
Hospital of Pittsburgh, Pittsburgh, PA,
USA

Tom Kalley
Harbor-UCLA Medical Center, David Geffen
School of Medicine, UCLA, Los Angeles, CA
USA

Marsha Kay
Department of Pediatric Gastroenterology,
Hepatology and Nutrition, The Cleveland
Clinic, Cleveland, OH, USA

Sara Koo
Pediatric Neurogastroenterology and Motility
Program, Anschutz Medical Campus, Denver,
CO, USA

Robert E. Kramer
Digestive Health Institute, Section of Pediatric
Gastroenterology, Hepatology and Nutrition,
Children's Hospital Colorado, Gastrointestinal
Eosinophilic Diseases Program, Department
of Pediatrics, Mucosal Inflammation Program,
University of Colorado School of Medicine,
Aurora, CO, USA

Thierry Lamireau
Centre of Pediatric Gastroenterolgy,
University of Bordeaux, Chu de Bordeaux,
Hopitaux de Bordeaux, Bordeaux, France

Kristina Leinwand
Pediatric Neurogastroenterology and Motility
Program, Anschutz Medical Campus, Denver,
CO, USA

Jenifer R. Lightdale
Division of Pediatric Gastroenterology,
UMass Memorial Children's Medical Center,
Department of Pediatrics, University of
Massachusetts, Worcester, MA, USA

Richard Lindley
Paediatric Surgical Unit, Sheffield Children's
Hospital NHS Foundation Trust, Sheffield,
UK

Markku Mäki
Faculty of Medicine and Health Technology,
Tampere University, Tampere, Finland

Michael Manfredi
Division of Gastroenterology, Hepatology
and Nutrition, Boston Children's Hospital,
Boston, MA, USA

Sean Marven
Sheffield Children's Hospital NHS Foundation
Trust, Sheffield, UK

Patrick McKiernan
Pittsburgh Liver Research Center, Children's
Hospital of Pittsburgh, Pittsburgh, PA, USA

Calies Menard-Katcher
Digestive Health Institute, Section of Pediatric
Gastroenterology, Hepatology and Nutrition,
Children's Hospital Colorado, Gastrointestinal
Eosinophilic Diseases Program, Department
of Pediatrics, Mucosal Inflammation Program,
University of Colorado School of Medicine,
Aurora, CO, USA

Erasmo Miele
Department of Digestive Endoscopy,
"Sapienza" University, Sant'Andrea Hospital,
Rome, Italy

Jean-François Mougenot
Médecin des Hôpitaux de Paris Honoraire,
Hôpital Robert Debré et Hôpital Necker-
Enfants Malades, Paris, France

Priya Narula
Centre for Paediatric Gastroenterology
and International Academy of Paediatric
Endoscopy Training, Sheffield Children's
Hospital NHS Foundation Trust, Sheffield,
UK

Natalia Nedelkopoulou
Centre for Paediatric Gastroenterology
and International Academy of Paediatric
Endoscopy Training, Sheffield Children's
Hospital NHS Foundation Trust, Sheffield,
UK

Andreia Nita
Centre for Paediatric Gastroenterology
and International Academy of Paediatric
Endoscopy Training, Sheffield Children's
Hospital NHS Foundation Trust, Sheffield,
UK

Salvatore Oliva
Maternal and Child Health Department,
Pediatric Gastroenterology and Liver Unit,
Sapienza – University of Rome, Rome, Italy

Rok Orel
Department of Gastroenterology, Hepatology
and Nutrition, University Children's Hospital,
University of Ljubljana, Ljubljana, Slovenia

Harpreet Pall
Section of Gastroenterology, Hepatology,
and Nutrition, St Christopher's Hospital
for Children; Drexel University College of
Medicine, Philadelphia, PA, USA

Simon Panter
Department of Gastroenterology, South Tyneside and Sunderland NHS Foundation Trust, Sunderland, UK

Alina Popp
"Alessandrescu-Rusescu" National Institute for Mother and Child Care and "Carol Davila" University of Medicine and Pharmacy, Bucharest, Romania

Antonio Quiros
Department of Pediatric Gastroenterology, Valley Health System, Paramus, NJ, USA

Prithviraj Rao
Centre for Paediatric Gastroenterology and International Academy of Paediatric Endoscopy Training, Sheffield Children's Hospital NHS Foundation Trust, Sheffield, UK

Luciana B. Mendez Ribeiro
Center for Pediatric Gastroenterology, Hospital Pequeno Príncipe, Curitiba, Brazil

Claudio Romano
Department of Human Pathology and Pediatrics, University of Messina, Messina, Italy

Shishu Sharma
Centre for Paediatric Gastroenterology and International Academy of Paediatric Endoscopy Training, Sheffield Children's Hospital NHS Foundation Trust, Sheffield, UK

Mike Thomson
Centre for Paediatric Gastroenterology and International Academy of Paediatric Endoscopy Training, Sheffield Children's Hospital NHS Foundation Trust, Sheffield, UK

Filippo Torroni
UOC di Chirurgia ed Endoscopia Digestiva, Bambino Gesù, Rome, Italy

Sabine Krüger Truppel
Center for Pediatric Gastroenterology, Hospital Pequeno Príncipe, Curitiba, Brazil

Dan Turner
Juliet Keidan Institute of Paediatric Gastroenterology and Nutrition, Shaare Zedek Medical Centre, Jerusalem, Israel; Faculty of Medicine, Hebrew University of Jerusalem, Israel

Arun Urs
Centre for Paediatric Gastroenterology and International Academy of Paediatric Endoscopy Training, Sheffield Children's Hospital NHS Foundation Trust, Sheffield, UK

Jorge H. Vargas
Ronald Reagan UCLA Medical Center, UCLA Mattel Children's Hospital, UCLA Medical Center, Santa Monica, CA, USA

Krishnappa Venkatesh
Centre for Paediatric Gastroenterology and International Academy of Paediatric Endoscopy Training, Sheffield Children's Hospital NHS Foundation Trust, Sheffield, UK

Gabor Veres
Deceased. Formerly Department of Paediatric Gastroenterology, University of Budapest, Budapest, Hungary

Jerome Viala
Department of Pediatric Gastroenterology, Robert-Debré Hospital, Paris, France

Mario Vieira
Center for Pediatric Gastroenterology. Hospital Pequeno Príncipe, Curitiba, Brazil

Catharine M. Walsh
Division of Gastroenterology, Hepatology and Nutrition and the Research and Learning

Institutes, Hospital for Sick Children,
Department of Paediatrics, and Wilson
Centre, University of Toronto, Toronto,
Canada

David Wilson
Department of Child Health,
University of Edinburgh, Edinburgh,
Scotland, UK

About the Companion Website

This book is accompanied by a website

www.wiley.com/go/gershman3e

- All figures from the book available to download in PowerPoint
- Videos chosen to show key components discussed in the chapters

Scan this QR code to visit the companion website

Part One

Pediatric Endoscopy Setting

1

Introduction

George Gershman and Mike Thomson

In the late 1960s, flexible gastrointestinal endoscopy emerged as a novel diagnostic tool but was not employed routinely in children until the mid-1970s when pediatric flexible esophagogastroduodenoscopes became commercially available. In the decade that followed, there was a significant expansion and application of this modality in children. As the result, many discoveries and improvements in diagnosis and treatment of various pediatric GI disorders have been made despite the limitations associated with light and image transmission through the fiberoptic cables – the technology which only allowed the operator to look down the scope through the eyepiece.

The advent of the microchip with a video camera sited at the tip of the endoscope has advanced the optical imagery significantly. The days of an operator's watery eye "glued" to the endoscope head and poor-quality images due to fiber breakage within the optic cables and condensation of water under the lenses at the tip of the instrument are long gone. The only "advantage" of fiberscopes was that no one else knew what you were looking at and there was a propensity for claims such as 'Oh yes, I got to the terminal ileum'! Nowadays, everyone can see where you are in the GI tract on the screens so there is no hiding . . .

Modern endoscopes include high-definition images, high magnification, confocal endomicroscopy with up to 1000× magnification, narrow-band imaging with focus on various light spectra to allow identification of dysplasia and polyp pit pattern, autofluorescence and other diagnostic modalities. Furthermore, the therapeutic capabilities of the modern endoscope are phenomenal and include up to 3.8 mm working channels and even scopes with two working channels to allow more sophisticated work. Very narrow (4.5 mm) scopes are now available to allow endoscopy in the smallest of infants/neonates and these are now applicable in older children for outpatient transnasal endoscopy without sedation. Three-dimensional imaging techniques are standard in most colonoscopes which enables identification of loops during ileocolonoscopy, speeding up the process and making it safer and less uncomfortable when it is done without general anesthesia. These concepts are now aided by the use of insufflation using carbon dioxide which is much more quickly absorbed than air.

In addition, endoscopic accessories have developed miraculously and allow many therapeutic procedures to occur which had previously been the domain of surgical options only.

Practical Pediatric Gastrointestinal Endoscopy, Third Edition. Edited by George Gershman and Mike Thomson.
© 2021 John Wiley & Sons Ltd. Published 2021 by John Wiley & Sons Ltd.
Companion website: www.wiley.com/go/gershman3e

These include endoscopic fundoplication, per-oral endoscopic myotomy for achalasia, percutaneous jejunostomy, duodenal stenosis treatment, fundal variceal ablation, pancreatic pseudocyst drainage and many others discussed in the corresponding chapters of the book.

In parallel with the advances in equipment, we have seen an enormous upskilling of the operators mainly due to the focus on training – this has been made possible by the greater availability of virtual models, hands-on animal training and more investment in one-to-one fellowships and short focused therapeutic endoscopic courses over the last 10–20 years. Online portfolios and direct observer procedure skill assessments are the cornerstones of these advances. Virtually every large GI meeting now has a hands-on endoscopy component and often a live endoscopy segment as well.

Virtually every year, a new endoscopic application is developed and many of the recent advances are included in this textbook – such as the over-the-scope clip for perforation closure, Hemospray® for diffuse GI bleeding, Stretta radioablation of the distal esophagus for reflux treatment, and then the concept of natural orifice transendoluminal surgery (NOTES) needs a mention as the newest kid on the block. This latter exciting technology is in some ways a modality looking for an appropriate application, especially in children, and is discussed at the end of the book.

We have tried to make this text the definitive one for pediatric endoscopy and we hope you enjoy reading it. No doubt more advances in technology will have been developed by the time this book hits the shelves but this is to be applauded. If the velocity of advances continues at the present pace, there is no barrier or horizon that is safe from endoscopy. It is reasonable to say that the gastrointestinal endoscopist should have the aim to make the GI pediatric surgeon virtually redundant. However, it has to be said that increasingly, the two disciplines are working more closely together and pediatric surgeons use endoscopy more and more themselves.

We hope that this book will enthuse the younger generation of trainees to follow the path of minimally invasive solutions to every problem that the GI tract produces in children. We may learn a lot from our adult colleagues but conversely, with our exposure to congenital abnormalities, we may be able to take a lead in these areas also. Imagination is our only barrier.

We would like to thank our colleagues who have kindly given up their valuable time to contribute some really fantastic chapters and images. We hope you really enjoy reading the book and that you gain a lot from it. The images and videos and webpage will allow knowledge to be disseminated widely. Most, if not all, of the world experts in pediatric endoscopy have contributed and we are truly grateful. We would like to thank the publishers, without whose guidance and help this would have been impossible.

This journey would not have been possible without the love and support of our families.

> *MIKE*: thanks to Kay, my wife, and Ella, Jess and Flo, my wondrous daughters who put up with their old dad – especially editing the chapters when on holiday!
>
> *GEORGE*: many thanks to Irina, my beloved wife and muse, and my two precious artists: my daughter Zhenya and granddaughter Nikka who continue to bring beauty to the world.

Thank you and hopefully those of you who are training now will be contributors in future editions and we will pass on the baton to you in due course. Remember – do no harm and have fun. It is the best specialty you can imagine.

Mike and George

2

History of pediatric gastrointestinal endoscopy

Samy Cadranel, Jean-François Mougenot, and Douglas S. Fishman

 KEY POINTS

- Rigid endoscopy as the proof of concept: invisible could be visible: the first step toward exploration of the esophagus and the proximal stomach.
- Semiflexible endoscopy as the next step toward correct diagnosis of gastric pathology beyond the gastric body and development of endoscopic target biopsy.
- Fiberoptic flexible gastrointestinal endoscopy as the foundation of modern diagnostic and therapeutic pediatric gastrointestinal endoscopy – more recently, videochip at the tip.

During the last half century, two achievements can be considered as major advances in the field of gastroenterology: the adaptation of fiberoptics to gastrointestinal endoscopy, and, as a consequence, the discovery of *Helicobacter pylori* [1,2]. Indeed, the role of *H. pylori* would not have been suspected without the pathologic and microbiologic study of biopsy material obtained with the endoscope. Attempts to inspect in vivo the internal cavities of the human body are probably as ancient as medicine itself. The challenge was to find a safe source of light that would not generate heat that could damage tissues.

The precursors

As early as the end of the 18th century, the Lichtleier, an ancestor of the modern proctoscope, paved the way with a system of lenses illuminated by candlelight. The name "endoscope" was coined as early as 1853 by A.J. Desormeaux for an instrument used in urology [3] while the first "gastroscope" was developed in Erlangen by A. Kussmaul [4]. These instruments were hampered by the fact that they could not direct enough light to the targeted site. With the invention of the electric bulb, a better insight became possible, but these instruments could not be used for prolonged periods of time because of the heat generated by the light bulb.

In 1881, Mikulicz performed the first gastroscopy in a human being using a rigid instrument of 65 cm long and 14 mm diameter [5]. This angulated instrument compensated for the anatomical angulations of the human esophagus and was equipped with a water circulation system to cool the light bulb and channels for the light source and to introduce air.

Practical Pediatric Gastrointestinal Endoscopy, Third Edition. Edited by George Gershman and Mike Thomson.
© 2021 John Wiley & Sons Ltd. Published 2021 by John Wiley & Sons Ltd.
Companion website: www.wiley.com/go/gershman3e

In 1932, the first semiflexible gastroscope was developed by instrument maker and technician George Wolf and gastroenterologist Rudolf Schindler who is widely rated as "the father of gastroscopy." This instrument allowed a greater range for examination, facilitating diagnosis and endoscopic treatments.

We cannot leave the discussion of semiflexible gastroscopy without mentioning one of the most decorated American gastroenterologists, Walter L. Palmer, who brought a new level of understanding to the diagnosis and treatment of digestive diseases, particularly peptic ulcer, gastrointestinal cancer, and ulcerative colitis. In 1934, he facilitated the release of Dr. Schindler from a Nazi concentration camp where he was held because of his part-Jewish blood. Eventually, Dr Schindler immigrated to the US. In 1941 he founded the Gastroscopic Club, now the American Society for Gastrointestinal Endoscopy, and became its first president.

The fiberscope

The development of fiberoptics led to the birth of modern gastrointestinal endoscopy.

In the hybrid semiflexible gastroscope built by the German instrument maker Storz in 1966, lenses were used for visualization while the electric light bulb was replaced by optical fibers made of either glass or plastic. Plastic fibers were more flexible and durable than glass; however, glass optical fibers could be manufactured with diameters smaller than their plastic counterparts, and the quality of light transmission was superior in glass optical fibers. The next improvements in fiberoptic technology were due to optical engineers who considered the possibility of fiberoptics transmitting not only light but also images. In 1954, two articles were published in the same issue of *Nature*, a brief note by van Heel on the "transport of images" and an extensive article on a flexible fiberscope by Harold Hopkins of London and his co-worker Narinder Singh Kapany [6]. Thanks to the collaboration between Basil Hirschowitz and the physicist Larry Curtiss who succeeded (with the aid of Corning Glass) in producing high-quality fiberoptics, clinical application of fiberoptics to gastrointestinal endoscopy became possible and was reported in *Gastroenterology* in 1958 [7].

Prototype fiberscopes were made by American Cystoscope Makers (ACMI) in 1960 and a commercial model was produced in 1961 with the first color images published in the *Lancet* [8]. Because of the high prevalence of gastric cancer in Japan, the Machida Company developed fiberendoscopy and soon the technicians at Olympus, led by the engineer Kawahara, produced many fine models of high optical quality with side- and front-viewing capabilities [9].

Following the adaptation of fiberoptics for medical instruments, endoscopy of the GI tract became a routine diagnostic and therapeutic tool in many gastroenterology units throughout the world. In the early 1970s, the curiosity of a few pediatric gastroenterologists and surgeons was stimulated by the growing interest in endoscopy and its diagnostic success in adult gastroenterology. At that time, gastrointestinal endoscopy in children was performed with the standard adult gastroscopes, bronchoscopes and prototypes of pediatric fiberscopes which were available in a few pediatric hospitals in Europe, United States and Japan [9–14].

During the middle and late 1970s, several publications demonstrated the safety, diagnostic and therapeutic value of pediatric GI endoscopy, contributing to our knowledge of many GI diseases in infants and children [15–23]. Although the literature was not readily accessible, similar skills were developing in Eastern Europe and Russia [24–27]. Less than 10 years after its introduction in pediatric gastroenterology, endoscopy was the subject of several books in Spanish, German, and English [28–30]. By middle and late 2000s, an extensive knowledge of pediatric GI endoscopy was summarized in additional books [31–33].

Today, training in pediatric gastroenterology is not complete without acquiring competence in diagnostic upper gastrointestinal endoscopy and colonoscopy and basic therapeutic endoscopic GI procedures [34]. Diagnostic endoscopy has become a routine part of pediatric gastroenterology, combining the advantage of direct visual observation of the GI tract with target mucosal biopsy and therapeutic procedures.

The arsenal of accessory instruments has been diversified and very much improved whether dealing with foreign body extraction, diathermic loops for polypectomy, sclerotherapy needles and bands (silicon or latex) for variceal eradication, dilation bougies and pneumatic balloons, hemostatic clipping devices and electro- and photocoagulation devices for hemorrhagic lesions, and gastrostomy kits. The reliable use of these tools needs constant maintenance by skilled staff and good training to guarantee a safe procedure.

Training

The great progress of the video endoscopic equipment has rendered teaching and training a simpler task through participation of the trainee in the procedure. A growing number of "train the trainer" courses has also been implemented worldwide, with focused programs in Australia, United Kingdom, and Canada. Computerized programs and simulators have been developed and are very useful to familiarize the trainee with the space distribution of organs and to learn to exert the right movements of the endoscope to reach the targeted organ or perform a delicate therapeutic procedure [35–38].

Also, several good "hands-on" courses with live demonstrations and training on porcine models have been developed in Belgium, France, Italy, the Netherlands, UK and United States. Finally, the trainee should complete their training in a reputed pediatric center, large enough to get the necessary experience and with support from an experienced pediatric gastroenterologist.

Evolution

The improvements that have occurred in instruments, sedation and anesthesia during the last 40 years have transformed pediatric endoscopy and gastroenterology. Pediatric gastroenterologists are now able to perform difficult diagnostic and therapeutic procedures that used to be left to the adult endoscopist, such as endoscopic ultrasonography. These procedures likely need to be concentrated in referral tertiary hospitals that can afford the costly equipment and specialized staff. These highly specialized units can safely count on such facilities as surgical and intensive care assistance, in case of adverse events because one should always bear in mind that endoscopy is an invasive procedure with inevitable risks. The constant progress in instrument quality has considerably enhanced the diagnostic power of endoscopy. Several instrument makers have implemented optical zooms but also more sophisticated methods such as dyeless virtual chromoendoscopy, Olympus Narrow Band Imaging (NBI®), Fujinon Flexible Spectral Imaging Color Enhancement (FICE®) and Pentax™ i-Scan®.

Mechanical improvements have enhanced the maneuverability of the endoscopes, for instance the adjustable stiffness of colonoscopes that facilitates access to the whole colon, insertion into the ileocecal valve and exploration of the terminal ileum. Exploration of the upper GI tract beyond the proximal jejunum and the terminal ileum is also possible with the double balloon enteroscope [39], which permits not only visualization of small bowel lesions but also biopsies and polypectomy. The most spectacular progress has been the wireless video capsule endoscopy (WCE) which allows exploration of the complete small bowel [40,41] matched with an array of enteroscopes which can traverse the deepest parts of the small intestine to complement findings seen on the WCE.

Conclusion

Endoscopy is undoubtedly an invasive technique and invasiveness is not welcomed in pediatrics. However, there is no doubt that GI endoscopy has a promising future in the field of therapeutic and interventional endoscopy with more improvements to come.

Gastrointestinal endoscopy in children has evolved from a rather confidential tool in the early 1970s, available to very few pediatric gastroenterologists with special skills and curiosity, to a routine diagnostic technique present in almost all pediatric gastroenterology units throughout the world. The stimulating adventure granted to the early "discoverers" has been replaced by less thrilling but probably more useful procedures since continuous improvement of the instruments allows deeper and more audacious therapeutic procedures.

 • See companion website for videos relating to this chapter topic: www.wiley.com/go/gershman3e

REFERENCES

1 Villardell F. *Cien Años de Endoscopia Digestiva. La Endoscopia Digestiva en El Segundo Milenio*. Aula Medica Ediciones, Madrid, 2003.

2 Janowitz HD, Abittan CS, Fiedler IM. A gastroenterological list for the Millenium. *J Clin Gastroenterol* 1999, **29**, 336–338.

3 Désormeaux AJ. De l'endoscope, instrument propre à éclairer certaines cavités intérieures de l'économie. *Comptes Rendus Acad SCI Paris* 1855, **40**, 692.

4 Kluge F, Seidler E. Zur Erstanwendung der Ösophago-und Gastroskopie. Briefe von Adolf Kussmaul und seinen Mitarbeitern. *Medizin Historisches J* 1986, **21**, 288–307.

5 Mikulicz J. Über Gastroskopie und Oesophagoskopie. *Centralbl Chirurgie* 1881, **43**, 673–676.

6 Hopkins NH, K apany NS. A flexible fiberscope using static scanning. *Nature* 1954, **173**, 39–41.

7 Hirschowitz BI, Curtiss LE, Peters CW, Pollard HP. Demonstration of a new gastroscope: the "fiberscope." *Gastroenterology* 1958, **35**, 50–53.

8 Hirschowitz BI. Endoscopic examination of the stomach and the duodenal cap with the Fiberscope. *Lancet* 1961, **1**, 1074–1078.

9 Kawai K, Murakami K, Misaki F. Endoscopical observations on gastric ulcers in teenagers. *Endoscopy* 1970, **2**, 206–208.

10 Freeman NV. Clinical evaluation of the fiberoptic bronchoscope (Olympus BF 5B) for pediatric endoscopy. *J Pediatr Surg* 1973, **8**, 213–220.

11 Cremer M, Rodesch P, Cadranel S. Fiberendoscopy of the gastrointestinal tract in children. Experience with newly designed fiberscopes. *Endoscopy* 1974, **6**, 186–189.

12 Rodesch P, Cadranel S, Peeters JP. Digestive endoscopy with fiberoptics in children. *Acta Paediatr Scand* 1974, **63**, 664.

13 Gleason PD, Tedesco FJ, Keating WA. Fiberoptic gastrointestinal endoscopy in infants and children. *J Pediatr* 1974, **85**, 810–813.

14 Gans SL, Ament ME, Christie DL, Liebman WM. Pediatric endoscopy with flexible fiberscopes. *J Pediatr Surg* 1975, **10**, 375–380.

15 Rodesch P, Cadranel S, Peeters JP, *et al.* Colonic endoscopy in children. *Acta Paediatr Belg* 1976, **29**, 181–184.

16 Mougenot JF, Montagne JP, Faure C. Gastrointestinal fibro-endoscopy in infants and children: radio-fibroscopic correlations. *Ann Radiol (Paris)* 1976, **19**, 23–34.

17 Vanderhoof JA, Ament ME. Proctosigmoidoscopy and rectal biopsy in infants and children. *J Pediatr* 1976, **89**, 911–915.

18 Forget PP, Meradji M. Contribution of fiberendoscopy to diagnosis and management of children with gastroesophageal reflux. *Arch Dis Child* 1976, **51**, 60–66.

19 Ament ME, Christie DL. Upper gastrointestinal endoscopy in pediatric patients. *Gastroenterology* 1977, **72**, 492–494.

20 Cadranel S, Rodesch P. Pediatric endoscopy in children: preparation and sedation. *Gastroenterology* 1977, **71**, 44–45.

21 Cadranel S, Rodesch P, Peeters JP, *et al.* Fiberendoscopy of the gastrointestinal tract in children and infants: a series of 100 examinations. *Am J Dis Child* 1977, **131**, 41–45.

22 Gyepes MT, Smith LE, Ament ME. Fiberoptic endoscopy and upper gastrointestinal series: comparative analysis in infants and children. *Am J Roentgenol* 1977, **128**, 53–56.

23 Graham DY, Klish WJ, Ferry GD, Sabel JS. Value of fiberoptic gastrointestinal endoscopy in infants and children. *South Med J* 1978, **71**, 558–560.

24 Rumi G, Solt I, Kajtar P. Esophagogastroduodenoscopy in childhood. *Acta Paediatr Acad Sci Hung* 1978, **19**, 315–318.

25 Isakova IF, Stepanov EA, Geraskin VI, *et al.* Fibroscopy in diagnosis of diseases of the upper digestive tract in children. *Khirurgiia (Mosk)* 1977, **7**, 33–37.

26 Mazurin AV, Gershman GB, Zaprudnov A, *et al.* Esophagogastroduodenoscopy of children at a polyclinic. *Vopr Okhr Materin Det* 1978, **23**, 3–7.

27 Gershman GB, Bokser VO. Fibrogastroscopy in the diagnosis of gastritis in children. *Vopr Okhr Materin Det* 1979, **24**, 25–30.

28 Beltran S, Varea V, Vilar P. *Fibroendoscopia en Patologia Digestiva Infantil.* Jims, Barcelona, 1980.

29 Burdelski M, Huchzermeyer H. *Gastrointestinale Endoscopie im Kindesalter.* Springer-Verlag, Berlin, 1980.

30 Gans S.L. (ed.). *Pediatric Endoscopy.* Grüne and Stratton, New York, 1983.

31 Gershman G, Ament ME (eds). *Practical Pediatric Gastrointestinal Endoscopy.* Blackwell, Oxford, 2007.

32 Ament ME, Gershman G. Pediatric colonoscopy. In: Waye JD, Rex DK, Williams C (eds). *Colonoscopy Principles and Practice.* Blackwell, Oxford, 2003, pp. 624–629.

33 Winter HS, Murphy MS, Mougenot JF, Cadranel S (eds). *Pediatric Gastrointestinal Endoscopy: Textbook and Atlas.* BC Decker, Hamilton, 2006.

34 Thomson M. Training in pediatric endoscopy. In: Winter HS, Murphy MS, Mougenot JF, Cadranel S (eds). *Pediatric Gastrointestinal Endoscopy: Textbook and Atlas.* BC Decker, Hamilton, 2006, pp. 34–41.

35 Ferlitsch A, Glauninger P, Gupper A, *et al.* Evaluation of a virtual endoscopy simulator for training in gastrointestinal endoscopy. *Endoscopy* 2002, **34**, 698–702.

36 Thomson M, Heuschkel R, Donaldson N, Murch S, Hinds R. Acquisition of competence in paediatric ileocolonoscopy with virtual endoscopy training. *J Pediatr Gastroenterol Nutr* 2006, **43**, 699–701.

37 Haycock A, Koch AD, Familiari P, *et al.* Training and transfer of colonoscopy skills: a multinational, randomized, blinded, controlled trial of simulator versus bedside training. *Gastrointest Endosc* 2010, **71**, 298–307.

38 Obstein KL, Patil VD, Jayender J, *et al.* Evaluation of colonoscopy technical skill levels by use of an objective kinematic-based system. *Gastrointest Endosc* 2011, **73**, 315–321.

39 Urs AN, Martinelli M, Rao P, Thomson MA. Diagnostic and therapeutic utility of double-balloon enteroscopy in children.

J Pediatr Gastroenterol Nutr 2014, **58**, 204–212.

40 Iddan G, Meron G, Glukhovsky A, Swain P. Wireless capsule endoscopy. *Nature* 2000, **405**, 417.

41 Oliva S, Di Nardo G, Hassan C, *et al.* Second-generation colon capsule endoscopy vs. colonoscopy in pediatric ulcerative colitis: a pilot study. *Endoscopy* 2014, **46**, 485–492.

3

The endoscopy unit

Harpreet Pall

 KEY POINTS

- Well-designed endoscopy units are essential to providing high-quality care in pediatric gastroenterology.
- Meticulous disinfection of the instruments is a vital component of patient safety.

- Appropriate staffing models are important to the safety and success of endoscopy.
- Process and quality improvement activities are a key component of unit management.
- Close attention to the equipment needed for pediatric endoscopy is necessary.

Unit design

Proper design of the pediatric endoscopy unit is crucial to the experience of the patient as well as the efficiency of the endoscopy team. Pediatric-focused facilities prioritize the child and family experience with the goal of reducing patient anxiety and providing age-appropriate analgesia [1,2]. Design and management of the endoscopy unit needs to be specialized for this unique patient population. A calming environment and smooth patient flow are critical. Ideally, encounters between preprocedure and postprocedure patients should be minimized.

In the United States, endoscopy procedures in children are performed in a variety of locations, including operating rooms, procedure rooms, dedicated endoscopy suites, and ambulatory surgery centers [1,2]. In low-volume centers, use of the operating room may be appropriate. For those units located in general hospitals, a combined adult/pediatric unit can offer cost savings in terms of equipment and facilities, as well as close proximity for pediatric endoscopists to adult therapeutic endoscopists. Recent survey data suggest up to 40% of centers in the United States currently perform endoscopy in a dedicated pediatric endoscopy unit [1]. Sharing space with other specialties such as pulmonology may be an option, but this can decrease the ability to customize the space for gastrointestinal endoscopy.

An endoscopy suite with at least two procedure rooms is desirable depending on the number of endoscopists and volume of procedures. Two rooms allow for concurrent procedures to take place and the ability to perform emergent inpatient procedures. Adult teaching hospitals are generally expected to do 1000 procedures per room per year [3]. In addition, the unit can include a motility room, capsule endoscopy viewing room, and advanced endoscopy room for fluoroscopic procedures. Plans

---

Practical Pediatric Gastrointestinal Endoscopy, Third Edition. Edited by George Gershman and Mike Thomson.
© 2021 John Wiley & Sons Ltd. Published 2021 by John Wiley & Sons Ltd.
Companion website: www.wiley.com/go/gershman3e

for designing a pediatric endoscopy unit should include anticipated volume, procedural complexity, and growth of the unit over time. Considerations of space are difficult and carry the greatest implications for overall construction costs [4].

All units should have a reception area and waiting room, where children and caregivers are greeted when they first arrive. The waiting areas should be child friendly. Bathrooms should be easily accessible, with special considerations for obese patients or handicapped patients in a wheelchair. Once escorted into the unit, patients require a clear area to be prepared for the procedure. From this area, the patient is transported directly to the procedure area. In general, a procedure room should be at least 400 square feet with more space often needed for advanced therapeutic cases involving fluoroscopy. Two separate doors should provide access to the procedure rooms: one to allow for the entry of the patient and clean supplies and the other for the removal of used equipment and specimens. Procedure rooms should be equipped to provide CO_2, oxygen, suction, and adequate electrical socket outlets for ancillary equipment. Ceiling-mounted booms may be helpful in keeping lines and equipment off the floor. One side of the room should be dedicated to nursing. Anesthesia and associated medications and supplies should be located at the head of the bed. After the procedure, a dedicated space for immediate and/or final recovery is needed.

A work area for physicians is an important consideration so endoscopists can complete procedure notes, enter patient orders, and coordinate care by phone. Including a room for consultation with patients and families to allow for confidential conversations is also important [1].

A major decision that must be made is where endoscopes will be stored and reprocessed between cases. Ideally, reprocessing is most efficient when it can be located directly adjacent to and shared with the other procedure rooms. Contaminated endoscopes have been linked to many outbreaks of device-related nosocomial infections. There have also been outbreaks recently related to the elevator mechanism of the duodenoscope [5]. Endoscopy staff should be well trained in disinfection procedures and skills should be annually assessed. Flexible GI endoscopes should first be comprehensively cleaned manually and then subjected to at least high-level disinfection (HLD). HLD can be performed in an automated endoscope reprocessor or using manual processes. Step-by-step guidelines on appropriate scope disinfection can be found in the multi-society guidelines originally published in 2011 [6] and updated in 2016 [7]. An understanding of how a specific reprocessor might be integrated into a unit under design is critical to avoiding last-minute space refitting, as well as potential breaches in patient safety once procedures are being performed.

When preparing plans for construction of the endoscopy unit, thorough discussion should take place with the hospital system facility management or a licensed architect familiar with healthcare facilities. The coding of these facilities will vary from state to state and country to country. To prevent future problems, the architect and licensing agencies should be consulted regarding all possible uses of the unit, as regulations vary depending on the use of the unit. Attention to these possibilities may prevent the possibility of retrofitting after the unit is already built.

Unit management

The Society of Gastroenterology Nurses and Associates (SGNA) has published guidelines suggesting the minimum number of qualified personnel who should be allocated to various positions during endoscopic procedures [8]. Running a cost-effective and safe endoscopic practice is a balance between appropriate staffing and the expense of maintaining that staff. Determining the number of staff needed to run the endoscopy unit is dependent on several factors. These include availability of equipment, time, types of procedures, complexity of patients, and presence of trainees. Maintenance of certification and licensing of endoscopy nurses are state specific in the United States (http://ce.nurse.com/RState Reqmnt.aspx). It would be prudent for the endoscopy unit to have annual assessments and training set up for all employees. A recent survey of pediatric centers suggests that more than 70% use an endoscopy RN and an endoscopy technician in the room during the performance of each procedure, and 100% use dedicated anesthesia staff [1].

Plans for after-hours coverage should be determined for weekend and after-hours emergencies. Based on a recent survey [1], 66% of US centers currently have a system in which a GI technician, a GI RN, or both are available on call. On-call staff should be cross-trained so that they can function well in all areas of the procedure. In some centers, general operating room staff assist with emergent after-hours cases. These staff may not be trained in endoscopic procedures. Assigning a unit director is important in ensuring a focus on process improvement activities, and ensuring that equipment and services remain competitive.

It is important to recognize that an endoscopy unit should not target 100% efficiency, as this will lead to scheduling conflicts and decreased patient satisfaction. Instead, standard efficiency rates should be considered to be 70–85% [9]. The unit may have a dual purpose of serving both inpatient and outpatient populations, as opposed to an outpatient endoscopy center. It should therefore provide easy access to both types of populations. Optimizing turnover time should be a target for quality improvement initiatives as it impacts unit productivity. Patient no-show may be an important barrier to improved efficiency. Preprocedure interventions have been shown to be effective in decreasing the no-show rate [10]. On-time starts and decreased turnover time can help maximize room efficiency [11]. Patient satisfaction surveys should be used as an indicator of quality of service. A recent study on patient experience in pediatric endoscopy identified important aspects from the patient and family perspective [12].

Documentation is an important aspect of endoscopy unit management. There are three broad areas of documentation: nursing documentation before and after procedure, the procedure itself, and sedation record. The Joint Commission on Accreditation of Healthcare Organizations provides guidance on components of documentation.

Equipment

Pediatric patients often have limitations in therapy due to size and approved measures. Endoscopic equipment can be purchased used or new or leased for a predetermined amount of time.

Purchasing or leasing endoscopy equipment represents a significant capital budget item for any setting in which pediatric endoscopy will be performed. Fewer endoscopes may be necessary to run concurrent rooms in smaller centers, compared with larger centers that feature more endoscopists and more endoscopy rooms. There are no data to guide how many scopes should be on hand at any endoscopy unit. To maximize efficiency, one light source and processor should be available per endoscopy room and one scope reprocessor allocated for each 1000 procedures per year. For adult units, one colonoscope and gastroscope per 350 procedures per year has been suggested as ideal [4], but this general recommendation may not apply to pediatric endoscopy in which there may be a need for endoscopes of various diameters and sizes to accommodate infants and children. The frequency of endoscope upgrades is also a major factor in determining how many endoscopes should be purchased.

In a recent survey, most centers reported replacing the endoscopes every 6–7 years [1].

An ideal endoscopy unit offers diagnostic endoscopy, including capsule endoscopy, small bowel enteroscopy, pH impedance testing, and motility testing. Therapeutic endoscopy should be available at pediatric centers or offered by an adult gastroenterologist in the area. If trained endoscopy staff are not always available to participate in emergent cases, having specific toolkits such as a bleeding or foreign body removal kit can ensure that correct endoscopic accessories are available.

Conclusion

Well-designed pediatric gastrointestinal endoscopy units are critical to the effective diagnosis and management of gastrointestinal disorders in children. A thoughtful approach to the design, management, and necessary equipment for the unit is essential.

 • See companion website for videos relating to this chapter topic: www.wiley.com/go/gershman3e

REFERENCES

1 Lerner DG, Pall H. Setting up the pediatric endoscopy unit. *Gastrointest Endosc Clin North Am* 2016, **26**(1), 1–12.

2 Pall H, Lerner D, Khlevner J, *et al.* Developing the pediatric gastrointestinal endoscopy unit: a clinical report by the Endoscopy and Procedures Committee. *J Pediatr Gastroenterol Nutr* 2016, **63**(2), 295–306.

3 Beilenhoff U, Neumann CS. Quality assurance in endoscopy nursing. *Best Pract Res Clin Gastroenterol* 2011, **25**(3), 371–385.

4 Petersen B, Ott B. Design and management of gastrointestinal endoscopy units. In: Cotton P (ed.). *Advanced Digestive Endoscopy: Practice and Safety*. Blackwell, Oxford, 2008, pp. 3–32.

5 FDA. *Design of Endoscopic Retrograde Cholangiopancreatography (ERCP) Duodenoscopes May Impede Effective Cleaning*. FDA Safety Communication, Montgomery, MD, 2015.

6 ASGE Quality Assurance in Endoscopy Committee. Multisociety guideline on reprocessing flexible gastrointestinal endoscopes: 2011. *Gastrointest Endosc* 2011, **73**(6), 1075–1084.

7 Peterson BT, Cohen J, Hambrick III RD, *et al.* Multisociety guideline on reprocessing flexible GI endoscopes: 2016 update. *Gastrointest Endosc* 2017, **85**(2), 282–294, e1.

8 SGNA. Position statement on minimal registered nurse staffing for patient care in the gastrointestinal endoscopy unit. *Gastroenterol Nurs* 2002, **25**(6), 269–270.

9 da Silveira EB, Lam E, Martel M, *et al.* The importance of process issues as predictors of time to endoscopy in patients with acute upper-GI bleeding using the RUGBE data. *Gastrointest Endosc* 2006, **64**(3), 299–309.

10 Mani J, Franklin L, Pall H. Impact of pre-procedure interventions on no-show rate in pediatric endoscopy. *Children* 2015, **2**(1), 89–97.

11 Tomer G, Choi S, Montalvo A, *et al.* Improving the timeliness of procedures in a pediatric endoscopy suite. *Pediatrics* 2014, **133**(2), e428–433.

12 Jacob DA, Franklin L, Bernstein B, *et al.* Results from a patient experience study in pediatric gastrointestinal endoscopy. *J Patient Exp* 2015, **2**(2), 23–28.

4

Pediatric procedural sedation and general anesthesia for gastrointestinal endoscopy

Tom Kallay, Rok Orel, and Jernej Brecelj

 KEY POINTS

- Uniform sedation guidelines should be in place when performing any level of procedural sedation for children.
- The sedation practitioner must be able to recognize the various levels of sedation in children of different ages, as it is common for children to pass from the intended level of sedation into a deeper state where physiologic compromise may occur.
- Use of end-tidal capnography during procedural sedation has been shown to reduce episodes of hypoxemia.

- New evidence regarding predictors of adverse events has emerged in the setting of upper respiratory infection, obesity, and raises questions about current nil per os guidelines.
- Open communication between the gastroenterologist and monitor provides an environment which allows for timely adjustments in medication titration or endoscopic technique.

Introduction

Sedation or general anesthesia is a prerequisite for safe and effective endoscopic procedures in the majority of pediatric patients. General anesthesia is always performed by an anesthesiologist. Ideally, deep sedation should be performed by an anesthesiologist too, but this depends on national or institutional organization and resources. Even in environments where sedation by nonanesthesiologists is the usual approach, this activity must be organized according to the highest safety standards with a skilled anesthesiologist team available for specific procedures, high-risk patients or possible complications.

The goals of procedural sedation are to (i) guard the patient's safety and welfare; (ii) minimize physical discomfort and pain; (iii) control anxiety and minimize psychological trauma (in the child and parents); (iv) control behavior and/ or movement to allow the safe completion of the procedure; and (v) return the patient to a state in which safe discharge from medical supervision is possible.

Practical Pediatric Gastrointestinal Endoscopy, Third Edition. Edited by George Gershman and Mike Thomson.
© 2021 John Wiley & Sons Ltd. Published 2021 by John Wiley & Sons Ltd.
Companion website: www.wiley.com/go/gershman3e

Definitions/spectrum of sedation to general anesthesia

There are four levels of sedation defined by the American Society of Anesthesiologists (ASA), and these may be thought of as a continuum: minimal sedation (anxiolysis), moderate sedation and analgesia (conscious sedation), deep sedation (unconscious), and general anesthesia.

Anxiolysis is a drug-induced state where motor and cognitive functions may be impaired, but the patient responds to verbal commands. Ventilatory and cardiovascular functions are largely unaffected with anxiolysis.

During moderate sedation, also known as conscious sedation, the child may respond purposefully to verbal commands (e.g., "open your eyes") with or without light tactile stimulation. Airway and cardiovascular function are unaffected; however, endoscopy presents a unique challenge as the tools employed for the procedure can predispose some patients to airway obstruction. This is especially relevant in smaller children, where the trachea is smaller and with soft cartilaginous rings, and more prone to obstruction than that of an older child with a larger, more rigid airway. In some cases where there is considerable risk of airway obstruction with endoscopy, intubation may be indicated. Due to the relative size of the endoscope and discomfort involved in its placement, moderate sedation is rarely successful in children when performing this procedure, unless the patient is old enough to cooperate.

Deep sedation refers to a state in which the child responds only to deep or repeated stimulation, and ventilation may be impaired. Patients may require assistance with ventilation or maintaining an airway, but cardiovascular function is usually maintained. One can anticipate a partial or complete loss of airway protective reflexes in this state, and preparations must be in place to accommodate for this.

General anesthesia describes a state in which there is no response to painful stimuli, and ventilation assistance is usually required due to depressed consciousness and neuromuscular function. Hemodynamic function may be compromised as well.

General anesthesia with endotracheal intubation is mandatory in patients graded III or higher according to the ASA physical status classification III (Box 4.1), in emergent procedures such as gastrointestinal bleeding or foreign body removal or more complex procedures such as endoscopic gastrostomy insertions or stenosis dilations. In interventional endoscopic procedures, a tracheal tube provides some airway protection against aspiration.

Sedation and analgesia for diagnostic and therapeutic endoscopy in children carries a number of considerations dependent on differences in age, developmental status, and presence of co-morbidities. One of the goals in sedating children is to control behavior, which is entirely dependent on their chronological and developmental age. Children younger than 6 or 7 years often require a deep level of sedation in order to safely complete an uncomfortable procedure, where respiratory drive, airway patency and protective reflexes may be compromised. Studies have shown that it is common for children to pass from the intended level of sedation into a deeper state in an effort to control their behavior, where physiologic compromise may occur. In order to provide the

---

Box 4.1   ASA physical status classification

Class I A normal healthy patient

Class II A patient with mild systemic disease (e.g., controlled reactive airway disease)

Class III A patient with severe systemic disease (e.g., a child who is actively wheezing)

Class IV A patient with severe systemic disease that is a constant threat to life

Class V A moribund patient who is not expected to survive without the operation

safest conditions for a child undergoing sedation, it is important to understand the definitions pertaining to level of consciousness, as well as having the ability to rescue a child from a deeper level of sedation than was intended.

Assessing risk in the pediatric patient

The Pediatric Sedation Research Consortium (PSRC) is a collaborative of 40 hospitals and universities in the United States and Canada with a mission dedicated to understanding and improving the process of pediatric sedation and sedation outcomes. Member institutions prospectively enroll pediatric patients receiving sedation for all procedures outside the operating room, and the data are entered into a central database. This rich database has contributed a great deal to pediatric procedural sedation literature over the last 10 years.

Predictors of adverse events for GI procedures

In 2015 a review was performed to assess the predictors for adverse events during esophagoduodenoscopy (EGD) and colonoscopies for pediatric patients. 12 030 procedures were examined: 7970 EGD, 1378 colonoscopies and 2682 were a combination of both. The majority of adverse events were desaturation (1.5%) and airway obstruction (1%); there were no deaths or CPR administered. This analysis revealed that ASA greater than or equal to II, receiving both procedures, obesity, presence of lower airway disease, and age were independent predictors of adverse events. The highest occurrence of adverse events (15%) occurred in those less than 1 year of age, with an occurrence of 8% in those between 2 and 5 years. While the adverse events did not result in permanent consequences, the findings do support a case for preemptive airway control with endotracheal intubation in young children undergoing GI procedures.

Obesity

In 2015 the PRSC database was examined to quantify the effect of obesity on rates of adverse events. The study included 5153 patients with a body mass index greater than the 95th percentile, and compared them to 23 639 non-obese patients. Comparison of the groups revealed that obese children have a higher incidence of adverse respiratory events and resulting airway interventions during procedural sedation (odds ratio [OR] 1.49, 95% confidence interval [CI] 1.31–1.7). The obese group had a higher incidence of the need for bag valve mask (BVM), use of nasopharyngeal (NP) airway, and head repositioning (OR 1.56, 95% CI 1.35–1.8). These findings provide further supporting evidence that obesity is an independent risk factor for adverse events, as well as the need for airway intervention.

NPO

Historically, the issue of fasting intervals before an elective procedure has generally followed those for elective anesthesia set forth by the ASA, yet recently these have come into question. Current ASA NPO guidelines state six hours is sufficient time for most foods, including infant formula, eight hours for a full meal and 4–6 hours for breast milk and clear liquids.

In 2016 the PRSC examined the effect NPO status had on aspiration, as well as major complications such as cardiac arrest or unplanned hospital admission. A total of 139 142 procedural sedations were reviewed. NPO status was known in 107 947 cases; 25 401 (23.5%) were not NPO. Aspiration occurred in eight of 82 546 (0.97 events per 10 000) who were made NPO per ASA guidelines versus two of 25 401 (0.79 events per 10 000) who were not NPO (OR 0.81, 95% CI 0.08–4.08; p = 0.79). Major complications occurred in 46 of 82 546 (5.57 events per 10 000) versus 15 of 25 401 (5.91 events per 10 000) (OR 1.06, 95% CI 0.55–1.93; p = 0.88). Overall, there were 0 deaths, 10 aspirations, and 75 major complications. Multivariate analysis revealed NPO status is not a predictor of either aspiration or experiencing a major complication.

Upper respiratory infection

The presence of URI is ubiquitous in pediatrics. The decision to cancel a procedure due to an upper respiratory infection can have impacts on patient care, as well as logistical problems for healthcare providers and parents. There are numerous studies suggesting that when anesthesia is administered to a patient with an active or recent URI, there is an increased frequency of airway events such as coughing or laryngo/bronchospasm.

In 2012 the PRSC evaluated this question. A total of 83 491 sedations were included; 70 830 without URI were compared to 13 319 patients with either recent or active URI, classified as having either thin or thick colored secretions. Data were examined for airway-related adverse events.

Occurrence of adverse events increased progressively from 6.3% for those with no URI, 9.3% for recent URI, 14.6% for URI with thin secretions, to 22.2% for those with URI and thick secretions ($p < 0.001$). The most common events were airway obstruction, oxygen desaturation, snoring, cough that interfered with the procedure, secretions requiring suctioning, stridor, or wheezing. The need for airway interventions followed an identical pattern, increasing from no URI through URI with thick secretions. The most common interventions were providing BVM, suction, or repositioning. There were no emergent airway interventions, unplanned admissions, or administrations of CPR.

The data suggest that in addition to a recent or active URI, the nature of the secretions is significant in assessing risk, with thick secretions carrying the highest risk. While the findings revealed a statistically significant difference, the nature of the events and consequences may not be clinically significant. Events such as laryngospasm, aspiration, emergent intubation, unplanned admission, and emergent call for anesthesia all remained <1% regardless of URI status. While there is a higher risk for adverse events in children with recent or active URI with thick secretions, these must be balanced against the acuity of the patient's condition and the urgency of procedure.

Preparation

A thorough presedation assessment is crucial in order to identify patients at risk for adverse events. Sedation for endoscopy must be tailored for each individual, yet preparations should be approached in the same stepwise fashion for every patient. The components of a presedation evaluation should include (i) informed consent, (ii) verbal and written instructions for postprocedure issues, (iii) the child's medical history, (iv) physical exam, and (v) a risk assessment.

Informed consent specific to the procedural sedation must be obtained and documented in accordance with institutional guidelines. Verbal and written instructions to the parent or guardian should include the objectives of the sedation as well as anticipated effects during and after the procedure. Patients must know whom to contact after the procedure if any medical issue arises after being discharged from the hospital

The medical history should focus on any current or past medical illnesses affecting the cardiovascular, respiratory, hepatic or renal systems, which may affect the child's response to the medications chosen. Consultation with a pharmacist may be necessary when there is a concern for drug interaction. Previous experiences with procedures should be elicited in order to uncover events that the child may be predisposed to, and a family history regarding anesthesia should be obtained. A thorough history of allergies to any medications or foods is important. As an example, propofol is manufactured in an oil-in-water base with egg and soybean oil, and therefore is contraindicated for use in a patient with egg or soybean allergy.

The physical exam must include a complete set of vital signs, which includes temperature, heart and respiratory rate, blood pressure, and pulse oximetry. A current weight is needed for appropriate medication dosing. Particular attention must be paid to the oropharynx for findings such as micrognathia, facial dysmorphism, loose teeth, tonsillar hypertrophy, or any other condition which could affect the airway. Heart exam should focus on the presence of murmurs or gallops which could indicate anatomical or functional issues. The airway exam should focus on the presence of stridor or wheezing.

Risk assessment includes assigning an ASA physical status classification level (Appendix I). Children who are Class I and II are considered appropriate candidates for minimal, moderate, and deep sedation. Situations which would indicate consultation with an anesthesiologist would be ASA class III or IV, children with congenital heart or pulmonary disease, significant upper or lower airway obstruction (such as tonsillar hypertrophy or poorly controlled asthma), or morbid obesity. Neurologic conditions such as poorly controlled seizures, central apnea, or severe developmental delay are also considered high risk, and warrant consultation with appropriate specialty services.

Staffing and environment preparation

At a minimum, the staff required for pediatric endoscopy with procedural sedation consists of four individuals. In addition to the gastroenterologist and endoscopy nurse, there must be an anesthesiologist (in case of general anesthesia or sedation provided by anesthesiologist) or another practitioner dedicated to monitoring the patient, whose sole responsibility is to continually observe and respond to the patient's vital signs, physiologic status, and level of sedation. The practitioner should be skilled in assessment of cardiopulmonary function: respiratory rate and depth, early recognition of

cyanosis, perfusion, and pulse assessment. Optimally, this individual would have a dedicated sedation nurse but this may not be possible at some institutions. Whether the sedation practitioner is a physician, physician assistant or nurse practitioner, they should be PALS certified and have adequate specialized training in pediatric procedural sedation and rescue techniques. Regular maintenance of these skills is recommended.

The majority of procedures are performed in endoscopy suites, which must be appropriately equipped to perform sedations safely. A crash cart or kit should include age- and size-appropriate equipment and medications necessary to resuscitate a child. Airway equipment must include size-appropriate BVM, airway delivery devices, and intubating equipment with age-appropriate endotracheal tube sizes and laryngoscope blades. Cardiorespiratory monitoring should include electrocardiography, respiratory tracing, pulse oximetry, capnography, and noninvasive blood pressure monitoring with size-appropriate cuffs. An oxygen source and suction with catheters must be available. A defibrillator, with pediatric paddles and adhesive pads, should be accessible. There should be a protocol for accessing a higher level of care such as a pediatric intensive care or step-down unit, and in nonhospital environments, a system for accessing ambulance services.

Anesthesia apparatus is essential for procedures in general anesthesia. It may be situated in the endoscopy suite or the endoscopy team may perform procedures in the operating theatre with a mobile endoscopic device.

During sedation and monitoring

Before the administration of medications, a baseline set of vital signs should be documented. The name, route, site, time, and dosage of all drugs administered should be recorded. Once medication administration has begun, level of consciousness and vital signs should be documented on a time-based flow sheet every five minutes. The vital signs documented should include heart and respiratory rate, oxygen saturation, and blood pressure. Once the procedure is complete and no more medications are to be administered, vital signs should be documented every 15 minutes until the child awakens.

Whether administration of medications is performed by the gastroenterologist or the sedation practitioner, good communication is crucial in order to provide optimal procedural sedation. It is important in order to anticipate physiologic changes or the conclusion of the procedure, which could affect a decision to administer a dose of medication or not. Timing of medication administration should be predicated on anticipating patient responses, which is best performed by maintaining an awareness of the procedure through observation and communication. It is the responsibility of the individual monitoring the patient to alert the gastroenterologist to physiologic deterioration, and to temporarily stop the procedure if rescue measures are required.

The nature of gastrointestinal endoscopy mandates a discussion of the specific physiological considerations inherent to the procedure. For example, esophageal intubation can induce apnea and bradycardia due to stimulation of the laryngeal branch of the vagus nerve. Infants or children with spastic neuromuscular disorders are especially prone to this, due to their small size and high cricopharyngeal tone, respectively. When air is insufflated into the gastrointestinal tract, it has the potential to cause respiratory insufficiency. Excess air in the stomach can elevate the left hemidiaphragm, impeding respiratory excursion and subsequently tidal volumes, which can be deleterious for ventilation and oxygenation. The loss of functional residual capacity can subsequently cause hypoxemia from loss of alveolar recruitment, and positive pressure ventilation, along with gastric decompression, may be necessary to recover adequate oxygen saturation.

Mesenteric stretch can cause various degrees of abdominal discomfort in some individuals, and adequate analgesia is needed to blunt this response. Intense pain during a colonoscopy, for example, is a sign of excessive mesenteric stretching and requires not only adequate analgesia but immediate adjustment of endoscopic technique. This situation highlights the need for constant communication between the gastroenterologist and monitor, as adjustments must be made by both individuals for the best procedural conditions.

The issue of standard supplemental oxygen use is controversial. Due to the nature of the procedure, supplemental oxygen is often needed to maintain adequate oxygen saturations. It must be kept in mind that failure in ventilation may be masked by supplemental oxygen, due to the law of partial pressures in the alveoli.

End-tidal capnography

Oxygen desaturation (i.e., oxygen saturation <90% in USA or <92% in Europe) in the setting of procedural sedation is a sign of suboptimal ventilation. Patients receiving supplemental oxygen can be 100% saturated with significantly elevated carbon dioxide levels, and be at risk for respiratory deterioration. Over the last 10 years, improved microstream capnographs have arrived which allow accurate, real-time measurement and continuous display of end-tidal carbon dioxide. This does not, however, obviate the need for continued close observation of respiratory function at all times.

In a prospective, randomized, controlled trial, integrating capnography into monitoring of nonintubated children receiving moderate sedation for pediatric endoscopy and colonoscopy was shown to reduce hypoxemia. Many hospitals have instituted mandatory use of end-tidal monitors for all procedural sedations.

Postsedation care

The child who has received moderate or deep sedation must be monitored in an appropriate environment which includes vital signs and pulse oximetry until they are awake. The period of wakefulness should be sustainable, as children emerging from sedation often drift between states of sleep and consciousness as the drugs are metabolized. The recovery area should include qualified staff to continuously record vital signs every 15 minutes, suction apparatus, and oxygen delivery devices including BVM. Patients who have received medications with a long half-life, or reversal agents such as naloxone or flumazenil, should be monitored for a longer period of time due to the risk of resedation.

The following are recommended discharge criteria.

- Cardiovascular function and airway patency are adequate and stable.
- The patient is easily arousable and protective reflexes are intact.
- The patient can talk (if age appropriate).
- The patient can sit up without assistance (if age appropriate).
- For patients who are very young or developmentally delayed, the presedation level of responsiveness or a level as close as possible for that child should be achieved.
- The state of hydration is adequate.

Conclusion

Procedural sedation in children carries a significant number of considerations which depend on the developmental and chronological age of the patient, history of previous experiences, and individualized response to medication. In order to avoid complications, the setting for the procedure must be well equipped, and the staff performing procedural sedation must be adequately trained in pediatric pharmacology and resuscitation. Good communication between all practitioners during the procedure contributes to a safe and efficient environment, and the likelihood of procedural success.

Societal guidelines must be adapted to specific national legislation and institutional protocols. Once established, sedation and general anesthesia protocols must be controlled subjected to constant quality monitoring.

 • See companion website for videos relating to this chapter topic: www.wiley.com/go/gershman3e

📖 FURTHER READING

American Academy of Pediatrics, American Academy of Pediatric Dentistry, Coté CJ, Wilson S, and the Work Group on Sedation. Guidelines for monitoring and management of pediatric patients during and after sedation for diagnostic and therapeutic procedures: an update. *Pediatrics* 2006, **118**, 2587–2602.

ASGE Standards of Practice Committee. Modifications in endoscopic practice for pediatric patients. *Gastrointest Endosc* 2014, **79**(5), 699–710.

Beach ML, Cohen DM, Gallagher SM, Cravero JP. Major adverse events and relationship to nil per os status in pediatric sedation/anesthesia outside the operating room: a report of the Pediatric Sedation Research Consortium. *Anesthesiology* 2016, **124**, 80–88.

Biber JL, Allareddy V, Allareddy V, *et al.* Prevalence and predictors of adverse events during procedural sedation anesthesia-outside the operating room for esophagogastroduodenoscopy and colonoscopy in children: age is an independent predictor of outcomes. *Pediatr Crit Care Med* 2015, **16**, e251–e259.

Brecelj J, Trop TK, Orel R. Ketamine with and without midazolam for gastrointestinal endoscopies in children. *J Pediatr Gastroenterol Nutr* 2012, **54**(6), 748–752.

Chung HK, Lightdale JR. Sedation and monitoring in the pediatric patient during gastrointestinal endoscopy. *Gastrointest Endoscopy Clin North Am* 2016, **26**, 507–525.

Gozal D, Gozal Y. Pediatric sedation/anesthesia outside the operating room. *Curr Opin Anaesth* 2008, **21**(4), 494–498.

Mallory MD, Travers C, Cravero JP, *et al.* Upper respiratory infections and airway adverse events in pediatric procedural sedation. *Pediatrics* 2017, **140**(1), e2017–0009.

Orel R, Brecelj J, Dias JA, *et al.* Review on sedation for gastrointestinal tract endoscopy in children by non-anesthesiologists. *World J Gastrointest Endosc* 2015, **7**(9), 895–911.

Saunders R, Struys M, Pollock R, Mestek M, Lightdale JR. Patient safety during procedural sedation using capnography monitoring: a systematic review and meta-analysis. *BMJ Open* 2017, **7**, e013402.

Scherrer PD, Mallor M, Cravero J, *et al.* The impact of obesity on pediatric procedural sedation related outcomes: results from the Pediatric Sedation Research Consortium. *Pediatr Anesth* 2014, **25**, 689–697.

Thomson M, Tringali A, Dumonceau JM, *et al.* Paediatric gastrointestinal endoscopy: European Society for Paediatric Gastroenterology Hepatology and Nutrition and European Society of Gastrointestinal Endoscopy guidelines. *J Pediatr Gastroenterol Nutr* 2017, **64**(1), 133–153.

van Beek E, Leroy P. Safe and effective procedural sedation for gastrointestinal endoscopy in children. *J Pediatr Gastroenterol Nutr* 2012, **54**, 171–185.

Wengrower D, Gozal D, Gozal Y, *et al.* Complicated endoscopic pediatric procedures using deep sedation and general anesthesia are safe in the endoscopy suite. *Scand J Gastroenterol* 2004, **39**(3), 283–286.

5

Pediatric endoscopy training and ongoing assessment

Catharine M. Walsh, Looi Ee, Mike Thomson, and Jenifer R. Lightdale

 KEY POINTS

- Endoscopic skill acquisition can be accelerated by recently available teaching models including virtual simulators.
- Formative and summative direct observational procedural skill (DOPS) assessments are integral.
- Use of a contemporaneous record of cases performed and assessment of competence should be mandatory. e.g.. www.jets.thejag.org.uk.
- Hands On Courses are a useful adjunct to ongoing training.
- Ideally trainers should have been trained in endoscopy training specific to pediatrics.

Introduction

Achieving proficiency in gastrointestinal endoscopy requires the acquisition of related technical, cognitive, and integrative competencies. Given the unique nature of performing endoscopy in infants and children, its training and assessment must be tailored to pediatric practice to ensure delivery of high-quality procedural care. This chapter outlines current evidence regarding pediatric endoscopy training and assessment.

Training

Learning to perform endoscopy largely occurs during formalized pediatric gastroenterology training programs of at least two years' dura-

tion. The traditional endoscopy teaching method is based upon the apprenticeship model, with trainees learning fundamental skills under the supervision of experienced endoscopists in the course of patient care. More recently, novel instructional aids have been utilized with the aim of accelerating learning, facilitating instruction, and helping trainees attain base levels of proficiency prior to performing procedures in the clinical environment.

Endoscopy skill acquisition

With regard to learning to perform procedures such as endoscopy, skill acquisition has been described by Fitts and Posner [1] as a sequential process involving three major phases: cognitive, associative, and autonomous. In the

Practical Pediatric Gastrointestinal Endoscopy, Third Edition. Edited by George Gershman and Mike Thomson.
© 2021 John Wiley & Sons Ltd. Published 2021 by John Wiley & Sons Ltd.
Companion website: www.wiley.com/go/gershman3e

cognitive stage, a learner develops an initial mental understanding of the procedure through instructor explanation and demonstration. Performance during this stage is often erratic and error filled, and feedback should focus on correct procedural technique and identifying common errors. Subsequently, in the *associative* phase, the learner translates knowledge acquired during the cognitive stage into appropriate motor behaviors, tasks are gradually executed more efficiently, and there are fewer errors and interruptions. Feedback during the cognitive stage should aim to help learners self-identify errors and their associated corrective actions [2]. Finally, with ongoing practice and feedback, the learner transitions to the *autonomous* stage, where motor performance becomes automated such that the skills are performed without significant cognitive or conscious awareness.

Endoscopy training aids

A relatively recent trend towards ensuring both quality of training and patient safety has prompted educators to seek complementary methods of teaching endoscopy to enhance apprenticeship approaches. In particular, magnetic endoscopic imaging has been developed to provide real-time images that display three-dimensional views of the colonoscope shaft configuration and its position within the abdomen during an endoscopic procedure [3]. A metaanalysis of 13 randomized studies found that use of magnetic endoscopic imaging during real-life colonoscopy is associated with a lower risk of procedure failure, reduced patient pain scores and a shorter time to cecal intubation, compared with conventional endoscopy [4]. With regard to training, research indicates that use of an imager may enhance learners' understanding of loop formation and loop reduction maneuvers [5].

Simulation-based training provides a learner-centered environment for learners to master basic techniques and even make mistakes, without risking harm to patients [6,7].

Mastery of basic skills in a low-risk controlled environment, prior to performance on real patients, enables trainees to focus on more complex clinical skills [6]. Additionally, within the simulated setting, learners can rehearse key aspects of procedures at their own pace, training can be structured to maximize learning, and errors can be allowed to occur unhindered, with the goal of allowing trainees to learn from their mistakes [8].

However, it is important to recognize that simply providing trainees with access to simulators does not guarantee that they will be used effectively. Instead, there are clearly a number of best practices in simulation-based education – including feedback, repetitive practice, distributed practice, mastery learning, interactivity, and range of difficulty – which must be employed by the educator to optimize learning [9–13]. Additionally, feedback must be carefully deployed at the end of the simulation with the intention of promoting successful procedural mastery [10,12]. Indeed, terminal feedback, defined as feedback given by a trainer to a trainee at the end of task completion, is more effective than both feedback given during task performance (which can lead to overreliance on feedback by the learner) and/or withholding feedback, which has been shown to handicap learning [14,15]. In short, the simulated setting allows educators to employ a number of strategies, including terminal feedback, which can be detrimental to patient safety when teaching in the clinical setting.

Training the pediatric endoscopy trainer

There is increasing recognition that teaching endoscopic skills should be performed by individuals with formal skills and learned behaviors, including awareness of principles of adult education, the components of good training, best practices in procedural skills education and appropriate use of beneficial educational strategies such as feedback [16,17]. The ability to teach endoscopy is an important skill that can be improved with instruction. In turn, "train the trainer" courses have been developed to enhance endoscopy teaching [18]. These courses are now mandatory for adult gastroenterology endoscopy trainers in the United Kingdom [19] and are increasingly being implemented across other jurisdictions such as Canada [20].

Assessment

Assessment of endoscopic procedural performance is ideally an ongoing process that should occur throughout the learning cycle, from training to accreditation to independent practice. This requires thoughtful integration of both formative and summative assessments to simultaneously optimize learning and certificate functions of assessment. Formative assessment is process focused. It aims to provide trainees with feedback and benchmarks, enables learners to self-reflect on performance, and guides progress from novice to competent (and beyond) [21,22]. In contrast, summative assessment is outcome focused. It provides an overall judgment of competence, readiness for independent practice and/or qualification for advancement [22]. Summative assessment provides professional self-regulation and accountability; however, it may not provide adequate feedback to direct learning [22,23].

Over the past two decades, there has been a profound shift in postgraduate medical education from a time- and process-based framework that delineates the time required to "learn" specified content (e.g., a two-year gastroenterology fellowship) to a competency-based model that defines desired training outcomes (e.g., perform upper and lower endoscopic evaluation of the luminal GI tract for screening, diagnosis, and intervention [24]) [25–27]. Assessment is an integral component of competency-based education as it is required to monitor progression throughout training, document trainees' competence

prior to entering unsupervised practice, and ensure maintenance of competence.

Nevertheless, procedural assessment in pediatric gastroenterology continues to focus predominantly on the number of procedures performed by a learner, as well as a "gestalt" view of their competence by a supervising physician [28]. This type of informal global assessment is fraught with bias inherent in subjective assessment and is not designed to aid in the early identification of trainees requiring remediation. A major limitation to using procedural numbers to determine competency is a demonstrated wide variation in the rate at which trainees acquire skills [29,30]. Furthermore, there are a host of factors which have been shown to affect the rate at which trainees develop skills, including training intensity [29], the presence of disruptions in training [31], the use of training aids (e.g., magnetic endoscopic imagers [3]), the quality of teaching and feedback received, and a trainee's innate ability [32]. Reflective of these concerns, current pediatric credentialing guidelines outline "competence thresholds" as opposed to absolute procedural number requirements. A "competence threshold" is the minimum recommended number of supervised procedures a trainee is required to perform before competence can be assessed [33].

There is tremendous variability in current credentialing guidelines with regard to competence thresholds for pediatric upper endoscopy and colonoscopy [34–36]. In large part, this variability reflects a current lack of evidence for determining competence thresholds for pediatric endoscopy. As such, today's guidelines for procedural numbers at which a learner can be assessed for competency in upper endoscopy are principally based on expert opinion [37]. In contrast, current colonoscopy guidelines are empirically based. However, most rely on an early study of competency by Cass et al. [38] that assessed 135 adult gastroenterology trainees from 14 programs and determined that performance of 140 supervised colonoscopies was required to achieve a 90% cecal intubation rate. More recent studies of adult colonoscopy competency have found that thresholds are achieved by 275 and 250 procedures when utilizing criteria including cecal intubation rate, time to intubation, and competency benchmarks on the Mayo Colonoscopy Skills Assessment Tool (MCSAT) [39] and the Assessment of Competency in Endoscopy (ACE) [40] tool, respectively, while it may take upwards of 400 procedures for some trainees to achieve competence. To date, the largest study to prospectively analyze this question examined 297 trainees over one year in the UK and found that it requires 233 colonoscopies to achieve a 90% cecal intubation rate [29]. In addition, a regression analysis of 10 adult studies, including 189 trainees, estimated that 341 colonoscopies are required to achieve a 90% cecal intubation rate [41].

Assessment based on quality metrics

Current pediatric endoscopy training programs are increasingly requiring learners to monitor quality measures, such as independent terminal ileal intubation rate and patient comfort, to be used as part of a global or summative assessment of trainees. Additionally, quality metrics are being used by practicing endoscopists as formative assessment tools to help promote improvement in care delivery [42]. However, the application of quality metrics to pediatric endoscopy requires pediatric-specific measures, which have yet to be formally developed. Currently, there are limited data on the applicability of adult-derived quality metrics to pediatric practice and their impact on clinically relevant outcomes. For example, with regard to cecal intubation rate, the reported successful completion rate for pediatric endoscopists varies from 48% to 96% [43–48]. Perhaps of even more pertinence to pediatric procedures, the reported terminal ileum intubation rate varies from 11% to 92.4% [43,45–49]. Additional research is required to help further delineate and define

pediatric-specific quality indicators that can be used for assessment and quality assurance purposes and validate them in a longitudinal prospective fashion [50].

Direct observational assessment tools

In recent years, accreditation bodies and endoscopy training and credentialing guidelines have all placed greater emphasis on the continuous assessment of trainees as they progress towards competence. To this end, direct observational assessment tools have emerged to support a competency-based education model that defines desired training outcomes. It is critical to ensure that assessment tools are psychometrically sound and have strong validity evidence.

A number of endoscopy assessment tools have been developed in the adult contex [51] but they are not pediatric specific and validity evidence for use in assessing pediatric endoscopists remains limited. Walsh et al. [52] developed the Gastrointestinal Endoscopy Competency Assessment Tool for pediatric colonoscopy (GiECAT$_{KIDS}$), a task-specific seven-item global rating scale that assesses more holistic aspects of the skill and a structured 18-item checklist that outlines key steps. Using Delphi methodology, the GiECAT$_{KIDS}$ was developed by 41 pediatric endoscopy experts from 28 North American hospitals, and addresses performance of all components of a colonoscopy procedure, including pre-, intra-, and postprocedural aspects. In one study of 116 colonoscopies performed by 56 pediatric endoscopists (25 novice, 21 intermediate and 10 experienced) from three North American academic hospitals, the GiECAT$_{KIDS}$ was found to be a reliable and valid measure that can be used in a formative manner throughout training [53]. The GiECAT$_{KIDS}$ has also been found to have strong interrater reliability, excellent test–retest reliability, evidence of content, response process and internal structure validity, discriminative validity (ability to detect differences in skill level), validity evidence of associations with other variables thought to reflect endoscopic competence (e.g., ileal intubation rate), and educational usefulness [53].

Ultimately, the integration of rigorously developed assessment tools, such as the GiECAT$_{KIDS}$, will provide a means to document progress throughout the training cycle. In addition, these tools can be used to support trainees' learning through the provision of instructive feedback, allow program directors to monitor skill acquisition to ensure trainees are progressing, facilitate identification of skill deficits, and help ensure readiness for independent practice [51,54]. Looking to the future, the universal adoption of robust assessment tools by pediatric gastroenterology training programs across jurisdictions would be useful, as it would generate aggregate data that could be used to develop average learning curves of pediatric endoscopists. These data could also be used to define milestones for pediatric endoscopists at different levels of training and help to establish minimal performance-based benchmark criteria for competence in pediatric endoscopy procedures to support competency-based training.

Conclusion

Differences between pediatric and adult endoscopic practice highlight the need for pediatric-specific approaches to training and assessment. Intense efforts have been made over the past decade to define the competencies required to carry out pediatric endoscopic procedures and to develop tools to support competency-based assessment. In addition, new instructional aids, such as magnetic imaging and simulation, have been introduced with the aim of enhancing training quality and accelerating skills acquisition. Ultimately, competency assessment metrics should be inextricably woven within a core endoscopy curriculum to ensure optimal integration of teaching, learning, feedback, and assessment throughout the entire spectrum of training in pediatric gastrointestinal procedures.

 • See companion website for videos relating to this chapter topic: www.wiley.com/go/gershman3e

REFERENCES

1 Fitts A, Posner M. *Human Performance.* Brooks-Cole, Belmont, CA, 1967.
2 Rogers DA, Regehr G, MacDonald J. A role for error training in surgical technical skill instruction and evaluation. *Am J Surg* 2002, **183**(3), 242–245.
3 Shah SG, Brooker JC, Williams CB, Thapar C, Saunders BP. Effect of magnetic endoscope imaging on colonoscopy performance, a randomised controlled trial. *Lancet* 2000, **356**(9243), 1718–1722.
4 Mark-Christensen A, Brandsborg S, Iversen LH. Magnetic endoscopic imaging as an adjuvant to elective colonoscopy, a systematic review and meta-analysis of randomized controlled trials. *Endoscopy.*2015, **47**(3), 251–261.
5 Shah SG, Thomas-Gibson S, Lockett M, *et al.* Effect of real-time magnetic endoscope

imaging on the teaching and acquisition of colonoscopy skills: results from a single trainee. *Endoscopy* 2003, **35**(5), 421–425.
6 Walsh CM, Sherlock ME, Ling SC, Carnahan H. Virtual reality simulation training for health professions trainees in gastrointestinal endoscopy. *Cochrane Database Syst Rev* 2012, 6, CD008237.
7 Singh S, Sedlack RE, Cook DA. Effects of simulation-based training in gastrointestinal endoscopy: systematic review and meta-analysis. *Clin Gastroenterol Hepatol* 2014, **12**(10), 1611–1623.
8 Ziv A, Wolpe PR, Small SD, Glick S. Simulation-based medical education: an ethical imperative. *Acad Med* 2003, **78**(8), 783–788.
9 Cook DA, Brydges R, Zendejas B, Hamstra SJ, Hatala R. Mastery learning for health

professionals using technology-enhanced simulation: a systematic review and meta-analysis. *Acad Med* 2013, **88**(8), 1178–1186.

10 Hatala R, Cook DA, Zendejas B, Hamstra SJ, Brydges R. Feedback for simulation-based procedural skills training: a meta-analysis and critical narrative synthesis. *Adv Health Sci Educ Theory Pract* 2014, **19**(2), 251–272.

11 Cook DA, Hamstra SJ, Brydges R, *et al.* Comparative effectiveness of instructional design features in simulation-based education: systematic review and meta-analysis. *Med Teach* 2013, **35**(1), e867–898.

12 Issenberg SB, McGaghie WC, Petrusa ER, Lee Gordon D, Scalese RJ. Features and uses of high-fidelity medical simulations that lead to effective learning: a BEME systematic review. *Med Teach* 2005, **27**(1), 10–28.

13 Grover SC, Scaffidi MA, Garg A, *et al.* A simulation-based training curriculum of progressive fidelity and complexity improves technical and non-technical skills in colonoscopy: a blinded, randomized trial. *Gastrointest Endosc* 2015, **81**(5S), AB324–AB325.

14 Walsh CM, Ling SC, Wang CS, Carnahan H. Concurrent versus terminal feedback: it may be better to wait. *Acad Med* 2009, **84**(10 Suppl), S54–57.

15 Grover SC, Garg A, Yu JJ, Ramsaroom A, Grantcharov T, Walsh CM. A prospective, randomized, blinded trial of curriculum-based simulation training in colonoscopy as a means to enhance both technical and non-technical skills. *Gastrointest Endosc* 2014, **79**(5S), Abstract 433.

16 Coderre S, Anderson J, Rostom A, McLaughlin K. Training the endoscopy trainer: from general principles to specific concepts. *Can J Gastroenterol* 2010, **24**(12), 700–704.

17 Walsh CM, Anderson JT, Fishman DS. An evidence-based approach to training pediatric gastrointestinal endoscopy trainers. *J Pediatr Gastroenterol Nutr* 2017, **64**(4), 501–504.

18 Waschke KA, Anderson J, Macintosh D, Valori RM. Training the gastrointestinal endoscopy trainer. *Best Pract Res Clin Gastroenterol* 2016, **30**(3), 409–419.

19 Anderson JT. Assessments and skills improvement for endoscopists. *Best Pract Res Clin Gastroenterol* 2016, **30**(3), 453–471.

20 Canadian Association of Gastroenterology. Skills Enhancement for Endoscopy Program. www.cag-acg.org/education/see-program.

21 Shute VJ. Focus on formative feedback. *Rev Educ Res* 2008, **78**(1), 153–189.

22 Epstein RM. Assessment in medical education. *N Engl J Med* 2007, **356**(4), 387–396.

23 Govaerts MJB, van der Vleuten CPM, Schuwirth LWT, Muijtjens AMM. Broadening perspectives on clinical performance assessment, rethinking the nature of in-training assessment. *Adv Health Sci Educ Theory Pract* 2007, **12**(2), 239–260.

24 Rose S, Fix OK, Shah BJ, *et al.* Entrustable professional activities for gastroenterology fellowship training. *Gastrointest Endosc* 2014, **80**(1), 16–27.

25 Frank JR, Mungroo R, Ahmad Y, Wang M, de Rossi S, Horsley T. Toward a definition of competency-based education in medicine: a systematic review of published definitions. *Med Teach* 2010, **32**(8), 631–637.

26 Long DM. Competency-based residency training: the next advance in graduate medical education. *Acad Med* 2000, **75**(12), 1178–1183.

27 Iobst WF, Sherbino J, Cate O Ten, *et al.* Competency-based medical education in postgraduate medical education. *Med Teach* 2010, **32**(8), 651–656.

28 Coyle WJ, Fasge F. Developing tools for the assessment of the learning colonoscopist. *Gastrointest Endosc* 2014, **79**(5), 808–810.

29 Ward ST, Mohammed MA, Walt R, Valori R, Ismail T, Dunckley P. An analysis of the learning curve to achieve competency at colonoscopy using the JETS database. *Gut* 2014, **63**(11), 1746–1754.

30 Dafnis G, Granath F, Påhlman L, Hannuksela H, Ekbom A, Blomqvist P. The impact of endoscopists' experience and learning curves and interendoscopist variation on colonoscopy completion rates. *Endoscopy* 2001, **33**(6), 511–517.

31 Jørgensen JE, Elta GH, Stalburg CM, *et al.* Do breaks in gastroenterology fellow endoscopy training result in a decrement in competency in colonoscopy? *Gastrointest Endosc* 2013, **78**(3), 503–509.

32 Cohen J. Training and credentialing in gastrointestinal endoscopy. In: Cotton PB (ed.). *Digestive Endoscopy: Practice and Safety*. Blackwell, Oxford, 2008, pp. 289–362.

33 Armstrong D, Enns R, Ponich T, Romagnuolo J, Springer J, Barkun AN. Canadian credentialing guidelines for endoscopic privileges, an overview. *Can J Gastroenterol* 2007, **21**(12), 797–801.

34 Leichtner AM, Gillis LA, Gupta S, *et al.* NASPGHAN guidelines for training in pediatric gastroenterology. *J Pediatr Gastroenterol Nutr* 2013, **56** Suppl 1, S1–8.

35 BSPGHAN Endoscopy Working Group. *JAG Paediatric Endoscopy Certification*. https://bspghan.org.uk

36 Conjoint Committee for the Recognition of Training in Gastrointestinal Endoscopy. *Requirements for CCRTGE Recognition*. www.conjoint.org.au

37 Walsh CM. Training and assessment in pediatric endoscopy. *Gastrointest Endosc Clin North Am* 2016, **26**(1), 13–33.

38 Cass O, Freeman M, Cohen J, *et al.* Acquisition of competency in endoscopic skills (ACES) during training: a multicenter study. *Gastrointest Endosc* 1996, **43**(4), 308.

39 Sedlack RE. Training to competency in colonoscopy, assessing and defining competency standards. *Gastrointest Endosc* 2011, **74**(2), 355–366.

40 Sedlack RE, Coyle W. Colonoscopy learning curves and competency benchmarks in GI fellows. *Gastrointest Endosc* 2015, **81**(5S), AB34 (Abstract Su 1550).

41 Cass OW. Training to competence in gastrointestinal endoscopy: a plea for continuous measuring of objective end points. *Endoscopy* 1999, **31**(9), 751–754.

42 Kramer RE, Walsh CM, Lerner DG, Fishman DS. Quality improvement in pediatric endoscopy: a clinical report from the NASPGHAN Endoscopy Committee. *J Pediatr Gastroenterol Nutr* 2017, **65**(1), 125–131.

43 Poerregaard A, Wewer AV, Becker PU, Bendtsen F, Krasilnikoff PA, Matzen P. Pediatric colonoscopy. *Ugeskr Laeger* 1998, **160**(14), 2105–2108.

44 Hassall E, Barclay GN, Ament ME. Colonoscopy in childhood. *Pediatrics* 1984, **73**(5), 594–599.

45 Dillon M, Brown S, Casey W, *et al.* Colonoscopy under general anesthesia in children. *Pediatrics* 1998, **102**(2 Pt 1), 381–383.

46 Stringer MD, Pinfield A, Revell L, McClean P, Puntis JW. A prospective audit of paediatric colonoscopy under general anaesthesia. *Acta Paediatr* 1999, **88**(2), 199–202.

47 Israel DM, McLain BI, Hassall E. Successful pancolonoscopy and ileoscopy in children. *J Pediatr Gastroenterol Nutr* 1994, **19**(3), 283–289.

48 Mamula P, Markowitz JE, Neiswender K, Baldassano R, Liacouras CA. Success rate and duration of paediatric outpatient colonoscopy. *Dig Liver Dis* 2005, **37**(11), 877–881.

49 Thakkar KH, Holub JL, Gilger MA, Fishman DS. Factors affecting ileum intubation in pediatric patients undergoing colonoscopy. *Gastrointest Endosc* 2014, **79**(5S), AB279–AB280.

50 Forget S, Walsh CM. Pediatric endoscopy, need for a tailored approach to guidelines on quality and safety. *Can J Gastroenterol* 2012, **26**(10), 735.

51 Walsh CM. In-training gastrointestinal endoscopy competency assessment tools:

types of tools, validation and impact. *Best Pract Res Clin Gastroenterol* 2016, **30**(3), 357–374.

52 Walsh CM, Ling SC, Walters TD, Mamula P, Lightdale JR, Carnahan H. Development of the Gastrointestinal Endoscopy Competency Assessment Tool for pediatric colonoscopy (GiECATKIDS). *J Pediatr Gastroenterol Nutr* 2014, **59**(4), 480–486.

53 Walsh CM, Ling SC, Mamula P, *et al*. The Gastrointestinal Endoscopy Competency Assessment Tool for pediatric colonoscopy. *J Pediatr Gastroenterol Nutr* 2015, **60**(4), 474–480.

54 Beard JD. Assessment of surgical competence. *Br J Surg* 2007, **94**(11), 1315–1316.

6

Recertification and revalidation as concepts in pediatric endoscopy

Priya Narula and Mike Thomson

 KEY POINTS

- Direct Operational Procedural Skills (DOPS) assessment, as occurs in training, will become standard in due course in peer review of maintenance of endoscopic skill.
- Ensuring ongoing competency in GI endoscopy in pediatrics will require monitoring of key performance indicators, reviewing outcome data and adverse event rates and evidence of engagement in educational and clinical activities.

Revalidation and/or recertification are processes whereby doctors demonstrate on a regular basis that they are up to date and fit to practice with the help of a portfolio of evidence or supporting information that can include continuous professional development, peer and patient feedback, quality improvement or audit and significant events [1]. They represent a shift towards a broader culture of accountability and a proactive approach. Medical revalidation was introduced in the UK in 2012 and is similar to New Zealand's practicing certificate and recertification and the American maintenance of licensure and certification [2]. Revalidation and recertification schemes seek to improve patient care by the ongoing review of individual medical practice [2].

Such processes, considered predominantly summative, are underpinned by a progressive, intrinsically motivated ambition to define and drive up quality standards [1]. As professionals engaged with implementation and experienced the realities of revalidation in practice in the UK, stakeholders found that dealing with concerns about poor practice (professional regulation) and seeking to improve professional standards (professionalism) were complementary processes [1].

Whilst these schemes are more generic, there are currently no established revalidation or recertification schemes for pediatric endoscopists.

The goals of recredentialing or recertification in GI endoscopy are to ensure continued clinical competency, promote continuous quality improvement, and maintain patient safety [3]. Ensuring ongoing competency in GI endoscopy in adults requires monitoring of key performance indicators (KPIs), reviewing outcome data and adverse event rates and evidence of engagement in educational and clinical activities with a focus on continuous quality improvement [4]. There are unlikely to be opportunities to directly observe practice for

Practical Pediatric Gastrointestinal Endoscopy, Third Edition. Edited by George Gershman and Mike Thomson.
© 2021 John Wiley & Sons Ltd. Published 2021 by John Wiley & Sons Ltd.
Companion website: www.wiley.com/go/gershman3e

independent endoscopists and therefore quality assurance is dependent on surrogates of performance such as KPIs. Upskilling and maintenance of competence for practicing endoscopists should be directed at technical (motor skills), cognitive (knowledge and recognition), and integrative skills, such as leadership and communication [5].

There is little in the pediatric literature on quality indicators or auditable KPIs tailored to pediatric endoscopy practice which can form the foundation of quality assured practice and can then be linked to a process that ensures accountability and improves and maintains professional standards of pediatric endoscopists. Auditing against an agreed set of KPIs and reviewing practice can help reduce variation in practice and standards between individual endoscopists and units.

The successful national pilot of a pediatric endoscopy Global Rating Scale (GRS) in the UK [6] is the first step towards a pediatric endoscopy quality improvement (QI) tool. Regular engagement with a QI tool like the P-GRS will help embed measures included in this tool, such as regular review of auditable outcomes and quality standards for individual endoscopists, use of electronic endoscopy reporting systems to capture immediate procedural and performance data to inform individual endoscopist

appraisal and professional revalidation requirements and help identify areas for any development, recording and reviewing adverse events with appropriate actions undertaken, etc. in clinical practice. In time, this will lead to a systematic approach to quality assurance.

There is likely to be scepticism about such processes and practical difficulties around resources but experience with medical revalidation in the UK suggests that normalization and familiarization with the process and the acknowledgment and experience of the benefits gradually help embed the process [7].

A formal process of certification and assessment of competence has been adopted for pediatric endoscopists (www.thejag.org.uk) but there remains a need to develop a robust and clear process for monitoring of KPIs relevant to pediatric practice, thus ensuring performance of a high-quality endoscopic examination and maintenance of endoscopic proficiency. Such processes are likely to drive up clinical standards and ensure all services provide high-quality and safe pediatric endoscopy care.

 • See companion website for videos relating to this chapter topic: www.wiley.com/go/gershman3e

REFERENCES

1 Tazzyman A, Feguson J, Walshe K, *et al*. The evolving purposes of medical revalidation in the United Kingdom: a qualitative study of professional and regulatory narratives. *Acad Med* 2018, **93**, 642–647.

2 Archer J, de Bere SR. The United Kingdom's experience with and future plans for revalidation. *J Contin Educ Health Professions* 2013, **33**(1), S48–53.

3 Rizk MK, Sawhney MS, Cohen J, *et al*. Quality indicators in gastrointestinal endoscopy. *Gastrointest Endosc* 2015, **81**(1), 1–16.

4 Faulx AL, Lightdale JR, Acosta RD, *et al*. Guidelines for privileging, credentialing, and

proctoring to perform GI endoscopy. *Gastrointest Endosc* 2017, **85**(2), 273–281.

5 Dube C, Rostom A. Acquiring and maintaining competence in gastrointestinal endoscopy. *Best Pract Res Clin Gastroenterol* 2016, **30**, 339–347.

6 Narula P, Broughton R, Bremner R, *et al*. Development of a paediatric endoscopy global rating scale: results of a national pilot. *J Pediatr Gastroenterol Nutr* 2017, **64**, 25–26.

7 Tazzyman A, Ferguson J, Hillier C, et al. The implementation of medical revalidation: an assessment using normalisation process theory. *BMC Health Serv Res* 2017, **17**, 749.

7

The role of the Global Rating Scale in pediatric endoscopy

Priya Narula and Mike Thomson

 KEY POINTS

- The whole patient/family journey contributes to the excellence of a pediatric endoscopy and is not limited to the simple technical excellence of the procedure.
- The Global Rating Scale (GRS) is a web-based, self-assessment quality improvement tool, that

enables units to assess how well they provide a patient-centered service, track their progress during quality improvement, and drive changes.
- A pediatric-specific GRS is now available.

Introduction

Variability in the quality, safety, and patient experience in endoscopy is well recognized and therefore quality assurance programs that have the potential to assess all aspects of care and support safe and high-quality patient-centered care are important. Even if a patient has a procedure which is technically excellent, adverse experiences such as poor communication can negatively influence patient experience and therefore there is a need for a holistic assessment. Whilst quality improvement is a process based upon cycles of measuring, planning, implementing, and further measuring, quality assurance is a process that ensures a predetermined set of standards is achieved.

The Global Rating Scale (GRS) is a web-based, self-assessment quality improvement tool, that enables units to assess how well they provide a patient-centered service, track their progress during quality improvement, and

drive changes. The GRS was initially developed and implemented in the adult endoscopy services in England in 2004. Adult experience demonstrated that although adult endoscopy services were encouraged to generate a continuous quality improvement cycle, it was insufficient to achieve sustained results. Quality assurance via the professionally led peer-reviewed accreditation process helped achieve the stepwise change in quality of endoscopy care [1,2]. All adult endoscopy units in the UK currently complete the GRS online census twice a year and after a unit achieves the required levels across all items, it can apply for accreditation.

Internationally, the GRS has been shown to be applicable in Dutch adult endoscopy units [3] and has been adapted for use in Canadian adult endoscopy units [4]. A Scottish study conducted focus groups with patients and concluded that the GRS did address quality issues that mattered to patients undergoing

Practical Pediatric Gastrointestinal Endoscopy, Third Edition. Edited by George Gershman and Mike Thomson.
© 2021 John Wiley & Sons Ltd. Published 2021 by John Wiley & Sons Ltd.
Companion website: www.wiley.com/go/gershman3e

endoscopy and validated its use as a quality assessment tool [5].

However, it is evident that the adult GRS is not applicable to pediatric endoscopy services and there has been a need for a pediatric-relevant and -applicable GRS.

Pediatric endoscopy GRS

The British Society of Paediatric Gastro-enterology, Hepatology and Nutrition (BSPGHAN) and Royal College of Physicians of London (RCP) collaborated to develop a pediatric GRS by adapting the established adult framework. This was successfully piloted nationally and ensured that the standards and measures were relevant to pediatric endoscopy services and fit for purpose [6].

The pediatric GRS provides a holistic assessment and consists of four domains, each of which refers to a broad aspect of care (Table 7.1): clinical quality, quality of patient experience, workforce, and training. Each domain is composed of qualitatively different items or standards covering all the aspects of endoscopy delivery and no standard is more or less important than any other.

Different levels can be achieved for each standard, ranging from D (Basic) to A (Aspirational). Levels create a more complete picture of what is going on by describing the different levels of achievement for a standard.

Each standard is composed of several measures which are unambiguous statements that have been designated a level from D to A. They would either have been achieved or not achieved by the service completing the assessment. To attain a level, the service must achieve all the measures up to and including that level. Based on the responses, levels for each standard are generated and provide a summary of the service. It is recommended that a core team consisting of clinical endoscopy lead, nurse endoscopy lead, and operational manager completes the GRS census.

The results of the national pediatric endoscopy pilot [6] were similar to the experience of the adult endoscopy units when they first started using the adult GRS in the UK [2] and to the Canadian adult endoscopy services when they first used the modified Canadian GRS [4]. It is important to highlight that this does not imply poor performance but is simply a starting point. This could occur because there may be areas where improvements are needed such as access to an electronic endoscopy reporting system or the unit is currently unable to measure, record, and review their performance. It did allow pediatric endoscopy units to identify what the quick wins for their unit were and in addition promoted collaboration

Table 7.1 Pediatric GRS domains and standards (www.thejag.org.uk)

Clinical quality	Quality of patient experience
1) Leadership and organization	8) Consent process including patient information
2) Safety	9) Patient environment and equipment
3) Comfort	10) Access and booking
4) Quality	11) Planning and productivity
5) Appropriateness	12) Aftercare
6) Results	13) Patient involvement
7) Respect and dignity	

Workforce	Training
14) Teamwork	17) Environment, training, opportunity, and resources
15) Workforce delivery	18) Trainer allocation and skills
16) Professional development	19) Assessment and appraisal

between units, sharing of good practice documents and pathways and supported greater patient involvement in pediatric endoscopy services (P. Narula, unpublished results).

When the adult GRS was first implemented in 2004, the majority of the adult endoscopy units were achieving a level C or D. Following the implementation of the GRS and development of a professionally led peer-reviewed accreditation process, there was an acceleration in service improvement and endoscopy units developed policies and processes to help meet the standards, resulting in a majority achieving the required level B across all standards [1,2]. A knowledge management system was also created which allowed services to share best practice pathways, policies, and guidelines [2].

The future

Adult experience has shown that the endoscopy GRS allows for continuous quality improvement as the endoscopy units are regularly reviewing practice, looking for opportunities to further improve care and putting in measures to help achieve the highest standards of quality and patient-cenetred care. The GRS also promotes benchmarking and collaborative working, allowing units to share solutions to common service problems or deficiencies. It is flexible in practice as it does not set specific outcomes but refers to current speciality guidelines and ensures adherence to these. As pediatric endoscopy services embed the use of the GRS in their clinical practice as a quality improvement tool, this will help not only to identify any gaps or improvements needed to deliver high-quality patient-centered care but also serve as leverage for clinicians to request the necessary support from their hospital management. It is envisioned that in time, quality assurance by a pediatric accreditation process will help sustain and accelerate service improvements triggered by the pediatric GRS.

 • See companion website for videos relating to this chapter topic: www.wiley.com/go/gershman3e

REFERENCES

1 Stebbing JF. Quality assurance of endoscopy units. *Best Pract Res Clin Gastroenterol* 2011, **25**, 361–370.
2 Valori R. Quality improvements in endoscopy in England. *Techn Gastrointest Endosc* 2012, **14**, 63–72.
3 Sint Nicolaas J, de Jonge V, de Man RA, *et al*. The Global Rating Scale in clinical practice: a comprehensive quality assurance programme for endoscopy departments. *Dig Liver Dis* 2012, **44**(11), 919–924.

4 MacIntosh D, Dube C, Hollingworth R, *et al*. The endoscopy global rating scale – Canada: development and implementation of a quality improvement tool. *Can J Gastroenterol* 2013. **27**(2), 74–82.
5 William T, Ross A, Stirling C, *et al*. Validation of the Global Rating Scale for endoscopy. *Scott Med J* 2013, **58**(1), 20–21.
6 Narula P, Broughton R, Bremner R, *et al*. Development of a paediatric endoscopy global rating scale: results of a national pilot. *J Pediatr Gastroenterol Nutr* 2017, **64**, 25–26.

FURTHER READING

Joint Advisory Group on GI endoscopy (JAG). Global Rating Scale. www.jagaccreditation. org

Joint Advisory Group on GI endoscopy (JAG). Global Rating Scale (GRS) – Paediatric. www. thejag.org.uk/AboutUs/DownloadCentre

8

Quality indicators as a critical part of pediatric endoscopy provision

Priya Narula and Mike Thomson

 KEY POINTS

- Safe, efficient, technically-competent endoscopy is only part of the story.
- A child and family-friendly environment, good pre-procedure preparation, accurate documentation and clear and concise communication between team members is essential.
- Appropriate after care and information with follow up complete an ideal endoscopic experience for a child and family.

Introduction

High-quality pediatric endoscopy occurs when a child or adolescent receives an indicated procedure safely and efficiently in an appropriate environment, with relevant and adequate communication and documentation occurring before, during and after the procedure among the involved health professionals and the patient and family or carer, a correct diagnosis is made or excluded and appropriate therapy is provided as indicated. Quality in endoscopy is not just limited to technical expertise but includes other elements such as clinical quality, quality of patient experience, workforce providing this service, and training, which can influence the overall quality of endoscopy provision.

A quality indicator or measure or metric can be used to compare actual performance against a standard defined by ideal performance or benchmark and enable potential quality improvement [1]. Clinically relevant measures should correlate with clinically relevant endpoints, be evidence based with demonstrable gaps in performance and be amenable to both measurement and improvement [1]. Quality indicators in adult endoscopy are well established and involve measures of structure, process, and outcome [2] (www.thejag.org.uk). However, there is a limited evidence base for pediatric endoscopy quality indicators.

Quality indicators may be flexible as evidence and practice evolve. In the UK, identified quality and safety indicators have been used to underpin the respective items of the Pediatric Endoscopy Global Rating Scale (P-GRS), a quality improvement tool launched in 2017 which, amongst other measures, assesses the extent to which the audit cycle has been applied to the quality and safety indicators (www.bspghan.org.uk; www.thejag.org.uk). Suggested pediatric procedural quality indicators include procedure completion rates

Practical Pediatric Gastrointestinal Endoscopy, Third Edition. Edited by George Gershman and Mike Thomson.
© 2021 John Wiley & Sons Ltd. Published 2021 by John Wiley & Sons Ltd.
Companion website: www.wiley.com/go/gershman3e

such as cecal intubation and terminal ileal intubation rates, appropriate diagnostic biopsies based on best evidence, adequate bowel preparation for colonoscopies, and safety indicators that relate to complication rates. These are auditable outcomes for which there is some evidence base to help recommend a minimum standard, for example, ileal intubation rates in pediatric colonoscopy. As confirmation or exclusion of inflammatory bowel disease is one of the main reasons for pediatric colonoscopy, ileal intubation is a clinically important and meaningful pediatric quality indicator compared to only using cecal intubation rates that are more relevant for adult endoscopists in the context of bowel cancer screening. Cecal intubation rates are generally recommended to be >90% (www.thejag.org.uk). Reported ileal intubation rates in recent pediatric literature vary from 84% to 98% [3–5].

A recent North American endoscopy clinical report proposed >90% ileal intubation rate as a quality metric for pediatric colonoscopy [6]. The pediatric colonoscopy certification criteria in the UK use terminal ileal intubation rates of ≥60% and cecal intubation rates of ≥90%, amongst other criteria, for certifying pediatric gastroenterology trainees to perform independent ileocolonoscopies (www.thejag.org.uk).

Access to an electronic endoscopy reporting system is essential in all pediatric endoscopy units as this allows reliable and accurate data collection. There are other quality and safety outcomes which are important to monitor and review but due to a limited evidence base, it can be difficult to assign a standard, for example the minimum number of procedures required to maintain competence or unplanned admissions or procedures within a fixed time frame such as eight days of a gastrointestinal endoscopy or need for ventilation post gastrointestinal endoscopy performed under general anesthetic or unplanned use of reversal agents if sedation used. Other quality indicators may relate to the structure, process or staffing in a pediatric endoscopy unit.

Quality and safety indicators relating to structure can include access to age-appropriate equipment, endoscopy reporting system, supportive anesthetic, pathology and radiology service with pediatric expertise, etc. Quality and safety indicators relating to process include having agreed policies such as for managing patients with diabetes, adherence to guidelines for endoscope decontamination, use of timeout or WHO checklists pre-procedure, an endoscopy user group that meets regularly, etc. Quality indicators relating to staffing include staffing levels and skill mix appropriate to the volume and types of procedures performed with pediatric competencies, identified medical and nurse leads for endoscopy with adequate managerial and clerical staff support, appropriate supervision of trainees, etc.

The National Endoscopy Database (NED), led by the Joint Advisory Group on GI Endoscopy (JAG), is a very exciting development in the UK. The NED is populated by data extracted automatically from the endoscopy reporting system at endoscopy services in the UK. It will make data available in user-friendly outputs for clinicians, services and research purposes and enable improved quality assurance in endoscopy (https://ned.jets.nhs.uk/KPI).

Conclusion

Development of quality improvement tools like the P-GRS, a robust quality assurance process and the regular audit of performance against quality indicators that are clinically meaningful for pediatric endoscopy will help define their importance, measure performance variability against these indicators and in time allow pediatric endoscopy units to achieve and demonstrate the highest standards of quality and patient-centered care through repeated cycles of measurement, intervention, and evaluation.

 • See companion website for videos relating to this chapter topic: www.wiley.com/go/gershman3e

REFERENCES

1 Petersen BT. Quality assurance for endoscopists. *Best Pract Res Clin Gastroenterol* 2011, **25**, 349–360.

2 Rex DK, Schoenfeld PS, Cohen J, *et al.* Quality indicators for colonoscopy. *Gastrointest Endosc* 2015, **81**(1), 31–53.

3 Thakkar K, Holub JL, Gilger MA, *et al.* Quality indicators for paediatric colonoscopy: results from a multicenter consortium. *Gastrointest Endosc* 2016, **83**, 533–541.

4 Singh HK, Withers GD, Ee LC. Quality indicators in paediatric colonoscopy: an Australian tertiary centre experience. *Scand J Gastroenterol* 2017, **52**(12), 1453–1456.

5 Thomson M, Sharma S. Diagnostic yield of upper and lower gastrointestinal endoscopies in children in a tertiary centre. *J Pediatr Gastroenterol Nutr* 2017, **64**(6), 903–906.

6 Kramer RE, Walsh CM, Lerner DG, *et al.* Quality improvement in paediatric endoscopy: a clinical report from the NASPGHAN endoscopy committee. *J Pediatr Gastroenterol Nutr* 2017, **65**(1), 125–131.

9

e-learning in pediatric endoscopy

Claudio Romano and Mike Thomson

 KEY POINTS

- Distance learning facilitated by online means can achieve faster competence not only in lesion recognition but in learning technical skills prior to hands-on training.

- Examination of knowledge and appropriate application of endoscopic techniques may be a feature of future postpandemic assessment.

Advances in pediatric endoscopy have been assured since 1960. Over the past decades, the number of endoscopies for pediatric gastrointestinal disease has increased rapidly. Diagnostic and therapeutic applications increase at a rapid pace. Hands-on courses are the primary learning tool, along with training in dedicated training units.

Recently, with the burgeoning of information technology, teaching procedures and modalities by which to provide infomration have changed. The introduction of e-learning platforms has led to questions arround the appropriateness of teaching methods, design of the technological infrastructure, and the interaction of students with the technology. e-learning can be defined as learning through electronic devices using technology as a medium for online interaction and to access information. e-learning is used as one of the learning styles together with computer-aided learning and remote learning. Pediatric endoscopists can now acquire detailed knowledge, techniques and experience in many pediatric endoscopic fields, including the role and indications of endoscopsy in pediatric gastrointestinal diseases; technique of upper gastrointestinal endoscopic examination; risk assessment; recognition of complications; application of sedation/GA; lesion recognition of gastrointestinal pathology; ideal ileocolonoscopy technique including resolution of loop formation.

Lesion recognition is an area which lends itself nicely to this technology as competency can be examined remotely. The techniques underlying competent endoscopy can be taught with videos in advance of hands-on teaching and in this respect e-learning or any platform allowing access to "distant" learning of techniques is superior to textbooks or other modalities. Furthermore, endotherapeutic techniques such as variceal and nonvariceal bleeding, gastrostomy insertion, balloon dilation of strictures etc. lend themselves to web-based video learning of the techniques prior to hands-on activity and training.

Practical Pediatric Gastrointestinal Endoscopy, Third Edition. Edited by George Gershman and Mike Thomson.
© 2021 John Wiley & Sons Ltd. Published 2021 by John Wiley & Sons Ltd.
Companion website: www.wiley.com/go/gershman3e

Various platforms have been devloped by organizations and societies such as ESPGHAN, ESGE, BSG, UEG, ASGE, etc, and these are readily available online.

The last and possibly most useful application of e-learning is the ability to use it as an objective test of the user's competency – particularly in lesion recognition and testing the individual's knowledge generally of when and how to apply various techniques in pediatric endoscopy. It is envisaged that this may then contribute to any formative, summative, and ongoing assessments of a pediatric endoscopist's ability.

Of course, many examples of lesions and best practice endoscopy also exist on the internet outside the formal concept of e-learning.

 • See companion website for videos relating to this chapter topic: www.wiley.com/go/gershman3e

USEFUL WEBSITES

www.e-lfh.org.uk
www.esge.com/elearning
www.asge.org/home/education-meetings/
products/endoscopic-learning-library

www.ueg.eu/education/online-courses
www.espghan.org/education/e-learning

Part Two

Diagnostic Pediatric Endoscopy

10

Indications for gastrointestinal endoscopy in childhood

Dalia Belsha, Jerome Viala, George Gershman, and Mike Thomson

---

 KEY POINTS

- Diagnostic and therapeutic endoscopy are as available now for children as they were in previous years for adults.
- Ideally, a pediatric practitioner would perform these although in adolescents, adult GI practititoners are sometimes involved.
- Updated diagnostic and management guidelines for common disorders including celiac disease (CD), gastroesophageal reflux (GER), eosinophilic esophagitis (EE), and inflammatory bowel disease (IBD) illustrate

- the central role for endoscopy in pediatric practice.
- It is also recognized that therapeutic endoscopic approaches are widely available now and further broaden the referral spectrum – these include treatment of GI bleeding, gastrostomy insertion, dilation of strictures, polypectomy, and many others.
- The advent of newer technologies allows the examination of hitherto inaccessible areas of the GI tract such as the mid-small bowel by wireless capsule videoendoscopy and enteroscopy.

Introduction

Endoscopic examination of the gastrointestinal tract (GIT) for diagnostics and therapy has evolved markedly over the last 20 or so years and is now usually undertaken by pediatric endoscopists. Updated diagnostic and management guidelines for common disorders including celiac disease (CD), gastroesophageal reflux (GER), eosinophilic esophagitis (EE) and inflammatory bowel disease (IBD) illustrate the central role for endoscopy. It is also recognized that therapeutic endoscopic approaches are widely available now and

further broaden the referral spectrum – these include treatment of GIT bleeding, gastrostomy insertion, dilation of strictures, polypectomy, and many others. Lastly, the advent of newer technologies allows the examination of hitherto inaccessible areas of the GIT such as the mid-small bowel by wireless capsule videoendoscopy and enteroscopy. This chapter is more symptom focused as the place of endoscopy in various pathologies is covered in the relevant chapters later on.

Changing indications for pediatric endoscopy over the last 25 years may have also influenced other disease detection rates such as that of IBD.

Practical Pediatric Gastrointestinal Endoscopy, Third Edition. Edited by George Gershman and Mike Thomson.
© 2021 John Wiley & Sons Ltd. Published 2021 by John Wiley & Sons Ltd.
Companion website: www.wiley.com/go/gershman3e

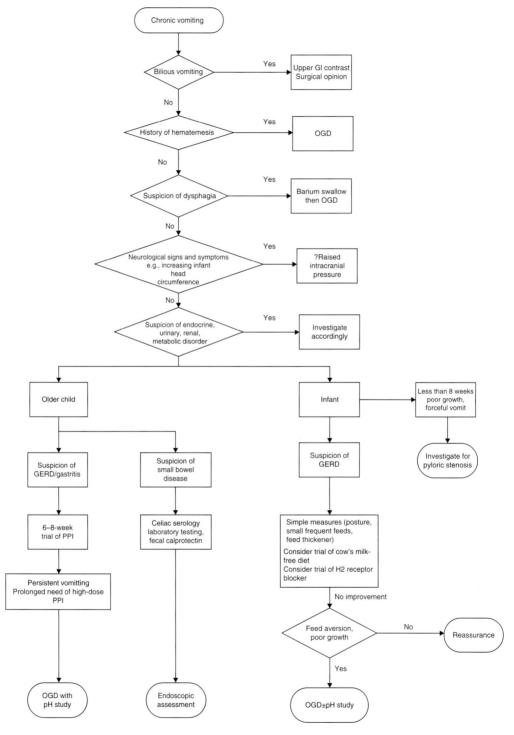

Figure 10.1 Suggested diagnostic algorithm of chronic vomiting. PPI, proton pump inhibitor. Source: BMJ Publishing Group Ltd and the Royal College of Paediatrics and Child Health.

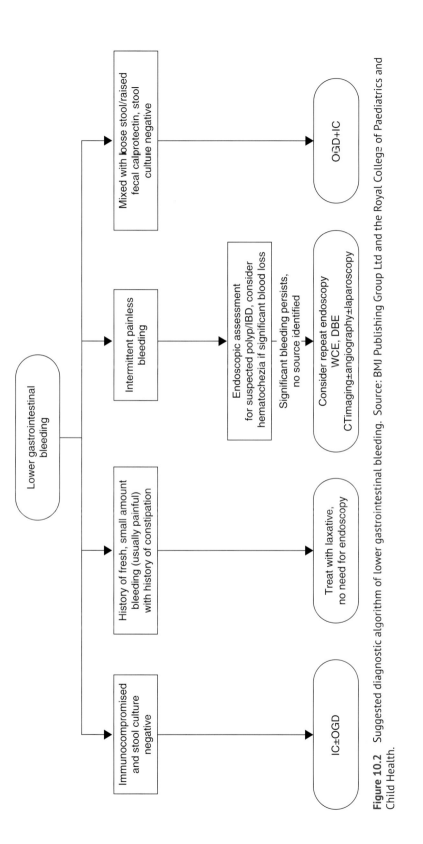

Figure 10.2 Suggested diagnostic algorithm of lower gastrointestinal bleeding. Source: BMJ Publishing Group Ltd and the Royal College of Paediatrics and Child Health.

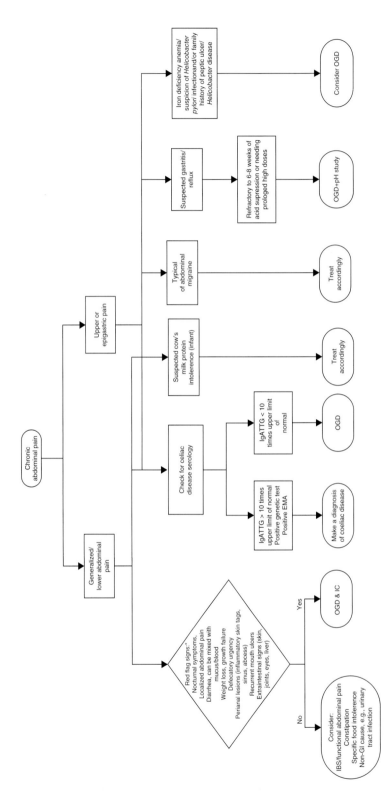

Figure 10.3 Suggested diagnostic algorithm for chronic abdominal pain. Source: BMJ Publishing Group Ltd and the Royal College of Paediatrics and Child Health.

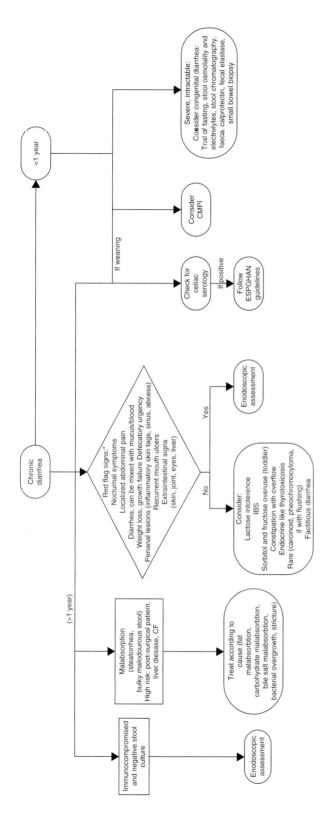

Figure 10.4 Suggested diagnostic algorithm of chronic diarrhea. Source: BMJ Publishing Group Ltd and the Royal College of Paediatrics and Child Health.

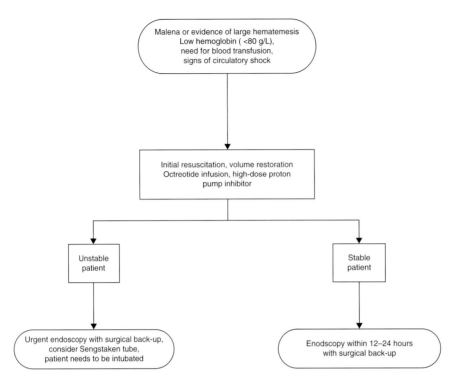

Figure 10.5 Suggested initial management of upper gastrointestinal bleeding. Source: BMJ Publishing Group Ltd and the Royal College of Paediatrics and Child Health.

Table 10.1 Therapeutic indications for EGD

Percutaneous endoscopic gastrostomy (PEG) insertion

Changing PEG tube to button/balloon gastrostomy

Naso-jejunal (NJ) or gastro-jejunal (GJ) tube placement

Foreign body removal

Food bolus impaction removal

Dilation of esophageal strictures ± topical application of antifibrotic mitomycin C

Esophageal stent placement – usually reserved for the palliative situation

Dilation of achalasia

Closure of esophageal fistulae with tissue glue and endo-clips

Upper GI polypectomy

Upper GI nonvariceal bleeding therapy

Esophageal varices banding (emergency or as prophylactic)

Injection of gastric fundal varices with histoacryl glue

Division of duodenal web/diaphragm/stenosis

Delivery of wireless video capsule

Laparoscopy-assisted percutaneous endoscopic jejunostomy (LAPEJ)

Endoscopic fundoplication

Endomucosal resection of sessile lesion (EMR)

Transgastric drainage of pancreatic pseudocyst

Endoultrasound-guided celiac plexus neurolysis

Endoscopic retrograde cholangiopancreatography (ERCP) – stent placement both biliary and pancreatic

ERCP – sphincterotomy and removal of biliary stones

Table 10.2 Indications for therapeutic colonoscopy in children

Polypectomy

Dilation of ileocolonic stenosis

Treatment of hemorrhagic lesions

Foreign body removal

Reduction of sigmoid volvulus (rare and usually not successful)

Stenting of strictures

Sigmoidostomy

Cecostomy

In prospective studies, pediatric IBD incidence rates are higher than had been reported previously, which might reflect a real increase but also may have been affected by acquisition bias secondary to wider availability of, and improvement in the quality of, endoscopic assessment

On the other hand and despite an increase in the number of GI endoscopies over recent years, diagnostic yield with abnormal histology results in overall endoscopic procedures remains constant at 62–76%. This suggests that the increase in number of pediatric endoscopies performed is due to increased demand rather than a lower threshold for the procedures.

In addition to IBD and EE, diagnosis of CD is increasing with increased awareness of the disease.

It is important to bear in mind that, in appropriately trained and experienced hands, endoscopy is very safe, it can be associated rarely with morbidity and it is not cheap compared to other less invasive diagnostic routes and hence a pragmatic approach is required in children.

Diagnostic endoscopy

Indications for diagnostic esophagogastroduodenoscopy (EGD) and/or ileocolonoscopy are provided in algorithms (Figures 10.1–10.5). The aim of these algorithms is to provide a guide to when the endoscopy might be necessary based on symptoms (chronic vomiting, dysphagia, chronic iron deficiency anemia, chronic abdominal pain, chronic diarrhea and lower GI bleeding).

Endoscopy is not usually indicated in older children in evaluation of functional GI disorders, including self-limited abdominal pain, constipation, and encopresis.

Esophagogastroduodenoscopy is not indicated in uncomplicated GER. In addition, it is not indicated for infants or children without overt regurgitation presenting with only one of the following: unexplained feeding difficulties (for example, refusing to feed, gagging or choking), distressed behavior, faltering growth, chronic cough or hoarseness. It is, however, to be considered for those in whom reflux-type symptoms persist after 1 year of age and in those presenting with dysphagia (a classic presentation of EE). Other considerations include patients with reflux-type symptoms and refractory iron deficiency anemia and those presenting with other complication factors such as faltering growth.

The reader is referred to the relevant chapters for the following diagnostic indications: eosinophilic esophagitis, *Helicobacter pylori*, CD, IBD, and less common pathologies (Chapters 20–24, 32, and 42).

Therapeutic indications for endoscopy

The reader is referred to the appropriate chapters dealing with the following: upper gastrointestinal bleeding; foreign body removal; stricture management; polypectomy; PEG placement, and less common interventions.

Indications for therapeutic applications of EGD are listed in Table 10.1 and for therapeutic ileocolonoscopy in Table 10.2.

 • See companion website for videos relating to this chapter topic: www.wiley.com/go/gershman3e

11

Diagnostic upper gastrointestinal endoscopy

George Gershman and Mike Thomson

 KEY POINTS

- An inspection of the equipment prior endoscopy is a simple way to avoid technical malfunction during the procedure.
- A key for a safe and successful EGD is adherence to proper preparation for the procedure, correct handling of the endoscope, an appropriate technique of esophageal intubation and navigation of the endoscope through the

esophagus, stomach and duodenum, and knowledge of the endoscopic landmarks of the upper gastrointestinal tract.
- Most complications of EGD are preventable with adequate sedation, appropriate patient selection, and proper technique tailored to patient age.

Introduction

This chapter is focused on practical aspects of esophagogastroduodenoscopy (EGD) in children with the goal of facilitating the learning curve of optimal and safe EGD techniques and also a brief description of some rare pathology of the upper GI tract. The detailed review of common disorders of the esophagus, stomach, and duodenum will be discussed in corresponding chapters.

Indications for EGD

Indications for EGD are covered in Chapter 10.

Assembling the equipment and preprocedure check-up

To ensure proper function of endoscopic equipment during endoscopy, the key elements of

the system should be checked prior to the procedure. This begins with turning the system on and establishing a white balance for a proper color scheme, and optimal brightness of the monitor. Proper function of the water delivery system is confirmed by water spurting vigorously from the nostril while pressing and holding down the air-water valve. If water is not running out at a decent pressure, check the status of the air pump, adjust the pressure level (medium level is optimal), check if the connecting tube from the water container to the endoscope is unclamped, confirm tight connection of the endoscope with the light source and the water container to the endoscope, tighten the cap of the water container and determine if the air-water valve is properly mounted. Consider sequential replacement of the air-water valve, water container and the endoscope, if all other options have been exhausted.

Practical Pediatric Gastrointestinal Endoscopy, Third Edition. Edited by George Gershman and Mike Thomson.
© 2021 John Wiley & Sons Ltd. Published 2021 by John Wiley & Sons Ltd.
Companion website: www.wiley.com/go/gershman3e

Check and adjust the intensity of the suction. If it is inadequate, check the suction system in a stepwise fashion: make sure that the wall-mounted suction valve is turned on and the suction canister is sealed off, and that the suction cable is tightly connected to the endoscope and the suction canister. If suction is still inadequate, reassemble the suction canister properly. Then, check the suction valve: pull it out for visual inspection, dip it in water and reinsert it back by pressing down into the suction nostril of the control panel until a soft click occurs. Replace the endoscope if all previous steps have failed.

Wipe the lens of the endoscope with an alcohol swab if the image is blurry.

Endoscope handling

The endoscopist holds the control panel of the endoscope in the left slightly extended palm by the fourth and fifth fingers with the connecting tube hanging behind the thumb (Figure 11.1). The index and middle fingers are positioned comfortably above the suction and air-water valves respectively (Figure 11.2). This allows the endoscopist to use the thumb for rotation of the large up/down (U/D) angulation knob in a clockwise or counterclockwise direction (Figure 11.3). An additional rotation

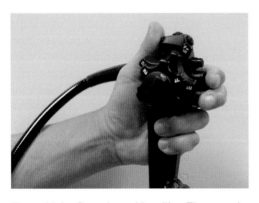

Figure 11.1 Control panel handling. The control panel is held by the left fourth and fifth fingers. The index and middle fingers control the air-water and suction valves respectively.

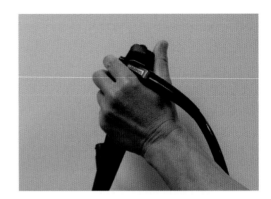

Figure 11.2 The connecting tube behind the thumb balances the weight of the control panel and further secures the correct grip.

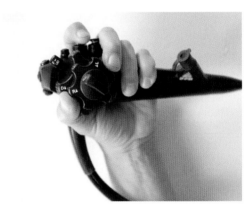

Figure 11.3 Manipulations with the R/L and U/D knobs. The thumb is the main tool for rotation of the U/D and R/L knobs.

can be achieved by "locking" the angulation knob from above by the middle finger and repositioning the thumb to the adjacent cog from below in a ratchet-wheel fashion (Figure 11.4).

The thumb can also be used for adjustment of the small right/left (R/L) angulation knob. However, the easiest way to produce lateral deflection of a flexed-up bending portion of the endoscope is to twist the left forearm in a clockwise or counterclockwise direction. The generated force is then transmitted from the control panel to the shaft of the endoscope and deviates the tip of the endoscope toward the target. The effectiveness of this technique is directly related to the degree of straightening

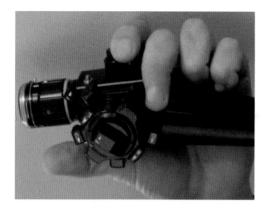

Figure 11.4 Technique of extensive rotation of the control knobs. The middle finger can function as the locker during extensive rotation of the knobs: ratchet-wheel technique.

of the working part of the endoscope between the control panel and the biteguard. However, the R/L angulation knob becomes very useful during target biopsy, the U-turn maneuver, and intubation of the second portion of the duodenum.

The endoscopist uses the right hand to advance, withdraw, and rotate the shaft of the endoscope. In addition, the right hand is in charge of manipulations with biopsy forceps or other accessories.

Preparation for esophageal intubation

A finely executed esophageal intubation is the key to a safe and successful EGD. Therefore, it is difficult to overestimate the importance of all steps involved in preparation to this phase of EGD.

This begins with proper positioning of the patient on the examination trolley. In children, this can usually be achieved only with adequate sedation. The patient should rest on the examination gurney on the left side with the spine supported by a folded pillow, preventing them from rolling back. The head should be in a neutral position or slightly flexed. Excessive flexion of the neck is counterproductive

because it increases the angulation of the endoscope on its way from the mouth to the esophageal orifice, requiring additional force to propel the shaft forward. It is usually associated with discomfort and irritability. On the other hand, excessive neck extension propels the endoscope toward the trachea and should also be avoided. Care should be taken to prevent lateral flexion of the neck and a predictable deviation of the bending portion sideways in the mouth and hypopharynx. Keeping the patient in the optimal position during EGD minimizes the risk of aspiration and facilitates proper localization of lesions within the stomach and duodenum and transition of the endoscope through the pylorus and into the distal duodenum.

The other important component of the preparation routine for EGD is straightening the shaft of the endoscope before inserting it into the mouth. This can be achieved by the examiner positioning themselves about a foot away from the gurney and about two feet away from the patient's head (the suggested distances are the subject of adjustments based on the actual height and length of a stretched right arm of the endoscopist). The straightening of the endoscope will facilitate its alignment with the esophageal axis, a midline navigation toward the esophagus and steering along the stomach and the duodenum.

Lastly, placement of a biteguard is mandatory for all children, except infants without teeth. The biteguard serves three important functions.

- Protection of the endoscope.
- Facilitation of proper positioning of the endoscope between the palate and the tongue.
- Anchoring of the suction catheter.

A modern biteguard consists of a plastic cylinder with a front hollow bumper and sideclips with an attached strip of ribbon, preventing it from sliding to the side.

Despite its clever design, close attention should be paid to the position of the biteguard to avoid mechanical damage of the endoscope when the child becomes more awake or agitated. To prevent accidental trauma, both lips should be gently pulled in corresponding directions (up or down), protecting them from entrapment between the teeth and the biteguard.

Techniques of esophageal intubation

Three different techniques can be used for esophageal intubations: direct vision insertion, blind, and finger assisted. The direct vision technique is the method of choice for pediatric upper GI endoscopy with forward-viewing endoscopes. Before insertion of the scope into the mouth, the proper function of the angulation mechanism is confirmed by corresponding deviation of the tip of the endoscope to the lateral and vertical movements of the angulation knobs. The bending portion is lubricated to the level of 20 cm and curved slightly downward to mark the vertical plane of the endoscope and to align it with the longitudinal axis of the pharynx by synchronous twisting of the control panel and the shaft. Then, the endoscope is passed through the bite block and advanced over the tongue. Direct observation through the biteguard is necessary to insure the correct/midline position of the scope within the mouth before further insertion. This is especially important in infants and toddlers due to the relatively small volume of the oral cavity and easy displacement of the tongue toward the pharynx by the biteguard.

If the tongue is flipped up or sticking out through the biteguard, attempts to insert the endoscope may push it toward the pharynx, increasing the risk of apnea and accidental trauma of the buccal or pharyngeal mucosa, due to lateral displacement of the instrument. A simple solution is to remove the biteguard from the mouth, fit it over and slide it along the shaft. This opens up more room for manipulation within the oral cavity. Once the bending portion is placed over the tongue, the biteguard is fitted back into the mouth.

From this moment on, attention should be switched to the monitor. While looking at the screen, it is worth remembering about the reverse nature of the endoscopic images which could explain the appearance of a relatively pale tongue with its papillae surface on the upper portion of the monitor and palatine raphe at the bottom (Figure 11.5).

These two structures are the landmarks of the midline approach to the pharynx. Gentle advancement of the endoscope along this pathway and bending it down guarantees a smooth transition into the pharynx and avoidance of accidental trauma. The lumen of the oropharynx may vanish briefly. Two structures, the root of the tongue in the upper portion of the screen (Figure 11.6) and the uvula at the bottom, may emerge just before appearance of the pharynx. The distant view of the epiglottis is

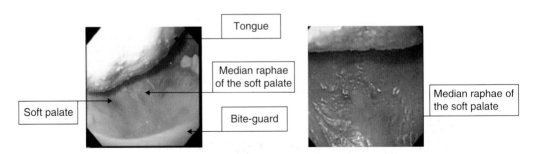

Figure 11.5 The initial phase of esophageal intubation. The endoscopist should concentrate on proper positioning of the scope in the oral cavity. On the right is a view of the tongue and soft palate through the biteguard.

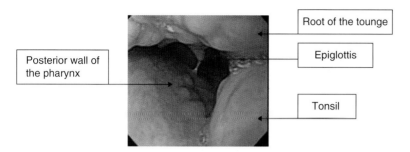

Figure 11.6 The root of the tongue appears as a cobblestone texture. It may be seen briefly or not at all during routine procedures. However, careful examination of this area and the tonsils should be attempted in children with suspected posttransplantation lymphoproliferative disorder.

the sign that the endoscope is in the pharynx. The epiglottis will occupy the upper part of the screen as a crescent-shaped structure (Figure 11.7). In approaching the epiglottis, the tip of the scope should be brought down toward the posterior wall of the pharynx. Failure to find the epiglottis indicates that the endoscope was advanced too far anteriorly (above the epiglottis), or too close to the crico-arytenoid cartilage, or was angled laterally.

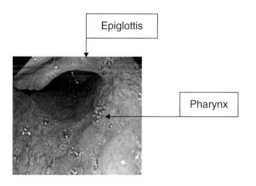

Figure 11.7 The initial view of the epiglottis. The epiglottis should be found and seen clearly before esophageal intubation is attempted.

Always follow the rule of thumb: pull the endoscope back until orientation is fully restored. A reappearance of the uvula pointed up from the bottom of the screen, the tonsils or the median raphe of the tongue at the top of the monitor is a sign that the scope is withdrawn too far back. Reposition the shaft along the midline and move it forward and down slowly until the larynx is approached.

The larynx has a triangular shape with the epiglottis above, two small spherical structures of arytenoid cartilage at the bottom, and the aryepiglottic fold on one side (Figure 11.8). The true vocal cords can be occasionally seen as a white/silver reversed letter "V" (Figure 11.9). A close view of the vocal cords is a warning sign of excessive deviation of the endoscope anteriorly. Remember that the esophageal orifice is hiding behind the crico-arytenoid cartilage, i.e. at the very bottom of the screen. In order to reach it, the tip of the endoscope should be angled downward toward the posterior wall of the pharynx.

Direct midline intubation of the esophagus is practically impossible due to significant

Figure 11.8 The endoscopic anatomy of the larynx: panoramic view.

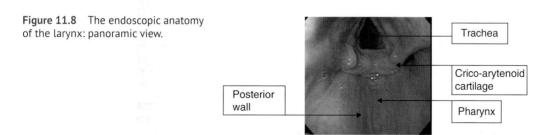

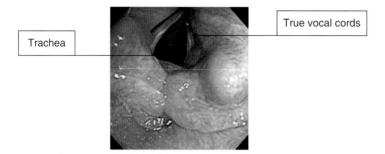

Figure 11.9 Endoscopic appearance of the vocal cords. A close capture of the vocal cords indicates that the tip of the scope is advanced too far anteriorly. The shaft must be pulled back a few centimeters and the tip should be deviated down toward the posterior wall.

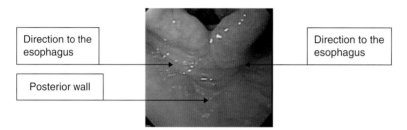

Figure 11.10 Close-up view of the crico-arytenoid cartilages. The esophageal orifice is hiding behind (posteriorly) and below the cliff of the cartilage.

resistance generated by the larynx toward the posterior pharyngeal wall. This force will push the endoscope either to the right or left of the larynx (Figure 11.10). If the scope has slipped to the right, rotate the shaft clockwise to about a one-quarter turn and, vice versa, twist the shaft counterclockwise if the scope slid to the left (Figure 11.11). Advance the shaft forward gently and angle the bending portion up simultaneously. Appearance of the vertical mucosal fold (Figure 11.12) is the sign to switch rotation in the opposite direction to avoid entering the piriform recess.

The final aspect of esophageal intubation could be simple, if the orifice of the cervical esophagus appeared open (a gentle push forward will propel the endoscope into the esophagus), or could be more challenging if the esophageal orifice is obscured by the tight crico-pharyngeal sphincter. In this case, direct the tip of the endoscope slightly down below the larynx into a narrow space between the larynx and adjacent

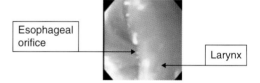

Figure 11.11 Side-view of the groove between the lateral wall of the larynx and pharynx. The shaft was rotated counterclockwise to approach the esophageal orifice. Direct intubation of the esophagus along the midline is impossible due to extensive pressure between the posterior wall of the larynx and anterior wall of the pharynx.

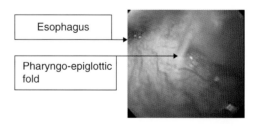

Figure 11.12 Appearance of the pharyngoepiglottic fold signals to reverse direction of rotation, flex the bending part upward and advance the scope forward.

pharynx, then deflect the bending portion up and advance the scope forward, guided by the diminishing resistance, toward the evolving cervical esophagus (Figure 11.13). In case of persistent resistance or loss of orientation, pull the endoscope back to the level of the crico-arytcnoid cartilage and repeat esophageal intu-bation from the opposite side of the larynx.

In neonates and infants under general anes-thesia, a gentle side-to-side wiggling helps to overcome a noticeable resistance within the cervical esophagus created by the endotracheal tube.

During swallowing, the larynx is moving upwards to protect the airways. It is useful to pull the endoscope back, wiggling with the swallow, and advance it quickly forward through the briefly opened esophagus. However, all upper GI endoscopy in children should ideally occur under GA so this should not be an issue. When the tip of the endoscope is submerged between the cricoid cartilage and posterior wall of the pharynx for longer than 10 seconds, it may induce irritability and agitation even in well-sedated patients. Apnea and/or bradycar-dia, especially in infants and toddlers, may also occur due to constant pressure on the larynx and irritation of the nearby superior laryngeal nerve. If intubation of the esophagus lasts more than 15 seconds, it is wise to pull the endoscope out until the child regains normal breathing.

Additional signs to abort esophageal intubation are significant resistance to the passage of the endoscope, the presence of light in the lateral neck, and loss of orientation. Again this should

not really be an issue for GA – there is no real excuse for unsuccessful esophageal intubation.

Exploration of the esophagus, stomach, and duodenum

Within the esophagus, the endoscope should be advanced strictly under direct observation of the esophageal lumen. A detailed visualization of the cervical esophagus is challenging due to a tonic contraction of the upper esophageal sphincter. An intense air insufflation is necessary to keep the cervical esophagus partially open.

The thoracic portion of the esophagus is nor-mally patent, except for brief peristaltic activity. It makes detailed examination of the entire tubu-lar esophagus quite easy without air insufflation. Distension of the esophagus with air is indicated only in a few situations such as extraluminal compression, foreign bodies, esophageal varices. and severe esophagitis. Intermittent clockwise or counterclockwise rotations of the endoscope help to keep the esophageal lumen fully visible.

The thoracic esophagus is tapered down at the area of the second physiological narrowing created by the left main bronchus. It is always unilateral (Figure 11.14). A bilateral narrowing of the thoracic esophagus is pathological and warrants further work-up to rule out a double aortic arch or aberrant subclavian artery.

A useful landmark in the distal esophagus is pulsation of the left atrium. The distal esopha-gus acquires a funnel shape right above the dia-phragm (Figure 11.15). It narrows down and

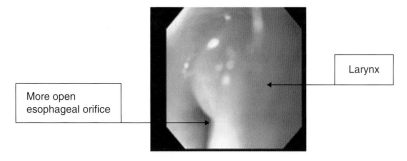

More open esophageal orifice

Larynx

Figure 11.13 Close-up view of the esophageal orifice.

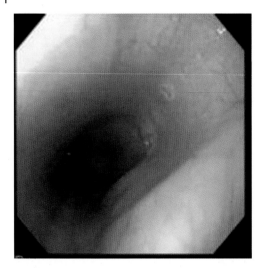

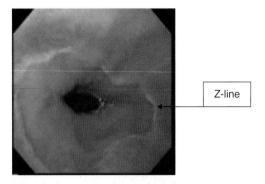

Figure 11.16 Z-line. The junction between the pale esophageal and richer colored gastric mucosa is slightly irregular. It is located at the level of or within 2 cm above the hiatal notch.

Figure 11.14 The second physiological narrowing of the esophagus. It does not have sharp borders and is always unilateral.

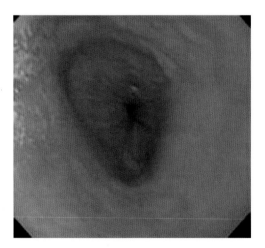

Figure 11.15 The distal esophagus. It tapers down toward the hiatal notch.

deviates to the left, passing through the diaphragmatic notch (third physiological narrowing). The border between the relatively pale esophageal and bright gastric mucosa, the so-called "Z-line," is slightly irregular (Figure 11.16). The location of the Z-line in relation to the hiatal notch varies. In general, elevation of the Z-line by 2 cm or more above the diaphragm is abnormal. The most reliable endoscopic marker of a diaphragm notch is a sequential constriction of the esophageal lumen during inspiration following by relaxation of the same segment with expiration. Respiratory excursion of the diaphragm is blunted in a deeply sedated child with shallow breathing, especially during antegrade approach. Location of the diaphragm in relation to the Z-line becomes more obvious during retrograde observation (U-turn maneuver).

To follow the natural course of the abdominal portion of the esophagus, the endoscope has to be slowly advanced and rotated counterclockwise with simultaneous elevation of the tip of the instrument. The straightforward approach to the stomach will result in a loss of orientation due to the close proximity of the posterior wall of the cardia or upper body. The stomach is recognized by the folds of the greater curvature between 5 and 7 o'clock as well as a pool of mucus (Figure 11.17). At this point, the endoscope should be rotated clockwise and bent downward until a panoramic view of the gastric body is achieved (Figure 11.18). Four slightly outlined folds between 1 and 3 o'clock highlight the lesser curvature. These folds disappear quickly during insufflation.

It is important to minimize pumping air into the stomach, especially in neonates and infants, who are quite sensitive to gastric distension and may become irritable, start retching and develop respiratory distress or bradycardia.

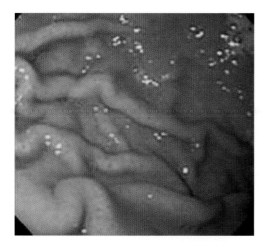

Figure 11.17 Prominent fold of the greater curvature of the stomach. Appearance of these folds is the sign of a successful intubation of the stomach.

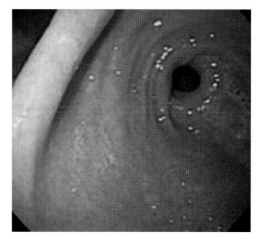

Figure 11.19 Gastric angularis. The detailed image of the angularis can be easily obtained during the withdrawal phase of the procedure. 1. Position the tip of the scope at the level of the distal body. 2. Rotate the scope counterclockwise and advance forward.

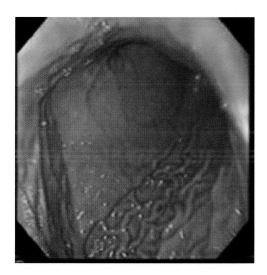

Figure 11.18 Panoramic view of the gastric body. It can be achieved by clockwise rotation of the shaft and elevation of the tip of the scope.

Exploration of the distal portion of the gastric body is facilitated by an additional clockwise rotation and upward deflection of the tip of the endoscope. The junction between the gastric body and antrum is marked by a prominent incisura angularis from above and loss of folds of the greater curvature from below (Figure 11.19). Further elevation of the tip

facilitates transition of the endoscope toward the antrum.

Resistance or loss of orientation warrants pulling back. In some cases, especially in infants and younger children, it is difficult to reach the pylorus just by pushing the endoscope forward. Instead, it is more productive to use a repetitive back and fore movement in combination with clockwise rotation and advancement of the endoscope slightly deeper each time until the pylorus is reached.

A normal pylorus looks like a ring, which disappears during peristalsis. The length of the normal pylorus channel during relaxation is approximately 3–5 mm. For successful intubation of the pylorus, the endoscope should be advanced along the prepyloric folds. The tip has to be bent slightly downward to avoid flipping into a retroflexed (U-turn) position (Figure 11.20).

If the pylorus is lost during peristalsis, it is useful to either wait until it opens up spontaneously or to pull the endoscope 3–4 cm backward to regain a panoramic view of the prepyloric antrum.

Gentle pressure is usually sufficient to navigate the endoscope through the pylorus. In some cases, attempts to bypass the pylorus will

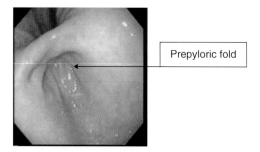

Prepyloric fold

Figure 11.20 Panoramic view of the antrum. At this stage of the procedure, the tip of the scope should be deviated down to prevent flipping of the shaft into a U-turn position. The prepyloric folds are pointed toward the pylorus.

move the endoscope away from the target. In such circumstances, pull the endoscope back into the gastric body, decompress the stomach and approach the pylorus as close as possible following the direction of prepyloric folds. Apply gentle pressure on the gastric wall and direct the tip toward the visible portion of the pyloric ring using the R/L angulation knob simultaneously until the endoscope is fully engaged within the pylorus. Sometimes, it is useful to pull the shaft back slightly to straighten the bending portion of the scope.

Passage of the pylorus is manifest by the disappearance of resistance and change of the mucosal pattern from smooth to villous/velvet type. The endoscopist must be careful to avoid blind trauma of the duodenal bulb due to rapid advancement of the endoscope. The duodenal bulb should be examined carefully before exploration of the second portion of the duodenum. The endoscope has to be pulled back toward the pylorus slowly and deviated to the right to achieve a panoramic view of the duodenal bulb (Figure 11.21).

There is a "blind" zone in the proximal part of the duodenal bulb between the 3 and 6 o'clock positions. Rotating the patient into the prone position facilitates exploration of this area.

The walls of the duodenal bulb are labeled traditionally as the anterior, posterior, lesser, and greater curvatures (Figure 11.22).

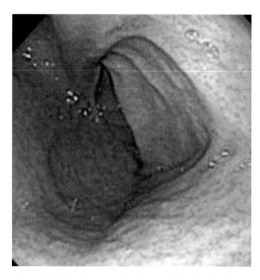

Figure 11.21 Panoramic view of the duodenal bulb. This is useful for correct engagement of the endoscope beyond the superior duodenal angle.

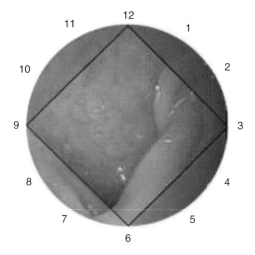

Figure 11.22 Endoscopic mapping of the duodenal bulb during the insertion phase of the procedure. The anterior wall is located between 6 and 9 o'clock; the posterior wall is located between 12 and 3 o'clock; the lesser curvature or medial wall is located between 9 and 12 o'clock; the greater curvature or lateral wall is located between 3 and 6 o'clock.

Certain corrections in orientation within the duodenal bulb should be made in relation to the stage of the procedure: the antegrade phase is always associated with coiling of the endoscope within the stomach and distortion of normal anatomy. Alternatively, the endoscope is more or less straightened during the retrograde stage of the procedure and the shape of the duodenal bulb regains its normal pattern (Figure 11.23).

Accurate mapping of lesions in the duodenal bulb is important, for example in patients with duodenal ulcers. Ulcers on the posterior wall of the distal portion of the duodenal bulb or the superior duodenal angle are associated with a high risk of severe bleeding due to intense blood supply to the area and close proximity of the pancreas.

The most efficient and safe way to intubate the second and third portions of the duodenum is the so-called "pull and twist" technique. The order and specific steps of this maneuver depend on the position of the mucosal folds which outline the transitional zone between the distal portion of the duodenal bulb and the superior duodenal angle: vertical versus horizontal (Figures 11.24 and 11.25).

In a "vertical" scenario, exploration of the second portion of the duodenum begins with advancement of the endoscope and positioning it just behind the AC line. The next step is

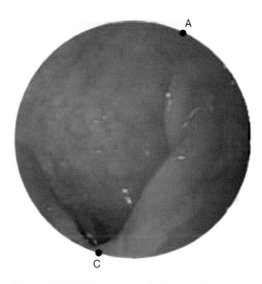

Figure 11.24 Appearance of the transitional zone between the duodenal bulb and the superior duodenal angle. AC line reflects the usual configuration of this transitional zone.

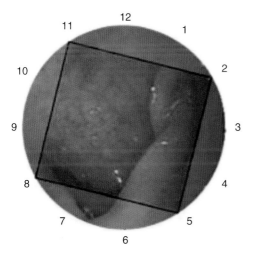

Figure 11.23 Mapping of the walls of the duodenal bulb after reduction of the gastric loop. The anterior wall is now located between 5 and 8 o'clock; the posterior wall is now located between 2 and 11 o'clock; the lesser curvature or medial wall is now located between 8 and 11 o'clock; the greater curvature or lateral wall is now located between 2 and 5 o'clock.

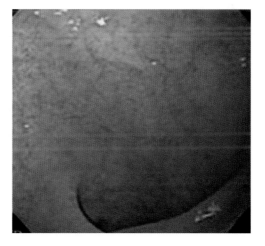

Figure 11.25 Horizontal configuration of the transitional zone between the duodenal bulb and the superior duodenal angle. Decompression of the stomach and reduction of the gastric loop should precede an exploration of the second portion of the duodenum. Counterclockwise rotation may facilitate intubation of the duodenum beyond the duodenal bulb.

bending the tip of the endoscope up and to the right into the 5 o'clock direction. This will anchor the scope to the superior duodenal angle. The final step is rotation of the shaft clockwise roughly 90° and pulling it back simultaneously until the duodenal lumen becomes clearly visible. If the duodenal folds are visible but the lumen is not, rotate the endoscope counterclockwise about a quarter turn and orient the tip in the 10–11 o'clock direction.

Intubation of the second portion of the duodenum can be challenging in a "horizontal" scenario. In this case, try a technique for a "vertical" scenario first. If unsuccessful, pull the endoscope back to the upper portion of the gastric body, decompress the stomach and intubate the duodenal bulb. Then, position the endoscope in the middle of the duodenal bulb and rotate it counterclockwise. The goal of this maneuver is to untangle the proximal duodenum and "unlock" the superior duodenal angle. Continue counterclockwise rotation and pull the endoscope back simultaneously until the second portion of the duodenum is reached.

In contrast to the majority of pediatric patients, a "pull and twist" technique has a limited role in intubation of the second portion of the duodenum in neonates and infants. Instead, a gentle push of the thin (less than 6 mm) instrument is safe and the preferred method. However, if this scope is unavailable, a regular 9 mm pediatric endoscope can be used but it is more stiff. Attempts to perform a "pull and twist" maneuver usually resuls in displacement of the endoscope back into the stomach. To overcome this obstacle, advance the endoscope toward the superior duodenal angle and move the tip to the right. If resistance is minimal, continue advancement. Rotate the endoscope counterclockwise about 15–20° as soon as the "crescent" of the duodenal lumen becomes visible. Direct the scope toward the lumen using the up/down angulation knob to achieve a panoramic view of the second portion of the duodenum. Advance the

endoscope forward until the duodenal lumen begins moving away due to increased resistance and looping of the endoscope in the stomach.

The hallmark of the second portion of the duodenum is the papilla of Vater (Figure 11.26). During the antegrade stage of the procedure, the major papilla is usually found between 9 and 11 o'clock on the medial wall of the second portion of the duodenum. During withdrawal of the endoscope from the distal duodenum, the location of the major papilla is shifted toward the 12 o'clock position.

Detailed images of the papilla of Vater can be obtained with a side-viewing duodenoscope (Figure 11.27).

The small duodenal papilla is located 3–4 cm proximal to the major one. It can be found in the right upper corner of the lumen between the 1 and 2 o'clock positions. It is a smooth, 4–5 mm structure, which resembles a sessile polyp.

The hallmark of the third portion of the duodenum is the superior mesenteric artery responsible for a prominent pulsation of the right part of the duodenal wall.

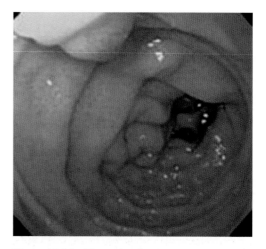

Figure 11.26 The major duodenal papilla, the hallmark of the second portion of the duodenum. It is seen more clearly during the withdrawal phase at the 11–12 o'clock location.

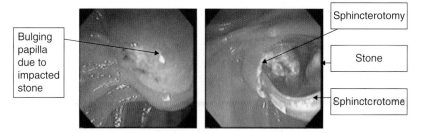

Bulging papilla due to impacted stone

Sphincterotomy

Stone

Sphinctcrotome

Figure 11.27 The major duodenal papilla. The side-viewing duodenoscope allows obtaining of a detailed image of the major duodenal papilla and performing endoscopic retrograde cholangiopancreatography (ERCP) and sphincterotomy.

The lumen of the fourth portion of the duodenum is narrowed at the level of the ligament of Treitz (Figure 11.28).

The withdrawal phase of upper GI endoscopy is the best for detailed observation of the entire duodenum, stomach, and esophagus. Retrograde inspection of the proximal stomach or the so-called U-turn maneuver is the best technique for careful exploration of the gastric cardia and fundus. It is reasonable to perform it at the end of the examination except for children with portal hypertension or acute bleeding from the stomach.

The U-turn technique consists of the following steps: first, position the tip of the endoscope in the middle of the gastric body and orient it toward the anterior wall in the 10 o'clock direction. Second, bend the tip of the endoscope further up and advance the shaft forward until the incisura angularis appears, separating the gastric body on the left from the antrum on the right part of the screen (Figure 11.29). Third, pull the endoscope back and rotate it clockwise to achieve a close-up view of the fundus (Figures 11.30 and 11.31).

For a detailed image of the cardia, target biopsy or precise hemostasis, find the grooves between the shallow folds of the lesser curvature during counterclockwise rotation and pull the endoscope back slowly. Recognition of the Z-line indicates the end of withdrawal (Figure 11.32). This part of the U-turn maneuver should be performed with caution to avoid

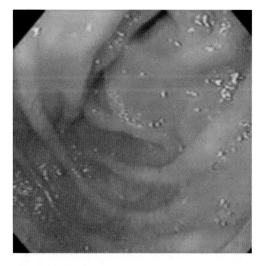

Figure 11.28 The endoscopic appearance of the duodenum at the level of the ligament of Treitz.

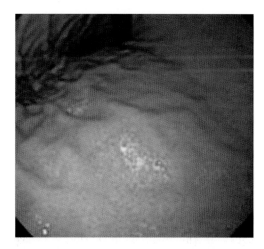

Figure 11.29 View of the gastric body during the initial phase of the retroflexion maneuver.

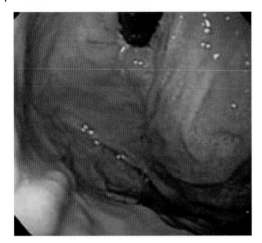

Figure 11.30 Appearance of the cardia after partial withdrawal of the shaft during the retroflexion maneuver (This is also referred to as the 'J manouver').

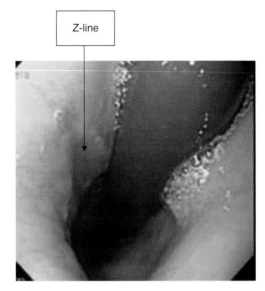

Figure 11.32 Appearance of the Z-line signals the end of the withdrawal part of the retroflexion technique.

Biopsy technique

Histological and histochemical analysis is crucial for definitive diagnosis of many diseases involving the GI tract, for example reflux or eosinophilic esophagitis, chronic gastritis, celiac disease, and chronic inflammatory bowel disease. Correct interpretation of regular microscopy slides is problematic without adequate tissue samples and virtually impossible without proper mounting of specimens in children with villous atrophy or dysplasia.

It is always feasible to obtain adequate tissue samples, even with small pediatric size biopsy forceps, if the endoscopist is familiar with the appropriate technique. There are three rules of endoscopic biopsy.

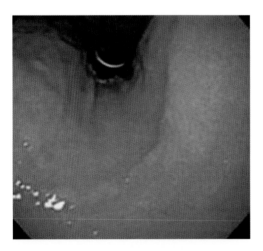

Figure 11.31 Detailed view of the cardia after further withdrawal of the scope.

accidental impaction of the sharply bent tip of the endoscope in the distal esophagus.

To get away from the cardia, safely push the endoscope forward, rotate it clockwise and return the control knobs to the neutral position. Check and unlock the control knobs if they lock accidentally to avoid blind trauma of the gastric mucosa. Decompress the stomach as much as possible before withdrawal. Careful examination of the esophagus should be carried out at the end of the procedure.

- It is not a blind procedure.
- The length of the biopsy forceps beyond the tip of the endoscope is in reverse correlation with the precision of the biopsy.
- Forceful pushing of the forceps up against the wall is a dangerous and ineffective way to obtain an adequate tissue sample.

The technique of esophageal biopsy is more complicated than either gastric or duodenal mucosal sampling. This is related to the tangential position of the forceps along the esophageal wall and the relatively narrow space within the tubular esophagus.

The proper technique of esophageal biopsy consists of the following steps. First, the endoscope is positioned 1–2 cm above the target. Then, the bending segment of the endoscope is configured into an L-shape by rotation of the control knobs upwards and to the right. The goal of this maneuver is orientation of the forceps perpendicular to the mucosa. The biopsy forceps should be advanced just enough to be fully open. Finally, suction is applied, forcing mucosa into the biopsy cap before it closes. The protocol of esophageal biopsy sampling for specific diseases will be discussed in the relevant chapters.

The larger volume of the stomach and duodenum makes the biopsy process less complicated, unless the target lesion is located in the gastric cardia or posterior wall of the proximal portion of the duodenal bulb, and the distal segment of the superior duodenal angle.

To obtain an adequate sample from the target lesion, the biopsy forceps should be positioned as much perpendicular to the surface of mucosa as possible. Application of excessive force to the forceps compromises safety, sample volume and quality of the biopsy, and should be avoided. In general, target biopsy for different areas within the stomach requires different approaches. Thus, biopsy of lesions within the gastric cardia and subcardia areas is more accurate during the U-turn maneuver. Biopsies from the antrum of the stomach are more efficient if taken when the endoscope is partially withdrawn into the distal portion of the gastric body with the tip deflected upwards.

Biopsy from the anterior wall of the duodenal bulb should be taken when the endoscope is positioned just beyond the pylorus. Biopsy from the distal portion of the duodenal bulb requires slightly deeper insertion of the scope.

Biopsy from the second and third portions of the duodenum provides better samples if taken from the edge of duodenal folds with minimal imbedding into the mucosa. A perpendicular orientation of the forceps to the mucosal folds

eliminates the need for deep and forceful imbedding of the biopsy cap into the tissue, prevents mucosal trauma and sampling artifacts, and guarantees the best tissue samples.

Proper orientation and mounting of tissue specimens is crucial for correct histological diagnosis of celiac sprue, inflammatory bowel disease, and dysplasia in patients with long-standing ulcerative colitis, Barrett's esophagus, and polyps. The proper tissue mounting technique on a fine synthetic mesh adds no more than 3–5 minutes to the endoscopic procedure. The orientation of tissue samples is more precise with a magnifying glass lamp.

Several steps are involved in proper mounting technique.

- Wearing of tight-fitting gloves free of talcum.
- Gentle transferring of a specimen from the open forceps to the index finger with or without the help of a dissecting needle.
- Uncurling of a specimen with a light touch of the side of the dissecting needle until the cleavage surface is exposed.
- Recognition of the surface area: the mucosal side of the specimen is more reddish and shiny.
- Complete uncurling of the specimen with the submucosal side facing up.
- Transferring the specimen from the index finger to the mesh, resting on the thumb of the same hand.
  - Touching the supporting mesh with half of the specimen.
  - Sweeping the visible part of the specimen to the mesh by placing one side of the dissecting needle between the biopsy specimen and the index finger.
  - Moistening the needle with water.
  - Pushing the remaining part of the specimen away from the index finger with the side of the needle.
  - Placing the mesh with mounted specimen upside down into the fixative solution to prevent it from floating off the supporting mesh.

The labeled bottle with fixative solution should contain no more than 2–3 biopsy specimens from each site of the GI tract.

pH and pH impedance probe placement

Catheter pH placement is standard and the tip position can be assessed with direct vision by the endoscopist. Care should be taken to not accidentally extract the catheter whilst removing the endoscope. Wireless Bravo and Alpha pH probe placement can occur in the distal esophagus and can also be positioned and confirmed under direct vision. This is particularly important when the patient is not intubated in order to ensure that the probe is placed in the esophagus.

Complications

Complications associated with EGD can be divided into mild, requiring no therapeutic intervention, and severe, mandating hospitalization. The true incidence of mild complications such as transient sore throat, bloating, and abdominal discomfort is unknown.

Serious complications include perforation, bleeding, and infections. The reported incidence of such complications is low across the pediatric and adult literature. According to American Society for Gastrointestinal Endoscopy (ASGE) and British Society of Gastroenterology (BSG) guidelines, perforations associated with EGD in adults are around 0.03–0.13%. Large cohort retrospective or prospective studies in pediatric patients who suffered from iatrogenic esophageal perforation during EGD are not available. However, a review of the pediatric literature supports the overall consensus that the incidence of perforation related to EGD in children is also low.

Moderate to severe bleeding during diagnostic EGD is extremely rare and usually occurs after biopsy in children with unrecognized coagulopathy.

Transient bacteremia is uncommon following diagnostic upper GI endoscopy and is rarely of clinical significance. According to revised guidelines from the American Heart Association and American Society for Gastrointestinal Endoscopy, antibiotic prophylaxis of infective endocarditis (ID) is not recommended for endoscopic procedures, except for patients with established GI tract infections in which enterococci may be part of the infecting bacterial flora, and one of the following conditions: a prosthetic cardiac valve, history of previous ID, cardiac transplant recipients, unrepaired cyanotic congenital heart disease (CHD), completely repaired CHD with prosthetic material, and repaired CHD with residual defects at the site of a prostatic patch or device.

Uncommon, incidental, and rare findings during EGD

Esophageal squamous papilloma (ESP)

Rare in children, ESP is asymptomatic and discovered incidentally during EGD for unrelated indications. It appears as a small, sessile or pedunculated verrucous polyp in the middle or distal portion of the esophagus (Figure 11.33). Biopsy confirms the diagnosis by documenting papillary projections of fibrovascular stroma covered by squamous epithelium.

Esophageal adenocarcinoma (EAC)

Esophageal adenocarcinoma is a rare finding in children. The youngest patient diagnosed with EAC was 8 years old. EAC should be considered in children or teenagers with progressive dysphagia and weight loss suspicious of a

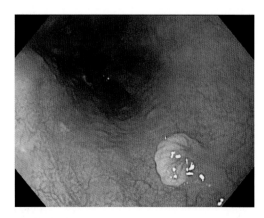

Figure 11.33 Small squamous papilloma of the middle esophagus.

(a)   (b)   (c)

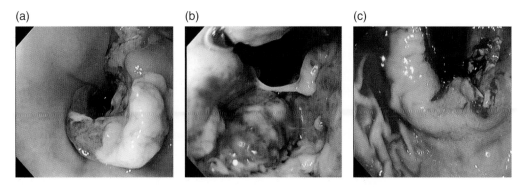

Figure 11.34 (a) Proximal edge of almost circumferential mass in the distal esophagus. (b) Deep ulceration of the esophageal tumor with necrotic tissue at the base and irregular edges. (c) Visual expansion of the tumor into the gastric cardia and subcardia.

mass or ulcerated lesion in the distal esophagus (Figure 11.34).

Collagenous gastritis

A rare disease characterized by marked subepithelial collagen deposition accompanied by mucosal inflammatory infiltrate. Abdominal pain and anemia are the two most common clinical features of the pediatric phenotype. Endoscopic findings are not specific (Figure 11.35). The histological hallmark of collagenous gastritis is inflammatory infiltration with thick collagen deposits.

Late sequelae of severe acid-induced corrosive gastritis

Although ingestion of household or industrial cleaning products containing strong hydrochloric or sulphuric acid occurs less frequently in Western compared to developing countries (<5%), the acute gastric injury, including

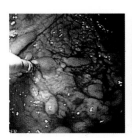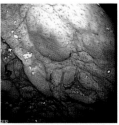

Figure 11.35 Highly unusual appearance of the gastric mucosa: prominent and irregular nodularity divided by deep grooves.

perforation, and the late sequelae, including gastric scarring and carcinoma, can be devastating for affected children and teenagers. A gastric outlet obstruction may occur as soon as 5–8 weeks after the accident. Scarring of the antrum and pylorus is the result of prolonged contact of acid with the stomach due to pyloric spasms. Endoscopic balloon dilation of the pyloric stricture can be effective but cannot guarantee sustained symptomatic relief (Figure 11.36).

Pyloric duplication cyst

Pyloric duplication cyst is an extremely rare congenital anomaly of the alimentary tract. The preoperative diagnosis is difficult but can be suspected when the cystic lesion is revealed by abdominal ultrasound or CT scan. EGD is rarely used as a primary diagnostic tool but can be useful in some cases (Figure 11.37).

Heterotopic pancreas

Heterotopic pancreas is asymptomatic in most children. It is always an incidental finding during EGD. True prevalence of ectopic pancreas in children is unknown. In the stomach, ectopic pancreas is located on the greater curvature of the antrum and appears as a small, less than 1 cm, dome-shaped lesion with a central depression (Figure 11.38). It is covered by normal gastric mucosa. Sometimes, the lesions may be less protruded toward the gastric lumen

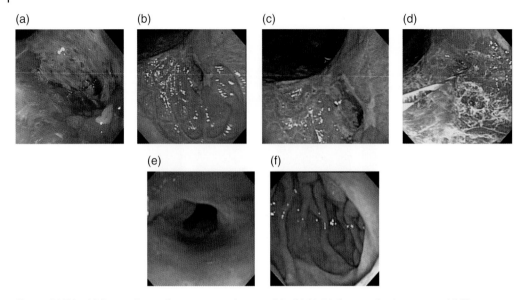

Figure 11.36 (a) Acute phase of severe corrosive gastritis. (b) Multiple scars in the antrum. (c) Close-up view of the scarred and narrowed pylorus. (d) First stage of balloon dilation: positioning the guidewire through the pylorus into the duodenum. (e) Pylorus after dilation. (f) Successful intubation of the duodenum after dilation.

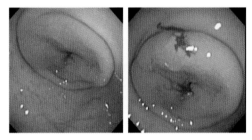

Figure 11.37 Pinpoint narrowing of the pylorus induced by the circular mass lesion bulging into the gastric lumen.

and appear as a "bagel" or "doughnut" structure. A biopsy is not indicated as ectopic tissue arises from the submucosal or subserosal layers.

Gastric polyps

Gastric polyps are rare in children. The predominant type is hyperplastic associated with chronic inflammation. In children such polyps are usually single, sessile, less than 1 cm, smooth, dome-shaped lesions located in the antrum (Figure 11.39a) or at the gastroesopha-

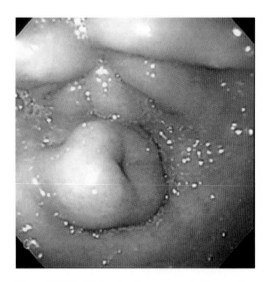

Figure 11.38 Heterotopic pancreas in the greater curvature of the prepyloric antrum.

geal junction, the so-called inflammatory polyp–fold complex (Figure 11.39b). Endoscopic polypectomy is indicated only if the patient is symptomatic or the polyp is pedunculated and bigger than 1 cm due to increased malignant potential. Endoscopic

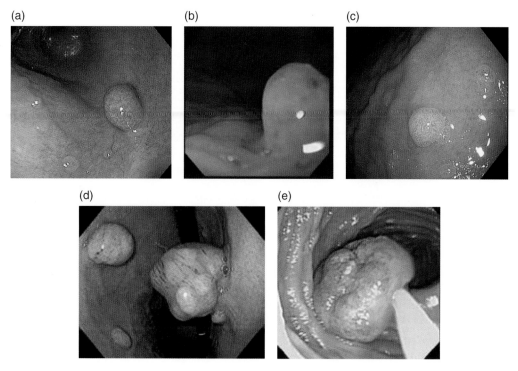

Figure 11.39 (a) Sessile hyperplastic polyp in the antrum. (b) Inflammatory polyp–fold complex. (c) Fundic gland polyps. (d) Multiple hamartomatous polyps in the gastric body in patient with Peutz–Jeghers syndrome. (e) Large duodenal hamartomatous polyp during polypectomy.

surveillance after polypectomy is unnecessary if the diagnosis is confirmed histologically.

The presence of multiple gastric polyps is the sign of polyposis syndrome. In children with Gardner's syndrome, small sessile polyps are usually located in the gastric fundus (Figure 11.39c). In generalized juvenile polyposis or Peutz–Jeghers syndrome, gastric polyps may be dispersed throughout the stomach (Figure 11.39d). The polyps can be removed in one or several endoscopic sessions. Sometimes, the number of polyps precludes complete eradication. In these cases, the largest polyps should be removed. In children with Peutz–Jeghers syndrome, gastric polyps co-exist with multiple hamartomas in the duodenum or proximal jejunum (Figure 11.39e). Some of these polyps can be quite large, reaching 4 or 5 cm. Such polyps are a common cause of chronic small bowel intussusceptions and the leading cause of intermittent abdominal pain.

Gastric malignancy

Malignant tumors of the stomach account for only 5% or less of all malignant neoplasms in children. The most common malignant gastric tumors in children are non-Hodgkin's or Burkitt's lymphoma or gastric involvement in lymphoproliferative disorder after solid organ or bone marrow transplantation (Figures 11.40 and 11.41).

Peptic ulcer disease

Peptic ulcer disease is relatively rare in children and affects less than 4% of children referred for EGD. It often affects middle and high school age children, especially male teenagers. The predominant location of ulcers is the duodenal bulb. Multiple ulcers (two or more) occur in more than 50% of patients. Exacerbation of the disease is often associated with prominent spasm of the duodenal bulb,

(a)

(b)

(c)

(d)

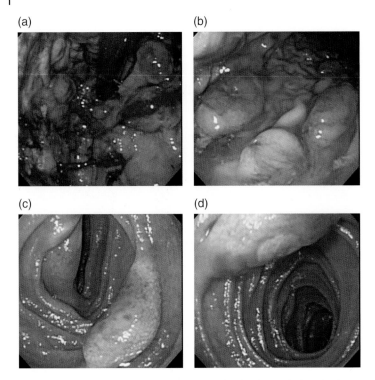

Figure 11.40 Burkitt's lymphoma: multiple ulcerated mass lesions in the stomach (a, b) and the duodenum (c,d).

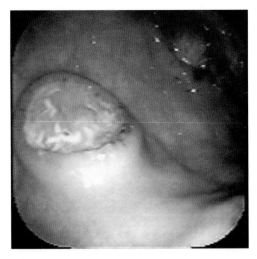

Figure 11.41 Razed, rounded ulcerated lesions with irregular base in the stomach.

which makes detailed assessment of the first portion of the duodenum challenging (Figure 11.42a). Changing the patient's position and intravenous administration of gluca-

gon may facilitate detailed inspection of the bulb. One of the visual clues to the "hiding" ulcer is the direction of the converging folds. It is not uncommon to see different combinations of scars and active (deep or shallow) ulcers (Figure 11.42b). GI bleeding could be the initial manifestation of peptic ulcer disease in affected children (Figure 11.42c).

Intestinal lymphangiectasia

Intestinal lymphangiectasia is a rare disorder characterized by dilated intestinal lacteals due to either a congenital defect in the lymphatic system or acquired diffuse or segmental lymphostasis within the enteric lymphatic vessels. It can be either primary (idiopathic) or secondary. Primary intestinal lymphangiectasia (PIL) is usually presented before 3 years of age with the symptom of protein-losing enteropathy, which in turn results in hypoalbuminemia, hypogammaglobulinemia, and lymphopenia.

(a)   (b)   (c)

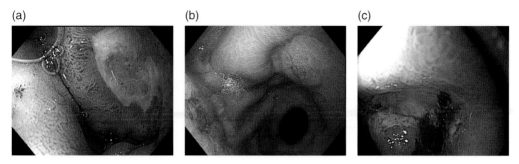

Figure 11.42 (a) A relatively large active ulcer on the posterior wall of the duodenal bulb associated with significant spasm of the first portion of the duodenum. (b) A combination of an active ulcer and scar. (c) Bleeding duodenal ulcer.

(a)   (b)

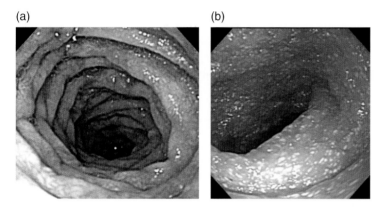

Figure 11.43 (a) Edematous and dilated folds of the duodenum. (b) Numerous whitish spots on the mucosal surface.

Secondary intestinal lymphangiectasia is more often seen in adults and is related to an elevated lymphatic pressure as may occur in lymphoma, constrictive pericarditis, cardiac surgery, inflammatory bowel disease, systemic lupus erythematosus, and malignancies.

Endoscopy with biopsy is the key for diagnosis of primary intestinal lymphangiectasia. The endoscopic signs of PIL are numerous white-yellowish spots on the surface of edematous small bowel mucosa and enlarged folds (Figure 11.43). Duodenal biopsies should always be taken when such abnormalities are seen.

 • See companion website for videos relating to this chapter topic: www.wiley.com/go/gershman3e

 FURTHER READING

Attard TM, Yardley JH, Cuffari C. Gastric polyps in pediatrics: an 18-year hospital-based analysis. *Am J Gastroenterol* 2002, **97**(2), 298–301.

Attard TM, Cuffari C, Tajouri T, *et al.* Multicenter experience with upper gastrointestinal polyps in pediatric patients with familial adenomatous polyposis. *Am J Gastroenterol* 2004, **99**, 681–686.

Bishop PR, Nowicki MJ, Subramony C, Parker PH. The inflammatory polyp-fold complex in children. *J Clin Gastroenterol* 2002, **34**(3), 229–232.

Biyikoglu I, Babali A, Çakal B, *et al.* Do scattered white spots in the duodenum mark a specific gastrointestinal pathology? *J Dig Dis* 2009, **10**, 300–304.

Brindley N, Sloan JM, McCallion WA. Esophagitis: optimizing diagnostic yield by biopsy orientation. *J Pediatr Gastroenterol Nutr* 2004, **39**, 262–264.

Christodoulidis G, Zacharoulis D, Barbanis S, *et al.* Heterotopic pancreas in the stomach: a case report and literature review. *World J Gastroenterol* 2007, **13**, 6098–6100.

Cohen J. The impact of tissue sampling on endoscopy efficiency. *Gastrointest Endosc Clin North Am* 2004, **14**(4), 725–734.

Contini S, Scarpignato C. Caustic injury of the upper gastrointestinal tract: a comprehensive review. *World J Gastroenterol* 2013, **19**(25), 3918–3930.

De Boissieu D, Dupont C, Barbet JP, *et al.* Distinct features of upper gastrointestinal endoscopy in the newborn. *J Pediatr Gastroenterol Nutr* 1994, **18**, 334–338.

Dina I, Braticevici CF. Idiopathic colonic varices: case report and review of literature. *Hepat Mon* 2014, **14**(7), e18916.

Dupont C, Kalach N, de Boissieu D, *et al.* Digestive endoscopy in neonates. *J Pediatr Gastroenterol Nutr* 2005, **40**, 406–420.

Fox VL. Patient preparation and general consideration. In: Walker WA, Goulet O, Kleinman RE, Sanderson IR, Sherman P, Shneider BL (eds). *Pediatric Gastrointestinal Disease*, 5th edn. BC Decker, Hamilton, Ontario, 2008, pp. 1259–1264.

Gershman G. Diagnostic upper endoscopy technique. In: Gershman G, Thomson M (eds). *Practical Pediatric Gastrointestinal Endoscopy*. Wiley Blackwell, Malden, MA, 2012, pp. 41–81.

Gershman G, Ament ME. Pediatric upper gastrointestinal endoscopy, endoscopic retrograde cholangiopancreatography, and colonoscopy. In: Lifschitz CH (ed.). *Pediatric Gastroenterology and Nutrition in Clinical Practice*. Marcel Dekker, New York, 2002, pp. 799–846.

Gershman G, Ament ME. Pediatric upper gastrointestinal endoscopy: state of the art. *Acta Paediatr Taiwan* 1999, **40**, 369–392.

Harris GJ, Laszewski MJ. Pediatric primary gastric lymphoma. *South Med J* 1992, **85**, 432–434.

Haycock A, Cohen J, Saunders BP, Cotton PB, Williams CB (eds). *Cotton and Williams' Practical Gastrointestinal Endoscopy: The Fundamentals*, 7th edn. Wiley Blackwell, New York, 2014.

Kamimura K, Kobayashi M, Narisava R, *et al.* Collagenous gastritis: endoscopic and pathologic evaluation of the nodularity of gastric mucosa. *Dig Dis Sci* 2007, **52**, 995–1000.

Khashab MA, Chithadi KV, Acosta RD. Antibiotic prophylaxis for GI endoscopy. *Gastrointest Endosc* 2015, **81**(1), 81–89.

Leung ST, Chandan VS, Murray JA, *et al.* Collagenous gastritis. Histopathologic features and associations with other gastrointestinal diseases. *Am J Surg Pathol* 2009, **33**, 788–798.

McGill TW, Downey J, Westbrook D, *et al.* Gastric carcinoma in children. *J Pediatr Surg* 1993, **28**, 1620–1621.

Murphy MS. Diagnostic upper gastrointestinal endoscopy. In: Winter HS, Murphy MS, Mougenot JF, Cadranel S (eds). Pediatric *Gastrointestinal Endoscopy: Textbook and Atlas*. BC Decker, Hamilton, Ontario, 2006, pp. 65–72.

Ormarsson OT, Gudmundsdottir I, Marvik R. Diagnosis and treatment of gastric heterotopic pancreas. *World J Surg* 2006, **30**, 1682–1689.

Ravicumara M, Ramani P, Spray CH. Collagenous gastritis: a case report and review. *Eur J Pediatr* 2007, **166**, 769–773.

Rebeuh J, Willot S, Bouron-Dal Soglio D, et al. Esophageal squamous papilloma in children. *Endoscopy* 2011, **43**, E256.

Rothbaum RJ. Complications of pediatric endoscopy. *Gastrointest Endosc Clin North Am* 1996, **6**(2), 445–459.

Schaeppi MG, Mougenot JF, Dominique CB. Upper gastrointestinal endoscopy. In: Walker WA, Goulet O, Kleinman RE, Sanderson IR, Sherman P, Shneider BL (eds). *Pediatric*

Gastrointestinal Disease, 5th edn. BC Decker, Hamilton, Ontario, 2008, pp. 1265–1284.

Sharma D, Bharany RP, Mapshekhab RV. Duplication cyst of pylopic canal: a rare cause of pediatric gastric outlet obstruction: a rare case report. *Indian J Surg* 2013, **75**(Suppl 1), S322–S325.

Suskind D, Wahbeh G, Murray K, *et al.* Collagenous gastritis, a new spectrum of disease in pediatric patients: two case reports. *Cases J* 2009, **2**, 7511.

Theilen TM, Chou AJ, Klimstra DS, LaQuaglia MP. Esophageal adenocarcinoma and squamous cell carcinoma in children and adolescents: report of 3 cases and comprehensive literature review. *J Pediatr Surg Case Rep* 2016, **5**, 23–29.

Vignes S, Bellanger J. Primary intestinal lymphangiectasia (Waldmann's disease). *Orphanet J Rare Dis* 2008, **3**, 5.

12

Pediatric ileocolonoscopy

George Gershman and Mike Thomson

 KEY POINTS

- Modern ileocolonoscopy is a procedure which combines examination of the entire colon and the terminal ileum.
- Pediatric ileocolonoscopy is a safe and high-yield procedure if performed by well-trained pediatric endoscopists in an adequately prepared colon.
- Knowledge of embryology and endoscopic anatomy of the large intestine helps to understand the concept of proper colonoscopy.

- Pediatric ileocolonoscopy requires adequate deep sedation or general anesthesia.
- The cornerstone of ileocolonoscopy is prevention of sigmoid colon and transverse colon loop formation by effective use of a torque steering technique.
- Adherence to the Thomson's 15 Golden Rules of Ileocolonosocpy makes it safe, effective and facilitates ileal intubation as the mandatory part of the procedure.

This chapter is focused on the key aspects of ileocolonoscopy to enable the reader to achieve a high level of skill with the goal of 100% ileocecal intubation and a proper recognition of common and rare pathology of the terminal ileum and the colon.

Bowel preparation for colonoscopy

Poor bowel preparation is a major factor that may prevent or complicate successful ileocolonoscopy. Emphasizing the importance of bowel preparation, in 2006 the American Society for Gastrointestinal Endoscopy and American College of Gastroenterology Taskforce on Quality in Endoscopy suggested

that every colonoscopy report should include an assessment of the quality of bowel preparation. Preparing infants and small children for colonoscopy can be challenging. The major obstacles are the volume and distasteful nature of laxatives and a restrictive diet.

The impact of inadequate or poor preparation for ileocolonoscopy in children is magnified by the necessity for deep sedation or general anesthesia and specifics of bowel preparation, especially in small children. Furthermore, multiple attempts to aspirate large amounts of semisolid stool often lead to clogging of the instrumental channel. Repeat efforts to restore adequate suction precipitate excessive insufflation and stretching of the large intestine and adjacent mesentery and, in conjunction with poor visibility, contribute to a

Practical Pediatric Gastrointestinal Endoscopy, Third Edition. Edited by George Gershman and Mike Thomson.
© 2021 John Wiley & Sons Ltd. Published 2021 by John Wiley & Sons Ltd.
Companion website: www.wiley.com/go/gershman3e

big loop formation, making the procedure more challenging. Therefore, despite a "natural" temptation to complete ileocolonoscopy, it is wise to terminate the procedure if the colon is not adequately prepped. This is especially relevant for patients with suspected or diagnosed chronic inflammatory bowel disease and children with anemia and/or rectal bleeding.

An adequate bowel preparation targets two important goals: maximum visibility and thorough examination of the entire colon and the terminal ileum, and prevention of complications.

Although administration of cleansing regimens is not always easy, modern protocols can be remarkably effective in cleaning the colon and ileum. Currently, three types of products are commonly used: polyethylene glycol (PEG) with electrolytes, PEG 3350 and sodium picosulfate/magnesium citrate (PICO). Large-volume PEG with electrolytes is generally less tolerable, especially in younger children. A combination of propulsion agents such as Senokot® and PICO (Pico-Salax® or Prepopik®, Ferring Pharmaceutical) has found favour because of increased tolerance and compliance. More recent low-volume PEG without electrolytes regimens are becoming increasingly popular in pediatric units and are well tolerated, with no observable electrolytic disturbance.

In general, large-volume PEG with electrolytes is less tolerable. especially for younger children as well as placement of a nasogastric (NG) tube which should be avoided if possible.

The key to successful bowel preparation for ileocolonoscopy is patient/parental compliance/cooperation and adherence to the chosen regimen tailored to the child's age. Several studies including prospective data collection from 14 pediatric US centers (almost 22 000 colonoscopies) published in 2016 reinforced the importance of differential approaches to bowel preparation based on the child's age. According to the Practice Committee of the American Society for Gastrointestinal Endoscopy (ASGE) and Israel Society for Paediatric Gastroenterology and Nutrition, a clear liquid diet for 24 hours and a normal saline solution enema (5 mL/kg) may suffice for infants younger than 2 years of age.

Our approach to bowel preparation for infants below 2 years of age is slightly different. Although it is debatable, we do not prep the colon in infants less than 4 months old. It is quite easy to irrigate and aspirate the small amount of liquid and semiliquid stool during the procedure.

In infants between 4 and 12 months of age, we achieve satisfactory results of colonic cleansing by using a liquid diet and milk of magnesia (1 mL/kg per dose twice a day) for two consecutive days prior to the procedure. For children 1–2 years of age, we recommend a combination of Senokot 0.5–1 mg/kg and sodium picosulfate ¼ sachet on two occasions the day before colonoscopy.

Based on the published data and our extensive personal experience, preferred methods of bowel preparation for children 2 years and older are PEG 3350 or PICO with Senokot in combination with a clear liquid diet (CLD) the day before colonoscopy. Liberal drinking is essential for successful cleansing and prevention of dehydration.

PEG 3350 solution is prepared as a mixture of 238 g of polyethylene glycol if purchased over the counter or 255 g if obtained by prescription. For older children, the suggested volume of PEG 3350 solution is 1.9 L. For younger children, it is recommended to take the PEG 3350 mixture until two consecutive clear stools are passed.

A recommended dose of PEG 3350 for one- and two-day regimens is 4 g/kg and 2 g/kg respectively for children with bodyweight below 50 kg or 238 g for patients whose weight is above 50 kg. The solution is prepared as a mixture of PEG 3350 with flavored sport drinks.

The quality of bowel preparation with PICO with Senokot is equal to PEG regimens but it is more tolerable for children. The age-specific doses are ¼ sachet (2.5 g) for children 1–6 years of age, ½ sachet for children 6–12 years of age, and one sachet for older children from 12 to 18 years of age, given twice with a 6–12 hour interval the day before colonoscopy. Each dose is diluted in 150 mL of cold water and taken twice at 4 pm and 6 hours later the day before colonoscopy. Intake of additional clear fluid after each dose (up to 1 L) should be encouraged.

If a large-volume lavage method (PEG with electrolytes) is chosen, the patient can eat and drink up until the afternoon of the day before the procedure. The patient is then asked to fast overnight. Flavored solutions are available. The cleansing agent (5–10 mL/kg up to 250 mL per dose) is given by mouth every 10 minutes until the rectal effluent is clear. There are some adolescents and teenagers who will accomplish this preparation readily but hospitalization for 24–48 hours. A nasogastric tube placement may be necessary for uncooperative patients. This is one reason why low-volume protocols are the preferred method in children and adolescents.

In recent years, serious side effects of oral sodium phosphate colonic lavage in adults have been reported. Among these were cases of fatal hyperphosphatemia with hypocalcemia, hypokalemia, dehydration and acute nephrocalcinosis with renal failure. Currently, we would not recommend sodium phosphate for colonic cleansing in children and teenagers.

Enemas are not routinely used for children, especially those with suspected inflammatory bowel disease, as they cause erythema, edema and petechiae of rectal and distal sigmoid mucosa, complicating the interpretation of endoscopic findings, but in certain circumstances they can help if the effluent is not clear two hours before the procedure.

The benefit of intravenous antispasmodic agents administered directly before the ileocolonoscopy has been demonstrated, for example hyoscine 20 mg administered intravenously. The use of such an agent given just prior to colonoscopy is determined by personal preference. Their use may facilitate luminal visualization but it may also increase the compliance of the colon, theoretically allowing a greater chance of loop formation. They are certainly of benefit in spastic colonic situations. It should be remembered that they work only for a short period of time, 5–10 minutes, and they may be readministered in certain situations, such as when one needs to relax a haustral fold if a polyp is just beyond and obscured by it, or to relax a spastic ileocecal valve. Glucagon is a longer-acting intestinal paralytic which can last for an hour or more; approximate dosing regimens are IV 0.5 mg under 20 kg body weight, IV 1 mg over 20 kg body weight. This is particularly useful in longer procedures such as enteroscopy (see Chapter 14). Clinically significant hyperglycemia is not seen.

Indications for ileocolonoscopy

Indications are covered in Chapter 10.

Contraindications for ileocolonoscopy

There are few absolute contraindications to attempting ileocolonoscopy in children (Table 12.1). In cases of fulminant colitis, careful examination of the rectum and distal sigmoid colon may be attempted by experts. Generally, ileocolonoscopy is delayed for at least 8 weeks following ileal pouch or other surgeries associated with colon exploration. Connective tissue disorders such as Ehlers–Danlos should be approached with care and understanding of the increased risk of perforation. Clearly, known intestinal perforation or peritonitis are absolute contraindications as well as absolute neutrophil count below 500.

Equipment

Three types of colonoscopies are available for routine diagnostic investigation in children: standard "adult" instruments with outer diameters 12.8–13.2 mm (Table 12.2), slim "pediatric" scopes with outer diameter 11.5–11.6 mm (Table 12.3), and ultra-slim scopes with outer diameter of 9.5–9.8 mm (Table 12.4). We would refer the reader to the manufacturers, however, as these specifications change and advance regularly.

Table 12.1 Contraindications to ileocolonoscopy

Peritonitis

Conditions with a high risk of perforation:

    Fulminant colitis

    Toxic megacolon

Recent surgical anastomoses (<8 weeks post surgery)

Some connective tissue disorders

Poor bowel preparation

Respiratory and cardiovascular distress

The extra stiffness of the adult version diminishes the likelihood of forming sigmoid loops, but extra care must then be taken, especially in younger children under general anesthesia, not to advance against undue resistance, to avoid the unlikely complication of colonic perforation. The large diameter of the adult colonoscope can also limit maneuverability within the smaller colonic lumen of a young child.

Slim pediatric and ultra-slim colonoscopes are more flexible and have a higher propensity to form loops. However, these instruments have an adjustable stiffness mechanism operated by a dial on the control section right below the biopsy channel, which allows the insertion tube to be made stiffer when passing through the sigmoid and transverse colon, decreasing the chance of sigmoid loops. Colonoscopes with adjustable stiffness should be standard in all pediatric centers conducting colonoscopy. In respect of

Table 12.2 Technical specifications of new regular adult colonoscopes

	Working length (mm)	Insertion tube diameter (mm)	Biopsy channel diameter (mm)
Olympus CF-HQ190L/I	1680/1330	12.8	3.7
Fujinon EC-6000 HL	1690	12.8	4.2
Pentax EC38-iL/F/M	1700/1500/1300	13.2	3.8

Table 12.3 Technical specifications of new slim colonoscopes

	Working length (mm)	Insertion tube diameter (mm)	Biopsy channel diameter (mm)
Olympus:			
PCF- H190L	1680	11.5	3.2
PCF- H190 I	1330	11.5	3.2
Fujinon EC-550 LS5	1690	11.5	3.8
Pentax:			
EC34-i10L[a]	1700	11.6	3.8
EC-3490LK Slim CD	1700	11.6	3.8
EC-3490TLi[b]	1700	11.6	3.2

[a] High-resolution image with close focus technology.
[b] High-resolution image system with RetroView™.

Table 12.4 Technical specifications of new ultra-slim colonoscopes

	Working length (mm)	Insertion tube diameter (mm)	Biopsy channel diameter (mm)
Olympus PCF- PH190L/I	1680/1330	9.5	3.2
Fujinon EC-580 RD/L/M	1690/1330	9.8	3.2
Pentax EC34-2990 Li	1700	9.8	2.8

training, the new generation of adult colono-scopes are equipped with electromagnetic coils incorporated within the shaft, which give the endoscopist a 3D view of the shape and position of the colonoscope within the patient's colon. This technology is now integrated into the standard hands-on colonoscopy courses offered in training centers and accelerates the learning curve especially in comprehension of loop formation and resolution (Scope Guide®, Olympus). A "through-the-scope" (via biopsy channel) version that is removable and reusable is also available.

There is a limited amount of published data to support the choice of colonoscope use in children. Recently, data from Japan suggest the use of a standard or pediatric colonoscope in patients weighing 12–15 kg or above, infant or standard adult gastroscopes in patients weighing 5–12 kg, and ultra-thin gastroscopes in patients weighing <5 kg.

Based on our large personal experience, the lower limit for the standard adult colonoscope is 3–4 years of age and/or 12–15 kg. A slim colonoscope can be used with care in children with bodyweight above 8 kg. Upper adult endoscope (under 10 mm) or ultra-thin colonoscope and ultra-thin gastroscope (5.8 mm) are suitable for infants from 5 to 8 kg and under 5 kg respectfully.

More recently, image-enhanced/magnifying colonoscopes have been developed, and their value in combination with dye spray or chromoendoscopy in various gastrointestinal diseases has been described (see Chapter 17). For instance, the decrease in the number of cryptal openings in ulcerative colitis can be observed and correlated to disease activity. Confocal colonoscopy is even more impressive in this regard (see Chapter 18) but this does not yet substitute for histologic assessment.

Informed consent and preprocedure preparation

Specific indications, risks and benefits of ileocolonoscopy must be the subject of a detailed discussion with the family. This should leave parents comfortable and confident about the need for and safety of the procedure before it is scheduled.

Ideally, both the child and parents should be offered a preparatory visit to the endoscopy unit to answer questions and defuse any potential concerns and anxieties regarding the procedure and admission. Younger children undoubtedly benefit from preadmission visits and the involvement of a play therapist to enable some understanding of what is to take place and why. Diagrams may help in explanations to older children. Preparatory online videos and child-friendly cartoons from webpages such as www.paediatricgastroenterologist.co.uk and www.moviegi.com are very useful for informing the patient and parent regarding what to expect and should be made available. Units can benefit from devising a sample videos specific to their own facility.

It is now considered best practice to obtain informed consent at the planning clinic visit rather than on the day of the procedure – further confirmatory consent can be signed for on the day also.

On the day of the procedure, the child, and parents are invited to the preprocedure area. Here, the patient changes clothes and is prepared for intravenous line placement. To minimize the discomfort of a venipuncture, EMLA® cream is applied to one or two potential intravenous sites 60 minutes before the procedure. Infusion of age-appropriate solution is started once the venous excess is established and secured. The patient is then transferred to the procedure area for the preparation of sedation or general anesthesia.

Specifics of sedation for colonoscopy

See Chapter 4.

Embryology of the colon relative to ileocolonoscopy

Abnormal rotation and fixation of the embryonic colon is probably the major reason for a "difficult" colon and incomplete colonoscopy.

A anticlockwise rotation around the superior mesenteric artery is the main mechanism of "packaging" the growing intestine in preparation for its return to the abdomen. Additional anticlockwise rotation is again crucial for proper relocation of the intestine into the peritoneal cavity.

As a result of a normal rotation, the colon acquires two zones of full fixation: the descending and ascending colon, as well as two areas of partial fixation: the cecum and rectum. In addition, the mobility of the splenic and hepatic flexure is somewhat limited by a phrenocolic and extension of the hepatorenal ligaments, respectively. Only the sigmoid and transverse colons possess their own mesentery and are fully mobile.

It is not surprising that they became a target of various endoscopic maneuvers preventing or minimizing stretching of these vulnerable segments of the intestine. It is easy to imagine

that abnormal rotation or fixation of the embryonic colon can multiply difficulties in navigating through the unusually mobile bowel.

Some of the anomalies can be suspected during a procedure, for example, fixation of the cecum in the right hypochondrium. The intrinsic propensity of the embryonic colon for anticlockwise rotation from the left iliac fossa to the right gives an important clue to the concept of a torque steering technique of a colonoscopy.

Endoscopic anatomy of the colon and terminal ileum

The only dependable and observer-reproducible anatomical landmarks in ileocolonoscopy are the anus, the appendiceal orifice, ileocecal valve, and terminal ileum. Everything between is guesswork! Many estimates of cecal intubation are incorrect due to confusion of the splenic or hepatic flexure with the cecum. Therefore, it is important to become accustomed to the nuances of endoscopic anatomy of the colon in order to achieve correct orientation during colonoscopy, accurate localization of lesions, and reassurance that the cecum has been reached.

The anal canal is less than 2 cm in a newborn, reaching an adult length of 3 cm by 4 years of age. It is normally closed due to tonic contraction of the anal sphincter but may be dilated in cases of chronic constipation or poor neurological control such as with spina bifida; beware that inference regarding possible sexual abuse is very difficult in a child under deep sedation or general anesthesia (Figure 12.1). It is important to remember that the axis of the anal canal is pointed anteriorly. Proper insertion of the colonoscope will minimize discomfort, eliminating excessive stretching of the anus and preventing embedding of the tip into the rectal mucosa.

The squamocolumnar junction or pectinate (dentate) line demarcates the proximal edge of the anal canal (Figure 12.2). A few longitudinal folds (columns of Morgani) run within the anal canal and terminate at the anal papillae (Figure 12.3). Occasionally, the anal papillae may be quite prominent, seen as cone-like grayish structures. The rectum becomes enlarged and fusiform between the upper edge of the columns of Morgani and the rectosigmoid junction. This part of the rectum is called the ampulla. It is marked by three semilunar folds referred to as the valves of Houston (Figure 12.4). There are two such folds on the left and one on the right lateral wall. The ampulla narrows at the level of the rectosigmoid junction, which is distanced from the anal verge by 9 cm in neonates and 15 cm in children 10 years and older. The rectal mucosa

is smooth and transparent, which allows good visualization of submucosal veins (Figure 12.5).

Multiple small lymphoid follicles in the rectal mucosa are normally present in infants and toddlers, but when excessive or surrounded by erythema they may indicate an allergic proctocolitis. The sigmoid colon is the most "unpredictable" part of the colon due to its long, "V"-shape mesocolon. Stretching during colonoscopy could double the length of the sigmoid colon. Therefore, an absolute length of the sigmoid colon is not important unless it is tremendously elongated.

The mobility and displacement of the sigmoid colon may be limited due to previous surgery, adhesions or shortening of the mesentery.

A relatively small sigmoid colon in infants and toddlers has some disadvantages for the endoscopist: first, it decreases the threshold for pain due to activation of stretch receptors. Second, it limits application the of alpha loop maneuver and use of standard pediatric colonoscopes, making the procedure more technically challenging.

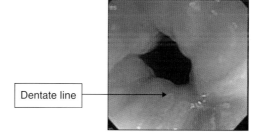

Figure 12.1 Unusually wide-open anus. This finding is suspicious for spina bifida, trauma, or sexual abuse.

Figure 12.2 Squamocolumnar junction or dentate line.

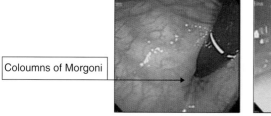

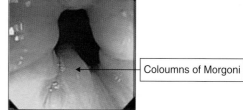

Figure 12.3 The longitudinal folds in the distal rectum (columns of Morgani) and prominent anal papilla. The U-turn maneuver in the rectum is useful for detailed observation of the distal rectum close to the anal canal.

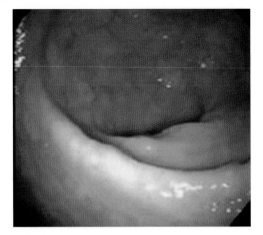

Figure 12.4 Semilunar folds of Houston in the rectum.

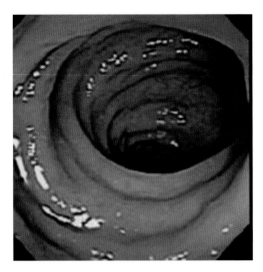

Figure 12.6 The sigmoid colon. The endoscopic markers of normal sigmoid colon are (i) rounded lumen, (ii) circular folds, and (iii) subtle vascular pattern.

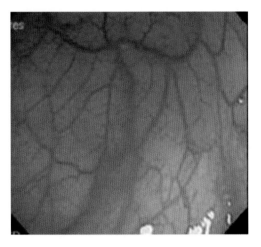

Figure 12.5 Typical vascular pattern of the normal rectum.

The normal sigmoid colon appears tubular because of the prominence of a circular muscle layer. The mucosa is less transparent than in the rectum. There are multiple circular folds throughout the sigmoid colon (Figure 12.6).

The taenia coli are not usually visible along the sigmoid colon except in the area adjacent to the sigmoid descending junction. The appearance of taenia coli in this area indicates significant stretching of the sigmoid colon.

During colonoscopy, the sigmoid colon is always stretched to some degree and becomes more spiral and twisted clockwise between the rectum and descending colon. The concave sacrum and a forward-projecting sacral promontory determine the initial anterior deviation of the sigmoid loop. At this stage of the procedure, a colonoscope can be palpated easily unless the sigmoid colon is extremely stretched.

The transitional zone between the sigmoid and descending colon is located posterior at the level of the pelvic brim and out of reach for transabdominal palpation. The angle between the sigmoid and descending colon is sharper when the descending colon extends down below the pelvic brim due to an unusually low fixation and/or when the sigmoid colon was stretched out extensively (Figure 12.7).

Normally, the descending colon is slightly wider and more oval than the sigmoid colon (Figure 12.8). It runs straight up toward the left hypochondrium to join the splenic flexure. The mucosa of the descending colon is slightly grayish. The stems of the vessels run along folds, i.e., perpendicular to the lumen. The small branches cross the folds in parallel to the lumen (Figure 12.9). The folds of the descending colon are spread more apart relative to the folds of the sigmoid colon. The taenia coli are

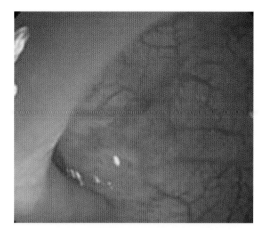

Figure 12.7 The angle is sharper when the descending colon extends down below the pelvic brim due to unusually low fixation and/or when the sigmoid colon was stretched out extensively.

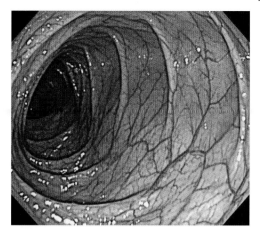

Figure 12.9 The vascular pattern of the descending colon. The stems of the vessels run along folds, i.e., parallel to the lumen. The small branches spread around and across the folds and along the lumen.

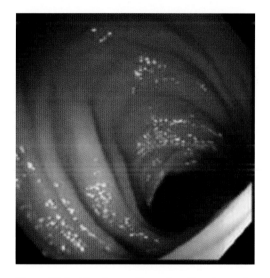

Figure 12.8 The descending colon. The shape of the descending colon is close to oval.

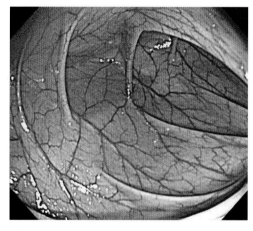

Figure 12.10 The splenic flexure. It is marked by bluish discoloration.

usually not visible. The splenic flexure is marked by the bluish color of the transilluminated spleen (Figure 12.10).

This area should occupy the right part of the lumen if the colonoscope was positioned properly inside the sigmoid and descending colon. The same color spot can be seen occasionally when the tip of the colonoscope is trapped within a very large sigmoid loop. Thus, this color mark does not definitively prove that the splenic flexure has been reached. The splenic flexure is firmly attached to the diaphragm by the phrenocolic ligament at the level of 10th and 11th ribs. That could explain occasional hiccups and transient hypoxia during exploration of the transverse colon due to excessive pressure and irritation of the phrenic nerve, especially in infants and young children.

The junction with the transverse colon is located along the upper aspect of the medial wall of the splenic flexure. It is angled by the mobile transverse colon, which hangs down from the elevated splenic flexure. The area is more sharply angled and even folded when the patient is in the left lateral position (Figure 12.11).

Relatively thin circular and thick longitudinal layers of the muscularis propria are responsible for the triangular shape of the transverse colon (Figure 12.12). The slope of the transverse colon is pointed toward the hepatic flexure, which is more voluminous

than the adjacent colonic segments and has a blue-gray color acquired from the neighboring liver (Figure 12.13). The folds become circular at both ends of the hepatic flexure. The junction with the ascending colon is located higher than the adjacent transverse colon. It points toward the right lobe of the liver and is sharply angled posteriorly (Figure 12.14). The area between the hepatic flexure and the ascending colon is always

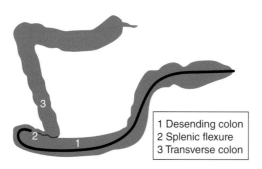

1 Desending colon
2 Splenic flexure
3 Transverse colon

Figure 12.11 The angle between the splenic flexure and transverse colon in relation to patient position during colonoscopy. The convoluted pathway through the splenic flexure is created by the transverse colon, which is sagging down when the patient is in the left lateral position.

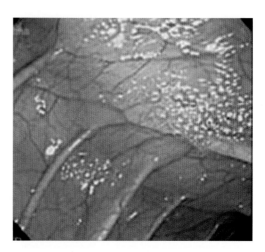

Figure 12.13 The hepatic flexure. The mucosa of this area is paler and has a light bluish tinge acquired from the adjacent liver.

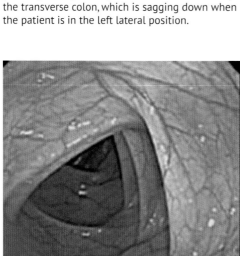

Figure 12.12 The transverse colon. The triangular shape is the endoscopic hallmark of the transverse colon.

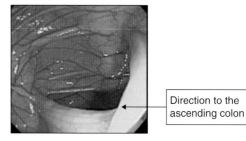

Direction to the ascending colon

Figure 12.14 The hepatic flexure, which is dome shaped. The junction between the hepatic flexure and the ascending colon is always hidden in the right upper corner of the screen behind the mucosal fold. Steering of the shaft anticlockwise, pulling it back, and elevation of the tip help to stretch the folded lumen. Subsequent clockwise rotation and deviation of the tip to the right and decompression of the colon facilitate exploration of the ascending colon.

hidden in the right upper corner of the screen behind the mucosal fold. Steering of the shaft anticlockwise, pulling it back, and elevation of the tip help to stretch the folded lumen. Subsequent clockwise rotation and deviation of the tip to the right and decompression of the colon facilitate exploration of the ascending colon.

The ascending colon is a short (5 cm in some young children), retroperitoneal and fixed segment of the right colon. It runs between the cecum anteriorly and the lower pole of the right kidney posteriorly. The lumen of the ascending colon is usually wide open. It extends into the cecum, a "blind" pouch outlined by the ileocecal valve at the top and the appendix orifice (the landmark of the cecum) at the bottom.

- the ileocecal valve
- the appendiceal orifice
- the triradiate fold.

The appendiceal orifice is usually oval or rounded and located at the intersection of the taenia coli at the cecal pole. The orifice can be thought of as a "bow" with an imaginary arrow pointing to the ileocecal valve (IV): "bow and arrow sign" (Figure 12.15). The IV is usually "hiding" on the upstream or "cecal" slope of the ileocecal fold but can be discovered by a focal bulging or widening of the medial aspect of the fold (Figure 12.16).

Torque steering technique – the key to successful ileocolonoscopy

A unique colonoscopy technique has been developed to overcome the high flexibility, elasticity, and multiple angulations of the large intestine (the sigmoid colon in particular).

It consists of two types of maneuver: loop prevention-torque steering and loop reduction.

The main principles of the torque steering technique are (i) substitution of lateral angulation control for torqueing the shaft clockwise or anticlockwise with the preceding up-and-down deflection of the bending section and two-corkscrew maneuvering around a sharply angled segment of the colon instead of application of linear force to push the endoscope forward (note that this technique works only when the shaft is straight).

A key element of the loop reduction technique is a combination of simultaneous clockwise or anticlockwise rotation and puling the shaft back, as explained below.

One important" trick" in learning ileocolonoscopy is to grasp the concept of the lumen as a clock face and the tip of the scope as a short hour hand. A simple angulation of the tip up or down is sufficient to reach the 12 or 6 o'clock sites. However, vertical angulation alone will not work if the target is anywhere on the left

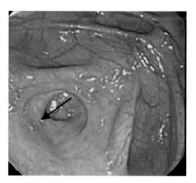 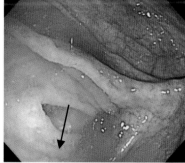

Figure 12.15 Appendiceal orifice and "bow and arrow sign": the imaginary arrow in the bow points the way to the ileocecal valve.

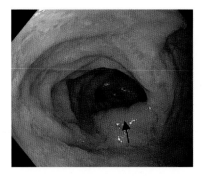 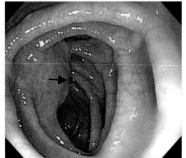

Figure 12.16 A focal widening or bulging of the circular fold at the upper aspect of the cecum is a sign of the hidden ileocecal valve.

side of the dial (between 12 and 6 through 9 o'clock) or the right side (between 12 and 6 through 3 o'clock). In this case, lateral deflection can be achieved by the shaft torque to the left/anticlockwise or to the right/clockwise direction with the tip deflected up or down respectively (Figure 12.17). This approach, which is the core of the torque steering technique, provides the best spatial orientation and control of the colonoscope by the left thumb and middle finger and "winding"-rotating the shaft up to 360° by the thumb, index, and middle fingers of the right hand.

Torque steering is the most important skill to acquire in the early days of a colonoscopist's career, especially in the rectosigmoid colon. Such skill acquisition and employment will markedly diminish the possibility of sigmoid loop formation.

Golden rules of ileocolonoscopy

1) Do not advance unless you know where the lumen is. Pushing blindly is useless and dangerous.
2) The direction of the luminal axis should be ascertained before pushing in.
3) Think before advancing the scop: each bend requires a conscious steering decision.
4) When searching for the lumen, the view must be clean; delicate insufflation and slow withdrawal with clockwise and anticlockwise rotation can help to identify the dark crescent which is nearest to the lumen.

5) Check scope for neutral position when in doubt of orientation.
6) Insufflate as little as possible: excessive air, especially in the sigmoid colon, makes it elongated and tortuous. The rule of insufflation is "as much as necessary, as little as possible."
7) Suction out excess air frequently to make the colon shorter and easier to navigate.
8) Suction fluid infrequently, only when it is necessary to clear the view.
9) Steer carefully and cautiously: initiate each angulation and torque slowly to be able to terminate the maneuver almost immediately if the tip is moving in the wrong direction.
10) Pull back frequently for shortening of the sigmoid colon and loop prevention.
11) Corkscrew around acute bends instead of pushing up against them.
12) Avoid forceful angulations of the bending portion while advancing the scope.
13) Avoid blind "slide-by" over the mucosa insertion for more than a few seconds. This maneuver is permissible as a last resort and if the scope slides easily over the surface with a clear view of the "slide-by" mucosal vascular pattern.
14) Change patient position when needed.
15) If you are stuck for more than 2–3 minutes, then change something – patient position, abdominal pressure, antispasmodic administration; do not just keep pushing and hoping!

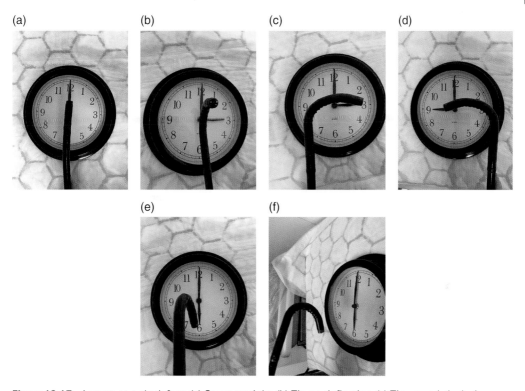

Figure 12.17 Lumen as a clock face. (a) Scope straight. (b) Tip up deflection. (c) Tip up and clockwise rotation. (d) Tip up and anticlockwise rotation. (e) Tip down to get to 6 o'clock. (f) Tip down to get to 6 o'clock side view.

Technique of ileocolonoscopy

Handling the colonoscope

There are three ways to perform an ileocolonoscopy.

- Single-handed one-person technique: the endoscopist handles the control panel with the left hand and the shaft of the colonoscope with the right hand.
- Two-handed one-person technique: the endoscopist uses both hands to control the angulation knobs while securing the shaft within the colon by fixing the shaft between the thigh and couch.
- Two-person technique: the endoscopist operates the control panel and guides the assistant with handling the shaft.

It is generally accepted that the single-handed one-person technique is the most effective way to conduct a colonoscopy. The benefits of this approach are as follows.

- Superior control of the colonoscope and feel as the shaft is interacting with the loops and bends.
- Precise control of bowel resistance.
- Quick adjustment of shaft position to the changes in the bowel lumen.

By choosing the single-handed one-person technique, the operator is committed to holding the control panel by the left third and little fingers, using the thumb for U/D knob adjustment with the help of the middle finger, leaving the index finger for handling the air-water and suction valves.

The shaft should be held between the thumb and fingers. The finger grip as opposed to the fist grip provides a better sensitivity to shaft insertion: smooth and easy when the scope is straight and firm and resistant when the bowel is bent or looped. In addition, the finger grip allows shaft rotation up to 360° compared with a maximum of 180° by the fist grip. The extra rotation is very useful for working around bends and loop reduction.

A colonoscope should be maximally straightened to optimize transmission of rotating force from the control panel to the shaft.

One of the most common mistakes of beginners is holding the scope too close to the anus. Grasping the shaft about 20–25 cm from the anus decreases the need for frequent hand changes and makes for a smooth insertion and easier application of torque and better feel of the force involved.

Getting started and patient positioning

The patient is usually positioned in the left lateral knee to chest position, although some operators prefer the right lateral position, citing easier sigmoid negotiation. Often the supine position is equally useful, and the patient may not require position change. Nevertheless, frequent and appropriate position change can be very useful in successful sigmoid colon passage; for example, if the operator is not gaining easy access to the splenic flexure, then patient repositioning from one side to the supine and then to the other side may be advantageous. In general, frequent turning of the patient is conducive to easier ileocolonoscopy and is to be advocated. An assistant applies abdominal pressure that may be deemed necessary to control, or try to prevent, loop formation in the sigmoid or transverse colon.

In handling the colonoscope, it is good practice to place the portion of the shaft that is not yet inserted on a flat unimpeded surface. This is important because then any resistance encountered by the operator to forward advancement of the scope can be attributed to loop formation within the child's colon. Hence, relatively quickly, the trainee can learn when to stop pushing the scope and proceed with loop preventing maneuvers.

Rectal intubation

Before insertion, the entire equipment and suction system should be checked for proper function. The gurney is lifted to a comfortable height for the endoscopist. The distal 20 cm of the shaft is lubricated.

A rectal exam prior to the procedure serves three purposes:

- lubrication of the anal canal
- reassurance that the patient has been adequately prepared and sedated
- detection of low-lying polyp which may be missed on endoscopic insertion.

The assistant gently lifts the right buttock to expose the anus. The endoscopist grips the shaft at 20–30 cm, positions the tip into gentle contact with the anus and aligns the bending portion of the shaft with the axis of the anal canal, which runs toward the anterior abdominal wall.

Insufflations of the anal canal facilitate sliding of the tip into the distal rectum with minimal pressure. This technique virtually eliminates accidental trauma of the distal rectum. Immediately after initial exploration of the rectum, the scope is pulled back slightly and angled upwards to establish a panoramic view of the distal rectum. Any liquid stool can easily be aspirated to simplify the approach to the proximal rectum. Do not aspirate semi formed stool at the beginning of colonoscopy to avoid clogging of the suction channel.

Three semilunar folds, or valves of Houston, appears on alternating sides of the rectal ampulla along the way to the rectosigmoid junction It is distant from the dentate line for about 10–15 cm.

This is the first but not the last time when the lumen may disappear.

Endoscopic clues to a hidden lumen

A constant search for a fully opened lumen is not a productive way to conduct ileocolonoscopy if the goal is to prevent development of a big sigmoid loop. It creates more problems than benefits for the endoscopist. First, it is not possible because many segments of the colon, especially the sigmoid colon, are angulated. Second, a long opened upstream segment of the sigmoid colon indicates a big loop formation and should be avoided. Third, an extensive search for a fully open lumen leads to over inflation of the colon, which makes it ridged and elongated.

Instead, the endoscopist should waste no time searching for a fully opened lumen but ascertain the direction of the upstream colon and the way to approach it. In general, intubation of the sigmoid colon creates clusters of angled bends, which have a corkscrew or spiral pattern. This means that the axes of two adjacent sigmoid bends run in opposite directions; for example, if the visible segment climbs up diagonally from 5 o'clock to 11 o'clock, the following segment falls in the opposite direction toward 5 o'clock.

Disappearance of the lumen can be explained by unequal shortening of the mesenteric and antimesenteric edges of the colon during rotation and pushing forward, and positioning of the tip too close to the mucosa. Two strategies are useful in these circumstances:

- search for a hidden lumen and colonic axis using endoscopic clues
- pulling the scope slowly and torque it gently clockwise and anticlockwise.

The first clue is the darkest site of the mucosal view. The second is the center of the converging folds. The third clue is the merging folds pointed to the slightly depressed or funnel-like area (Figure 12.18).

It is worth remembering that the main submucosal vessels are parallel to the circular folds. However, their small branches usually spread around between the folds and can highlight the axis of the lumen (Figure 12.19).

Lastly, a crescent-like or dimpled lumen of a twisted sigmoid colon is usually located in three areas: between 10 and 12 o'clock, 1 and 3 o'clock, or 4 and 6 o'clock (Figure 12.20).

When the tip is close to the sigmoid–descending junction, a prominent longitudinal fold or the center of a convex fold indicates the direction of the colonic axis and the location of the next segment (Figure 12.21).

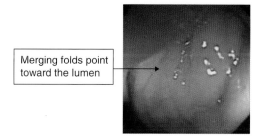

Merging folds point toward the lumen

Figure 12.18 Slightly depressed groove-like area and merging folds are the signs of the hidden lumen.

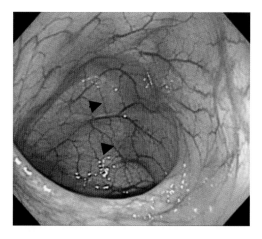

Figure 12.19 The main submucosal veins and their branches. The main vessels are parallel to the circular folds. The small branches are pointed toward the lumen. This endoscopic clue may be useful when the tip of the scope is distant from the mucosa for at least 1–2 cm.

(a)   (b)   (c)

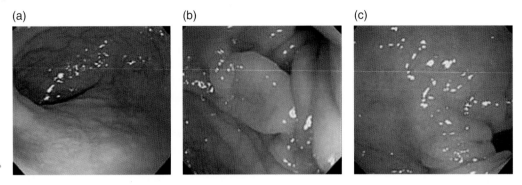

Figure 12.20 Common locations of the lumen. (a) The lumen is located at 9 o'clock. (b) The lumen is between 1 and 2 o'clock. (c) The lumen is located at 5 o'clock.

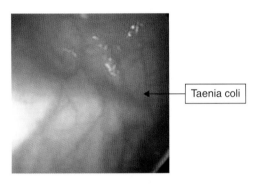

Taenia coli

Figure 12.21 Prominent taenia coli. An appearance of the taenia while approaching the sigmoid–descending junction indicates the direction of the lumen but also is the sign of the large sigmoid loop.

Exploration of the sigmoid colon and sigmoid–descending junction

The sigmoid colon is not as long in children as in adults. A relatively short sigmoid mesocolon in infants and young children typically prevents significant stretching. Nevertheless, an unexperienced endosocopist can create a giant loop in a deeply sedated child which is not palpable through the abdominal wall because it occupies both lateral gutters and hides under the liver and left diaphragm. This may produce a false impression of a properly performed procedure. The clinical clues to this dangerous condition are sudden changes in oxygen saturation, hiccups, shallow breathing, and irritability of the patient followed by signs of respiratory distress. Immediate

reduction of the loop and interruption of the procedure is mandatory until the child becomes stable.

Small loops are unavoidable during exploration of the sigmoid colon. However, development of large loops should be prevented.

The following is a description of the torque steering technique, which is particularly useful for sliding through the sharply angled segments of the sigmoid colon and sigmoid–descending junction.

- Orient the tip towards the narrowed lumen and advance the shaft slowly. If the lumen is located at 11 o'clock, rotate the shaft anticlockwise and angle the tip up.
- As soon as the edge of the lumen is approached, rotate the shaft clockwise and pull it back.
- If the lumen is located between 4 and 6 o'clock, rotate the shaft clockwise and pull it back. This will untwist the lumen and facilitate sliding of the tip into the proximal segment of the colon.
- If the next segment is open, advance the shaft forward a few centimeters. Rotate it clockwise and pull it back to telescope (shorten) the colon.
- Repeat this maneuver several times until the sigmoid–descending junction is reached.
- Transabdominal pressure by the assistant may be necessary just before an attempt to advance the scope into the descending colon

This technique is equally applicable to the rectosigmoid area and the junction between the splenic flexure and transverse colon.

The initial sigmoid fold can usually be passed by 90–120° of anticlockwise torsion.

The different loops encountered in the sigmoid are demonstrated in Figure 12.22.

Formation of a loop is suspected when the operator begins to feel more resistance to advancement with a visualized lumen. Another clue is loss of "one-to-one" movement; in other words, when the distance moved by the scope *outside* the patient is not mirrored by the colonoscope tip advancement *inside* the patient. Thirdly, if "paradoxical" movement is observed. This is when the operator advances the colonoscope and the tip starts to migrate distally. This usually indicates a large loop.

A so-called N loop may be overcome by transabdominal pressure by an assistant on the apex of the loop pushing toward the feet. This often allows a so-called alpha loop to form, which can usually be tolerated as the instrument advances toward the splenic flexure.

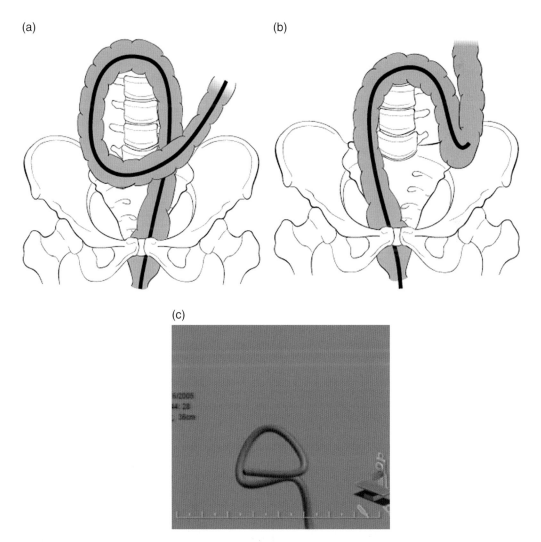

Figure 12.22 Schematic images of: (a) alpha loop, (b) N-loop and (c) Scope Guide® image of reverse-alpha loop.

An alpha loop (Figure 12.22a) may be suspected if the scope is running in very easily without acute bends. In this scenario, continue advancing the scope up to the proximal descending colon or even the splenic flexure (about 50–70 cm in older children) whilst one-to-one advancement is maintained. Reduction of an alpha loop is accomplished by extensive (at least 90°) clockwise rotation and then slow removal of the colonoscope, keeping the lumen in the center of the field of vision. *Remember that the rotation required to resolve a loop may be 360° or more (usually unsuccessful loop resolution is due to an inadequate degree of rotation).*

Changing the patient position and application of transabdominal pressure by the assistance may be necessary. Unsuccessful attempts of a loop reduction are the sign of reverse-alpha loop. *In this scenario, the loop can only be resolved by anticlockwise rotation.*

If using a variable stiffness scope, it is helpful to stiffen the scope after 15–20 cm of insertion. Eliminate extra stiffness before loop reduction maneuvers and restiffen the shaft afterwards. Abdominal pressure in the left iliac fossa may be helpful. Turning the patient into the supine position reduces the sharp angle of the sigmoid–descending colon junction.

To prevent recurrence of the loop after successful reduction, follow the same torque direction while advancing the scope forward: a gentle clockwise and anticlockwise steering in case of N or alpha loop and reverse-alpha loop respectively.

Descending colon

The lumen of the descending colon is more oval compared to the sigmoid colon although the difference can be subtle. The folds are less frequent, the color is more grayish, and the vascular pattern is more prominent. Once the descending colon is reached, advance the shaft quickly toward the splenic flexure. This is one of the easiest steps of a colonoscopy because loops are reduced and the shaft is fully straightened

within the descending colon which is fixed in the retroperitoneum. However, the external portion of the shaft is often twisted. To untwist the external portion of the colonoscope, the shaft should be rotated anticlockwise. Attention should be paid to the lumen of the descending colon, to avoid mucosal trauma by the tip of the colonoscope. This maneuver facilitates exploration of the splenic flexure.

Splenic flexure and transverse colon

The splenic flexure can be reached by the 40 cm mark on the straight shaft in older children and even 20–25 cm in children under 4 years if the sigmoid loop has been avoided or reduced.

When negotiating the splenic flexure:

- pull the shaft back usually with clockwise torque, until the feeling of resistance or slippage of the tip back occurs
- deangulate the tip to avoid over angulation within the splenic flexure and prevent resistance to sliding the scope forward
- deflate the colon
- consider hand pressure to the low abdomen to avoid sigmoid looping
- rotate the shaft clockwise and adjust the tip to keep the lumen view
- increase stiffness of adjustable colonoscopes to prevent relooping of the sigmoid colon and push the shaft forward slowly.

Changing the patient into the right lateral (ideal) or supine position facilitates bypassing of the splenic flexure.

Suspect reverse splenic flexure after failure of a few attempts and follow the new algorithm: pull the shaft back and rotate it anticlockwise and aim toward 11 o'clock. The lumen of the transverse colon will appear as a slot along the line between 7 and 1 o'clock. An additional angulation in the same direction and anticlockwise rotation will make the lumen wider. At this point, stiffen the shaft and rotate it clockwise a quarter turn and bring the tip down slowly. It is necessary to turn the shaft anticlockwise again and elevate the tip up before advancing the shaft into the transverse colon by "staccato" repetitive gentle pushing-in movements.

The triangular shape is common for the transverse colon but in smaller children is not always a reliable sign.

Exploration of the transverse colon does not require forceful advancement of the colonoscope. In the absence of visible progress or in case of increasing resistance, pull the shaft back a few centimeters while keeping the lumen opened, then elevate the tip and push it forward, applying clockwise torque simultaneously. Repeat this maneuver two or three times. If no significant progress has been made, rotate the patient into the right lateral position, straighten the colonoscope by pulling it back, apply external pressure to stabilize the sigmoid colon and advance the shaft forward. Decreased resistance and progression of the tip forward indicate successful exploration of the transverse colon, which has a distinctive triangular lumen. At this point, the hepatic flexure can be reached by either pulling the shaft back with simultaneous anticlockwise rotation or pushing it gently forward.

Creation of a so-called "gamma" loop (Figure 12.23) is an uncommon element of pediatric colonoscopy. It is revealed by increasing resistance and paradoxical movement of the proximal transverse colon away from the tip with attempts to push the shaft forward. Successful reduction of a gamma loop can be challenging. First, rotate the patient to supine, then pull the shaft back and rotate it anticlockwise. If the tip remains stable during the withdrawal phase of the maneuver, continue pulling back until the shaft is straightened.

Hepatic flexure, ascending colon, and cecum

The hepatic flexure can be reached by the 60 cm mark in older children and even 40 cm in children under 4 years if the sigmoid and

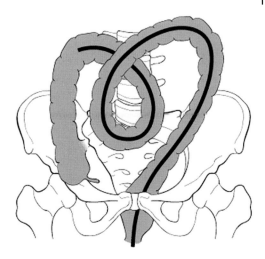

Figure 12.23 Gamma loop in the transverse colon.

transverse colon loops have been prevented or reduced. The hepatic flexure is recognized by the dark, usually blue, discoloration seen through the bowel wall (see Figure 12.13). It consists of a few sharply angled folds, making the negotiation into the ascending colon like a "chicane" movement. Left lateral position is best to allow this opening to reveal itself. The entrance to the area is always located at the 11 o'clock position.

The approach and transition through the hepatic flexure consist of the following steps.

1) *Orientation.* The transitional area between the transverse colon and the hepatic flexure often appears as a blind pouch, a source of confusion for inexperienced colonoscopists. The right part of the pouch is convex with a few circular folds creating an illusion of the "correct" direction. The left wall of the pouch is short due to its rotation and the spiral configuration of the bowel. Attention should be focused on the upper portion of this area.
2) *Withdrawal.* Pull the shaft back slowly and orient the tip to the 11 o'clock direction. Continue withdrawing and deflecting the tip in the same direction until appearance of a groove-like lumen.
3) *Decompression.* Decompress the bowel until the lumen begins to collapse.

4) *Switching direction and advancement.* Rotate the shaft clockwise and move the tip to the 4–5 o'clock direction (use the R/L knob if necessary or if the operator has small hands) once the lumen of the hepatic flexure is half opened (see Figure 12.14). Additional suction and abdominal pressure may be needed to advance the shaft beyond this point. Do not be discouraged if the scope bounces back.

5) *Final advancement.* Steer the shaft forward and keep it in the center of the lumen by gentle anticlockwise rotation and elevation of the tip.

It is important to remember that the ascending colon, which in children is of variable length, may be as short as 5 cm in some younger patients.

On some occasions, a deep gamma loop can occur before engagement with the hepatic flexure and the operator must put up with a "long scope." The scope should be pushed toward the hepatic flexure, the tip angulated around it and the scope pulled back with simultaneous strong anticlockwise and then clockwise torque until the loop is reduced. Suction is always helpful. Often, the scope itself will dictate the direction of rotation: a correct direction of the twist will be rewarded with decreased resistance and advancement of the tip forward. It is not unusual to find oneself then looking at the appendiceal orifice and hence the cecum because the scope will have travelled down rapidly into the ascending colon. This can be achieved if the operator "plays" with the shaft gently and sensitively, like a cellist with a bow. On some occasions, positioning the patient on the right side can be helpful. Confirm completion of colonoscopy by a close-up look at the appendiceal orifice.

Less specific signs of reaching the cecum are (i) transillumination: the presence of light in the right iliac fossa, which may be useful in some obese adolescents and (ii) indentation of the colonic wall with digital pressure over the right iliac fossa. Any doubts that the cecum has been reached should be resolved by finding the appendiceal orifice or intubation of the terminal ileum. If you are not sure that the scope is in the cecum, then most likely you are right, and the scope is probably in the hepatic or even splenic flexure.

If colonoscopy is performed properly, the cecum can be reached by the 70–80 cm marks on the shaft in older children and teenagers and 40–50 cm in children under 2–5 years, depending on their size.

Terminal ileum intubation

Two conditions guarantee successful intubation of the terminal ileum: reduction and straightening of any colonic loops and finding of the ileocecal valve. As mentioned above, the hallmark of the straightened shaft at the level of the cecum is 70–80 cm or 40–50 cm mark at the anus in older children/teenagers and children under 5 years old respectively. This ensures that the scope is under proper control when tackling the terminal ileum.

In general, the ileocecal valve is situated between 9 and 5 o'clock (Figure 12.24) and best seen as the bulging or flattened area on the last and most prominent haustral fold within 1–4 cm from the cecal pole. However, finding the precise location of the ileocecal valve is the key.

Three are three ways to enter the terminal ileum.

- *"Bow and arrow" technique*: find the appendix with the typical "bow" appearance; aim an arrow at the "bow" showing the direction where the appendix is pointing toward the center of the abdomen and the ileum is coming from (see Figure 12.16); steer in the direction of the arrow; pull back slowly and watch for the lip of the valve sliding by over the lens and enjoy the appearance of the terminal ileum.

- *"Straight-on" technique*: pull the scope back 5–7 cm from the cecal pole and look at the first prominent circular fold and search

(a) (b)

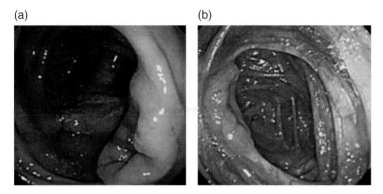

Figure 12.24 The ileocecal valve. It is usually located between the 5 o'clock (a) and 9 o'clock (b) position of the cecum.

for the portion which is not perfectly concave or appears as a thickened or bulged area (see Figure 12.17). Suction can often make the valve looks more noticeable. Torque the shaft clockwise or anticlockwise to rotate the view so that the valve bulge is at the bottom of the screen at 6 o'clock (the down angulation is the easiest steering movement for entry to the terminal ileum). Push the scope inwards over the bulge, angle it down toward the opening and pull back slowly to impact the tip into the valve. Continue to angle the tip down and insufflate to open the ileum and steer to find the direction of the lumen. Consider intravenous glucagon (0.5 mg under 20 kg bodyweight and 1 mg over 20 kg) or Buscopan (hyoscine butylbromide) to relax the haustral fold or a spastic ileocecal valve. If finding the valve or entering the terminal ileum failed, changing the patient's position to supine or right lateral and moving the valve to the 9 or 12 o'clock location by rotating the shaft may help.

- *Biopsy guidance technique* (reserved for the experienced endoscopist): position the scope as close to the identified or suspected ileocecal valve as possible; advance the forceps a few millimeters beyond the tip of the scope; apply gentle pressure to the upper lip of the valve to open it up; advance the forceps forward as far as allowed by the visible lumen of the terminal ileum, decompress the cecum and slide the shaft into the ileum guided by the forceps. Transabdominal pressure and position change may facilitate alignment of the forceps with the ileal axis.

A more experienced colleague should be sought after three or four unsuccessful attempts.

Successful exploration of the terminal ileum is manifested by the change in color and texture of the mucosa; while the cecum appears pink-grayish and smooth with prominent vessels, the mucosa of the terminal ileum is light pink or yellowish, velvet, with multiple small (less than 3 mm) lymphoid follicles (Figure 12.25).

Based on our extensive experience of about 20 000 ileocolonoscopies in children, these techniques will allow an ileal intubation rate of 100% in the absence of strictures or significant inflammation of the ileocecal valve.

Withdrawing

The withdrawing phase of colonoscopy is the best for detailed assessment of the colonic mucosa as some stretching of the bowel during advancement of the colonoscope makes the circular folds more flat and easy to explore. It is useful for detection of small lesions such as sessile polyps.

Complications

Routine use of colonoscopy in children would be impossible without solid proof that the procedure is safe. This does not mean, however, that it is free from complications (Table 12.5). This issue should be fully disclosed and explained to the parents or legal guardian as part of informed consent.

Complications associated with colonoscopy in children can be classified according to:

- the need for hospitalization
- absence or presence of structural damage to the intestine and/or adjacent organs.

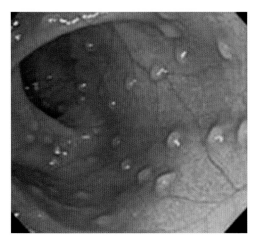

Figure 12.25 The terminal ileum. Velvety texture, yellowish tinge, and lymphoid follicles are the main endoscopic characteristics of the mucosa of the terminal ileum in children.

The incidence of minor complications is difficult to estimate. First, it is unlikely that all minor complications are going to be counted. Second, some complications are clinically silent: serosal tears and small mesenteric hematomas have been accidentally discovered during unrelated surgery soon after colonoscopy in adults.

The reported frequency of complications linked to pediatric colonoscopy (diagnostic and therapeutic combined) is under 0.8%, which is similar to the data from large-scale multicenter studies in adults. The most common adverse event related to diagnostic colonoscopy falls into the category of minor complications. Perforation is a rare complication associated with diagnostic colonoscopy. It can occur due to four reasons:

- excessive pressure created by forcefully advancing forward or withdrawing the shaft of a colonoscope
- embedding of the colonoscope into the bowel wall
- excessive air pressure
- inappropriate technique of polypectomy, hemostasis or balloon dilation of a benign stricture.

Three types of perforations related to diagnostic colonoscopy have been described. Shaft-induced perforations are the result of big loop formation. These are usually larger than expected and located on the antimesenteric

Table 12.5 Complications associated with pediatric colonoscopy

	Minor complications: no need for hospitalization	Major complications: requirement for hospitalization
Structural damage of the intestine or adjacent organs	Small, nonobstructing mucosal or submucosal hematomas, small mucosal lacerations, petechiae	Perforation Bleeding requiring blood transfusion and endoscopic or surgical hemostasis; post polypectomy syndrome
Absence of structural damage	Transient abdominal pain, bloating, abdominal distension resolving after passing gas, mild dehydration secondary to bowel preparation, transient hypoxia	Cardiovascular and respiratory distress, prolonged episode of hypoxia requiring resuscitation and/or endotracheal intubation

wall. Tip perforations are smaller and typically occur when the "sliding by" technique is used inappropriately, or a tip is embedded into mucosa when orientation is lost. Excessive air pressure perforation has been documented primarily with strictures of the left colon. Attempts to bypass the narrowed area create intermittent obstruction of the colon, accumulation of air in the upstream colon and increased hydrostatic pressure, which could reach a critical level of 81 mmHg for the cecum. This could explain the fact that most air pressure-related perforations have occurred in the cecum and even in the ileum after so-called uneventful colonoscopies. Hydrostatic perforations have not been described in children.

Most large traumatic perforations are immediately obvious. The presenting symptoms include a sudden onset of irreducible abdominal distention, decreased resistance to insertion of a colonoscope, failure to insufflate the collapsed colon, visible organs of the peritoneal cavity and severe and progressively increasing abdominal pain. Immediate discontinuation of the procedure and a request for plain abdominal films are mandatory. Closed perforations are less dramatic.

Almost 10% of patients with a perforated colon can initially be symptom free. In addition, another 10–15% may develop mild to moderate abdominal pain or discomfort. Absence of free air in the peritoneal cavity does not rule out perforation. High level of suspicion and careful postprocedure observation are important for early recognition of complications.

Persistent abdominal pain and/or low-grade fever should be considered as signs of perforation until proven otherwise. Early diagnosis in these circumstances is crucial to prevent or decrease morbidity and mortality associated with perforation of the colon.

Treatment of colonic perforation can be nonoperative or surgical. Patients with a well-prepared colon and therefore decreased risk of significant contamination of the peritoneal cavity, absence of peritonitis and who are oth-erwise stable can be treated medically with bowel rest, broad-spectrum antibiotics, and parenteral nutrition. Deterioration of a patient's condition, signs of peritoneal irritation, or suspicion of a large spillage of intestinal contents into the peritoneal cavity mandate surgical exploration. According to large-scale studies in adults, the frequency of colonic perforation after polypectomy is usually higher by two- or threefold. It results from excessive thermal coagulation of the tissue either due to an inappropriate power setting and current mode (more often when a "blended" mode is used), cutting a large sessile polyp more than 2 cm without a piecemeal technique, or accidental contact of the adjacent mucosa with the head of an excised polyp. These perforations are often small and subtle and cause late onset of abdominal pain a few hours after the procedure. Severity of pain usually increases with time. Fever is another common sign of deep tissue necrosis. The treatment of these complications (polypectomy syndrome) is similar to uncomplicated diverticulitis – aggressive treatment with broad-spectrum antibiotics, bowel rest, and good hydration.

Bleeding after diagnostic colonoscopy is quite rare and can be prevented by proper patient screening before the procedure, which should be focused on family history of bleeding diathesis, frequent nasal bleeding, oozing from gums after teeth brushing, and easy bruising without obvious trauma. A simple question about recent treatments with aspirin and/or NSAIDs is an effective way to prevent bleeding secondary to platelet dysfunction.

Bleeding disorders are not a contraindication to pediatric colonoscopy. Even patients with moderate to severe hemophilia could undergo successful colonoscopy with biopsy or polypectomy after special preparations have been made by a pediatric hematologist.

According to ASGE, colonoscopy and colonoscopic polypectomy are classified as low risk for bacteremia. In recent publications, transient bacteremia has been reported in less than 4% of patients after uneventful colonoscopy. The

100 | *Diagnostic Pediatric Endoscopy*

patients usually remain asymptomatic without requiring any medical treatment. If a patient becomes febrile, flat abdominal and cross-table films, blood culture and empirical treatment with broad-spectrum antibiotics are mandatory. Careful observation in a recovery room (until the child is fully awake and ready to leave), and next-day telephone follow-up should be a routine part of the postprocedure protocol.

Common pathology: rectal bleeding

Inflammatory bowel disease

The role of colonoscopy in patients with suspected or established inflammatory bowel disease is to define the extent of inflammation, obtain tissue samples, establish the specific diagnosis, and assess the efficacy of therapy and mucosal healing and screening for malignancy.

Common findings in children with untreated ulcerative colitis include continuous and circumferential mucosal inflammation with diffuse erythema, edema, increased mucosal friability, disappearance of vascular pattern, whitish-grayish exudate, erosions, or shallow ulcers (Figure 12.26).

Rectal involvement is universal. Inflammation can be restricted to the rectum and left colon or extend though the entire large intestine. A focal inflammation surrounding the appendiceal orifice's so-called "cecal patch" may co-exist with left-sided colitis (Figure 12.27). Signs of "back-washed" ileitis consist of diffuse mild to moderate erythema, edema and petechiae within 5–10 cm of the ileum adjacent to the ileocecal valve.

The hallmark of severe ulcerative colitis is striking edema and secondary narrowing of the colon and extreme friability of the rectal and colonic mucosa (Figure 12.28), making it reasonable to limit the procedure to proctoscopy and a few biopsies.

Deep ulcers are not typical for ulcerative colitis even with the severe form of the disease. A chronic and relapsing course of ulcerative colitis leads to unequal distribution of inflammation,

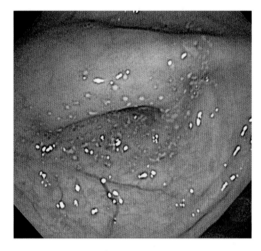

Figure 12.27 The "cecal patch": a focal inflammation of the appendiceal orifice with whitish dots – microabscesses – in a child with left-sided ulcerative colitis.

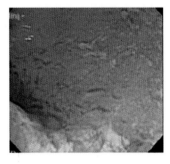
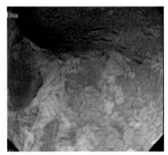
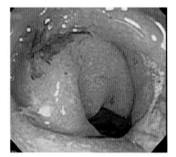

Figure 12.26 Ulcerative colitis. Diffuse inflammation is typical for ulcerative colitis: erythema, exudates, loss of vascular pattern.

(a)

(b)

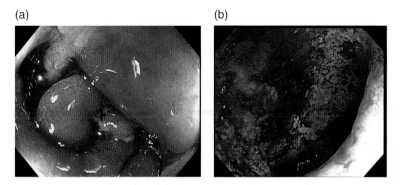

Figure 12.28 Severe form of ulcerative colitis. (a) Narrowing of the lumen due to severe edema. (b) Extreme friability.

(a)

(b)

(c)

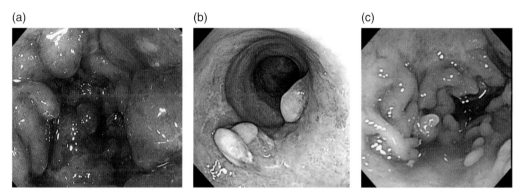

Figure 12.29 Multiple pseudopolyps. (a,b) Acute phase. (c) Endoscopic remission.

appearance of pseudopolyps, and attenuation of vascular pattern (Figure 12.29).

Colitis in patients with Crohn's disease is patchy with so-called "skip lesions" rather than being diffuse or uniform. It can be mild or intense and may involve the entire colon or just a part of it. Fifty percent of patients with Crohn's colitis have rectal sparing. At least half of children with Crohn's disease have ileocecal involvement.

Narrowing of the lumen, strictures, mucosal bridging and deep, longitudinal and aphthous ulcers are common findings in children with Crohn's disease (Figures 12.30–12.32).

Allergic proctocolitis

Allergic proctocolitis is characterized by inflammatory alterations of the colon and rectum, secondary to an immune reaction triggered by the ingestion of foreign proteins. The prevalence and natural history of allergic proctocolitis are unclear, although its frequency appears to be increasing even in infants who are exclusively breastfed. The most allergenic protein is mu-lactoglobulin. Clinical manifestations occur in the first weeks or months of life. The common symptoms are rectal bleeding frequently associated with diarrhea and mucus in stool. The endoscopic findings consist of patchy edema and erythema, nodular lymphoid hyperplasia and occasional erosions or superficial small ulcers. The most affected area is the sigmoid colon, although the rectum and descending colon could be involved (Figure 12.33).

It should be distinguished from isolated petechiae or small ulcerations in the sigmoid

(a) (b)

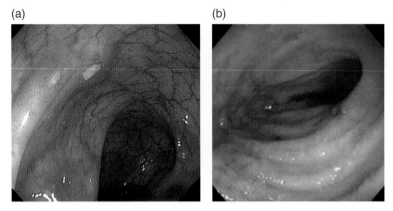

Figure 12.30 Aphthous ulcer. A small, 4–5 mm, shallow lesion with the rim of erythema. (a) Aphthoid ulcers of the colon. (b) Aphthous ulcers in the terminal ileum.

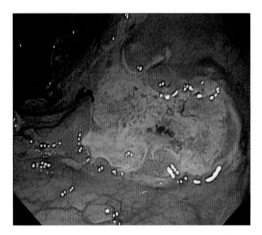

Figure 12.31 Deep longitudinal ulcers in a patient with Crohn's disease.

or descending colon induced by bowel preparation (Figure 12.34).

Pseudopolyps, juvenile polyps, and polyposis syndromes

Small lymphoid aggregates in the colon are common in infants and toddlers. They appear as light pink polypoid or umbilical-like lesions less than 3 mm (Figure 12.35). The rectum and sigmoid colon are the most involved.

Intestinal lymphoid hyperplasia of the terminal ileum is defined as presence of multiple lymphoid follicles more than 3 mm in size (Figure 12.36). It is a frequent finding in infants with abdominal pain and recurrent rectal bleeding due to food allergy or unrelated processes.

Occasionally, intestinal lymphoid hyperplasia can be the source of recurrent ileocolic intussusception (Figure 12.37).

Juvenile polyps are the most common type of polyps in children. They have distinctive cystic architecture, mucus-filled glands, prominent lamina propria, and dense infiltrations with inflammatory cells. They are most prevalent in children under 6 years of age. Recurrent painless rectal bleeding is a typical presenting symptom. Other manifestations include prolapsing rectal mass and an occasional presence of mucus in stool.

A typical juvenile polyp is a 1 cm pedunculated structure. Polyps less than 1 cm are usually sessile and have a raspberry or smooth-appearing "head" (Figure 12.38).

Although autoamputation occurs frequently, some polyps grow longer, reaching a significant size of up to 3 or even 4 cm. A large juvenile polyp is usually located in the sigmoid colon (Figure 12.39). In rare cases, it might be found in the descending or transverse colon (Figure 12.40). Such a polyp may induce intermittent pain due to colonic intussusceptions. The appearance of pale light yellow-speckled mucosa, a so-called chicken skin mucosa (Figure 12.41), should alert the endoscopist to an adjacent large juvenile polyp. The hallmark of "chicken skin" mucosa is an accumulation of lipid-laden macrophages in the lamina propria.

(a)   (b)

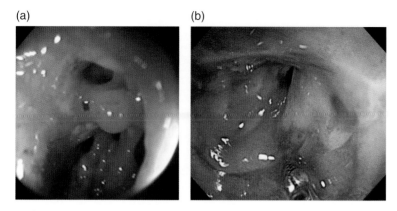

Figure 12.32 (a) Mucosal bridging. (b) Colonic stricture.

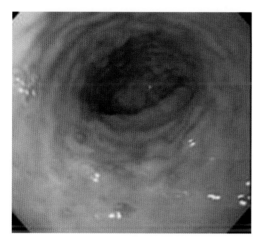

Figure 12.33 Allergic colitis. Multiple lymphoid follicles with rim of erythema: the "halo" sign and edema of the sigmoid colon.

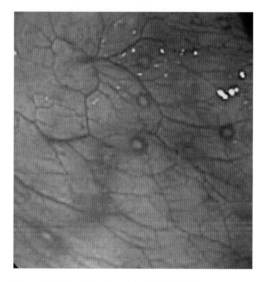

Figure 12.34 Small aphthoid-like lesions can occasionally be induced by bowel preparation.

The co-existence of juvenile polyps in both sites of the colon has been documented in at least one-third of children. For this reason, colonoscopy with polypectomy is the procedure of choice for children with recurrent painless rectal bleeding.

Rare pathology

Polyposis syndromes

Different types of hereditary polyposis syndromes can be revealed during a pediatric colonoscopy. Diagnostic criteria for juvenile polyposis include the presence of five or more juvenile polyps in the colon (Figure 12.42). Surveillance colonoscopy is indicated due to an increased risk of colon cancer.

Peutz–Jeghers syndrome

Peutz–Jeghers syndrome (PJS) is a unique form of hamartomatous polyposis associated with distinctive mucocutaneous pigmentation. It is caused by a germline mutation in the STK11 (LKB1) gene. The incidence of this condition is estimated to be between 1:50 000 to 1:200 000 live births. The polyps in patients with PJS display arborizing smooth muscle

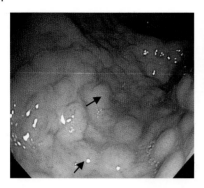 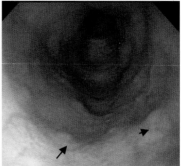

Figure 12.35 Numerous lymphoid follicles in the sigmoid colon.

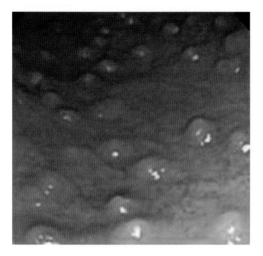

Figure 12.36 Multiple enlarged (more than 3 mm) lymphoid follicles in the terminal ileum is the sign of intestinal lymphoid hyperplasia, a nonspecific reaction of the intestinal immune system to various food or bacterial/viral antigens.

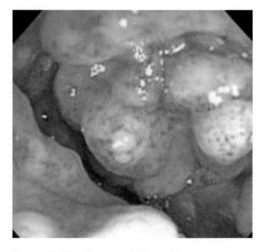

Figure 12.37 Six-year-old boy with recurrent ileocolonic intussusceptions. Intraoperative ileoscopy revealed highly enlarged (more than 4 mm) lymphoid follicles with multiple petechiae in the terminal ileum. Four-week treatment with oral prednisone was successful with complete resolution of lymphoid nodular hyperplasia and recurrent abdominal pain.

proliferation, distinguishing them from polyps in other forms of juvenile polyposis syndromes.

The diagnosis of PJS is based on the presence of one of the following clinical criteria: any number of hamartomatous polyps detected in an individual who has a family history of PJS in close relatives, characteristic mucocutaneous pigmentation in patients with close relatives diagnosed with PJS, and any number of polyps in individuals with characteristic mucocutaneous pigmentation.

Polyps occur more commonly in the small intestine. At least half of the patients have additional polyps in the colon and stomach. Polyps in children with PJS vary from a few millimeters to more than 5 cm. They are firmly anchored to the bowel wall by arborized smooth muscle bundles, preventing spontaneous amputation and predisposing to small bowel intussusception. Surveillance protocols in PJS target two goals: detection and removal of sizeable polyps preventing intussusception and detection of cancers at an early stage.

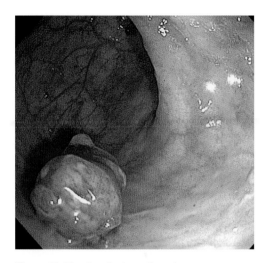

Figure 12.38 Sessile juvenile polyp.

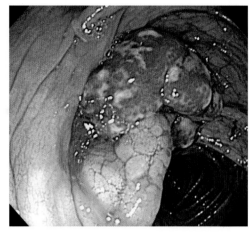

Figure 12.40 Large juvenile polyp in the descending colon.

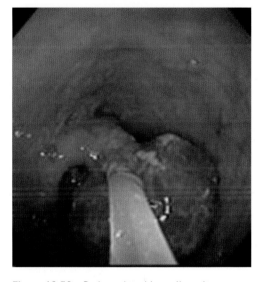

Figure 12.39 Pedunculated juvenile polyp.

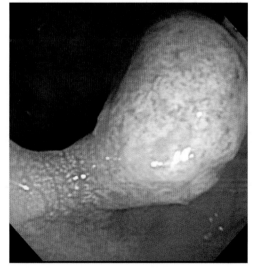

Figure 12.41 The "chicken skin" sign. The mucosa around a large juvenile polyp has a specific pattern induced by lipid-loaded macrophages.

A baseline EGD, colonoscopy and capsule endoscopy is indicated at the onset of clinical manifestation or at 8 years of age in asymptomatic children. All significant polyps (1 cm or bigger) should be removed. Children with significant polyps should be scheduled for a surveillance endoscopy every three years or sooner if symptoms occur. Double balloon enteroscopy is the procedure of choice for treatment of symptomatic children with small bowel hamartomas.

Familial adenomatous polyposis

Familial adenomatous polyposis (FAP) is a group of hereditary polyposis syndromes including autosomal dominant forms: familial adenomatous polyposis, attenuated familial adenomatous polyposis (AFAP), and autosomal recessive MYH-associated polyposis (MAP). Germline mutations of the adenomatous polyposis coli (APC) gene are present in

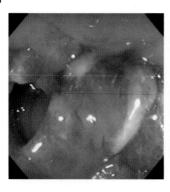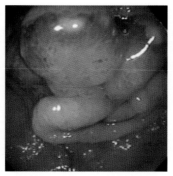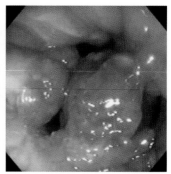

Figure 12.42 Juvenile polyposis. Multiple juvenile polyps in the rectum and the colon.

60–80% of classic FAP and 10–30% of AFAP patients. Mutations of the base excision repair (MYH) gene are likely to account for about 10%, 20%, and 25% of individuals with FAP, AFAP, and MAP respectively.

Mutations associated with classic FAP inevitably lead to colorectal cancer before the age of 39 in affected individuals without colectomy.

There is some correlation between specific mutation and clinical phenotype. Mutations between APC codons 1250 and 1464 cause severe polyposis, generally with >5000 polyps, and the recurrent codon 1309 mutation is associated with early onset and development of thousands of polyps.

Mutations linked with AFPC are responsible for different phenotypes as well: a late onset of polyps and cancer, a smaller number of polyps (less than 100; average 30), and predisposition toward involvement of the proximal colon and extracolonic manifestations.

Most children with FAP do not have any gastrointestinal manifestation of polyposis. The exception is a group of young children without a family history of FAP who tend to have an earlier onset of hematochezia. In this scenario, colonoscopy should not be delayed. Once the diagnosis of FAP is confirmed, upper GI endoscopy is reasonable for early detection of adenomatous polyps in the duodenum.

The main endoscopic feature of FPC in children is usually dozens or hundreds of small sessile polyps (Figure 12.43).

Multiple biopsies and polypectomies of the largest polyps are essential for diagnosis of adenomatous polyps and low- or high-grade dysplasia.

Genetic testing and surveillance sigmoidoscopy for asymptomatic children with family history of FAP usually begin between 11 and 15 years of age. Once the patient is diagnosed with FAP, prophylactic colectomy should be planned. According to recommendations of the American Society of Colon and Rectal Surgeons, for patients with mild disease and low cancer risk, prophylactic colectomy can be done in the mid-teens (15–18 years). When severe disease is found or if the patient is symptomatic, surgery is performed as soon as convenient after diagnosis.

Colon cancer

Sporadic adenocarcinoma of the colon in children is extremely rare. The presenting symptoms include progressive weight loss, changes of bowel habits, fatigue, anemia, and intermittent rectal bleeding. Despite the warning signs, the diagnosis is typically delayed by a few months due to a low level of suspicion. Tumors are equally distributed between the left and right colon. During colonoscopy, adenocarcinomas appear as discolored masses (Figure 12.44). It is quite difficult to examine the entire lesion due to an almost complete obstruction of the intestinal lumen and severe edema of surrounding tissue. Usually, the

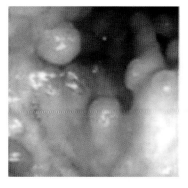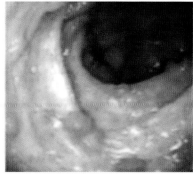

Figure 12.43 Multiple colon polyps in a 5-year-old boy with FAP.

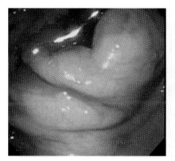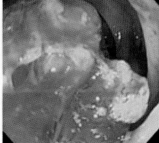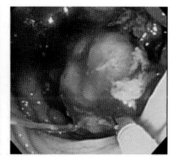

Figure 12.44 Adenocarcinoma of the right colon in an 11-year-old boy with significant weight loss, anemia, and ascites. Colonoscopy revealed severe edema of the distal part of the ascending colon. Further exploration of the ascending colon showed an ulcerated large tumor. The biopsy confirmed the diagnosis of mucinous adenocarcinoma.

tumor edge is firm and easily fragmented during biopsy. Most tumors are mucinous adenocarcinomas.

Adenocarcinoma of the colon in ulcerative colitis

The determining factor of malignancy in patients with ulcerative colitis seems to be the severity of the original disease as well as the extent of mucosal involvement and duration of colitis.

The cancer risk for patients with pancolitis is 3% in the first decade of disease and 1–2% per year thereafter. Patients with pancolitis should begin bi-yearly colonoscopies, 10 years after the onset of the disease. Multiple biopsies taken at intervals of a few centimeters of each other are recommended. Any flat or elevated lesions should be additional targets. Chromoendoscopy has been found useful to increase the yield of finding high-grade dysplasia in adults. More recently, confocal endomicroscopy has allowed greater accuracy in biopsy targeting.

Non-Hodgkin's lymphoma of the terminal ileum

Non-Hodgkin's lymphoma of the terminal ileum can be discovered during colonoscopy in children with intermittent abdominal pain and weight loss. Pain is usually a result of ileocolonic intussusception. During colonoscopy, irregular masses occupying the intestinal lumen may be found in the cecum or ascending colon (Figure 12.45). Care should be taken to avoid deep embedding of the forceps into

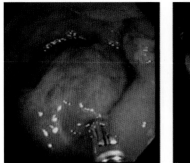 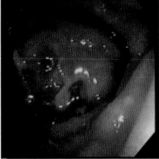 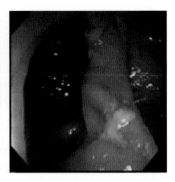

Figure 12.45 Non-Hodgkin's lymphoma of the ileum. The indications for a colonoscopy were intermittent severe right low quadrant pain, weight loss, and anemia. The intussusception was found in the descending colon. It was gently reduced after the tissue samples were cautiously obtained.

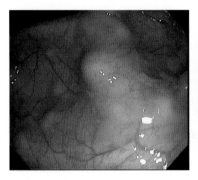 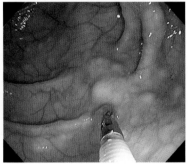

Figure 12.46 Langerhans cell histiocytosis of the colon: multiple yellowish sessile polypoid lesions in the colon.

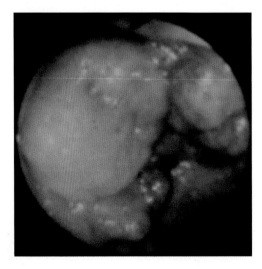 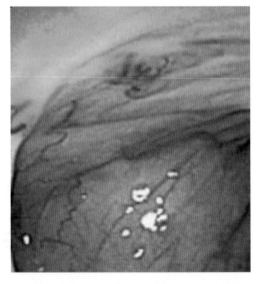

Figure 12.47 Large hemangioma of the sigmoid colon in a 3-year-old girl with recurrent episodes of low GI bleeding.

Figure 12.48 Angiodysplasia of the colon in a child with recurrent low GI bleeding. Tortuous, engorged small vessels are quite different from the normal colonic vasculature on the background of the image.

the tumor in order to prevent peeling of a large tissue fragment. Proper fixative solution is important for correct morphological and cytogenetic diagnosis.

Isolated Langerhans cell histiocytosis of the colon

Well-documented colon involvement in Langerhans cell histiocytosis is very rare. Initial symptoms are not specific and may include

diarrhea, sometimes with blood or mucus, malabsorption, failure to thrive, and edema secondary to protein-losing enteropathy. Colonoscopy may reveal yellowish sessile polypoid lesions throughout the colon or rectum (Figure 12.46).

Vascular malformation of the colon

Vascular malformation of the gastrointestinal tract is a rare finding in children. Three types of vascular malformation of the colon have been described in children: hemangiomas (Figure 12.47), angiodysplasia (Figure 12.48) and congenital/idiopathic colonic varices (Figures 12.49 and 12.50). The hallmark of these lesions is lower GI bleeding, which could be life-threatening. Angiodyplastic lesions in children have a predisposition to the left side of the colon and rectum. Endoscopic hemostasis of bleeding angiodysplasis can be achieved using argon plasma coagulation.

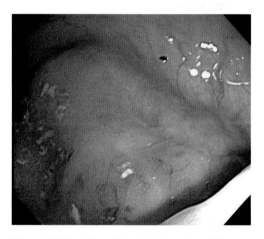

Figure 12.49 Idiopathic colonic varices of the right colon in a 9-year-old boy with recurrent low GI bleeding.

 • See companion website for videos relating to this chapter topic: www.wiley.com/go/gershman3e

(a) (b) (c)

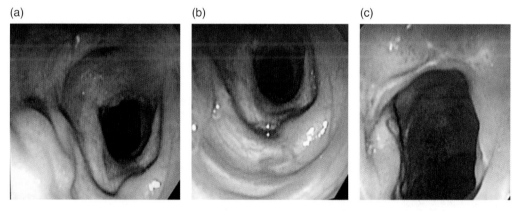

Figure 12.50 Congenital colonic varices in a 3-week-old baby with hematochezia and severe anemia. (a,b) Panoramic and close-up view of the colonic varices. (c) Ischemic ulcers at the site of the varices.

FURTHER READING

Adamiak T, Altaf M, Jensen MK, *et al.* One-day bowel preparation with polyethylene glycol 3350: an effective regimen for colonoscopy in children. *Gastrointest Endosc* 2010, **71**(3), 573–577.

Ament ME, Gershman G. Pediatric colonoscopy. In: Waye JD, Rex DK, Williams CB, *et al.* (eds). *Colonoscopy: Principles and Practice.* Blackwell Publishing, Oxford, 2003, pp. 624–629.

Arain Z, Rossi TM. Gastrointestinal bleeding in children: an overview of conditions requiring non-operative management. *Semin Pediatr Surg* 1999, **8**, 172–180.

ASGE Technology Committee, Barth BA, Banerjee S, Bhat YM, *et al.* Equipment for pediatric endoscopy. *Gastrointest Endosc* 2012, **76**(1), 8–17.

Begs AD, Latchford AR, Vase HFA, *et al.* Peutz–Jeghers syndrome: a symptomatic review and recommendations for management. *Gut* 2010, **59**, 975–986.

Berger T, Classen M, Engelgardt H, *et al.* Bowel preparation in pediatric colonoscopy: results of an open observational study. *Endosc Int Open* 2016, **4**, E 820–827.

Berkelhammer C, Caed D, Mesleh G, *et al.* Ileo-cecal intussusception of small-bowel lymphoma: diagnosis by colonoscopy. *J Clin Gastroenterol* 1997, **25**, 358–361.

Bousvaros A, Antonioli DA, Coletti RB, *et al.* Differentiating ulcerative colitis from Crohn's disease in children and young adults: report of a working group of the North American Society for Pediatric Gastroenterology, Hepatology, and Nutrition and the Crohn's and Colitis Foundation of America. *J Pediatr Gastroenterol Nutr* 2007, **44**, 653–674.

Cotton PB, Williams RH, *et al.* (2014) *Practical Gastrointestinal Endoscopy. The Fundamentals*, 7th edn. Wiley Blackwell, Oxford, pp. 78–152.

De La Torre L, Carrasco D, Nora MA, *et al.* Vascular malformations of the colon in children. *J Pediatr Surg* 2002, **37**, 1177–1200.

Di Nardo, G, Aloi M, Cucchiara S, *et al.* Bowel preparations for colonoscopy: an RCT. *Pediatrics* 2014, **134**(2), 249–256.

Durno CA. Colonic polyps in children and adolescents. *Can J Gastroenterol* 2007, **21**, 233–239.

Elitsur Y, Teitelbaum LE, Rewalt M, *et al.* Clinical and endoscopic data in juvenile polyposis syndrome in preadolescent children. *J Clin Gastroenterol* 2009, **43**, 734–736.

Farley DR, Bannon MP, Scott PZ, *et al.* Management of colonoscopic perforations. *Mayo Clin Proc* 1997, **72**, 729–733.

Garbay JR, Suc B, Rotman N, *et al.* Multicenter study of surgical complications of colonoscopy. *Br J Surg* 1996, **83**, 42–44.

Goldin E, Libson E. Intussusception in intestinal lymphoma: the role of colonoscopy. *Postgrad Med J* 1986, **62**, 1139–1140.

Gordon M, Karlsen F, Isaji S, *et al.* Bowel preparation for elective procedures in children: a systematic review and meta-analysis. *BMJ Paediatr Open* 2017, **1**, e000118.

Gupta SK, Fitzgerald JF, Croffie JM, *et al.* Experience with juvenile polyps in North American children: the need for pancolonoscopy. *Am J Gastroenterol* 2001, **96**, 1695–1697.

Haens GD, Rutgeerts P. Endoscopy of inflammatory bowel diseases. In: Waye JD, Rex DK, Williams CB (eds). *Colonoscopy. Principles and Practice*. Blackwell Publishing, Oxford, 2003, pp. 573–581.

Hill DA, Furman WL, Billups CA, *et al.* Colorectal carcinoma in childhood: a clinico-pathological review. *J Clin Oncol* 2007, **25**, 5808–5814.

Hoppin A. Other neoplasms. In: Walker WA, Durie PB, Hamilton JR, *et al.* (eds). *Pediatric Gastrointestinal Disease: Pathophysiology, Diagnosis and Management*, 3rd edn. BC Decker, Hamilton, Ontario, 2000, pp. 810–820.

Huang SC, Erdman SH. Pediatric juvenile polyposis syndromes: an update. *Curr Gastroenterol Rep* 2009, **11**, 211–219.

Hyar W, Neale K, Fell J, *et al.* At what age should routine screening start in children at risk of familial adenomatous polyposis? *J Pediatr Gastroenterol Nutr* 2003, **31**(Suppl 2**)**, 135.

Iacono G, Ravello A, Di Prima L, *et al.* Colonic lymphoid nodular hyperplasia in children: relationship to food hypersensitivity. *Clin Gastroenterol Hepatol* 2007, **5**, 361–366.

Iqbal CW, Askegard-Giesmann JR, Pham TH, *et al.* Pediatric endoscopic injuries: incidence, management, and outcomes. *J Pediatr Surg* 2008, **43**, 911–915.

Iqbal CW, Chun YS, Farley, DR. Colonoscopic perforations: a retrospective review. *J Gastrointest Surg* 2005, **9**, 1229–1236.

Jerkis S, Rosewich H, Scharf JG, *et al.* Colorectal cancer in two pre-teenage siblings with familial adenomatous polyposis. *Eur J Pediatr* 2005, **1**, 306–310.

Ker TS, Wasseberg N, Bear, RW Jr. Colonoscopic perforation and bleeding of the colon can be treated safely without surgery. *Am J Surg* 2004, **70**, 922–944.

Kokkonen J, Kartunen TJ. Lymphonodular hyperplasia on the mucosa of the lower gastrointestinal tract in children: an indication of enhanced immune response? *J Pediatr Gastroenterol Nutr* 2002, **34**, 42–46.

Kravarusic D, Feigin E, Dlugy E, *et al.* Colorectal carcinoma in childhood: a retrospective multicenter study. *J Pediatr Gastroenterol Nutr* 2007, **44**, 209–211.

Lightdale JR, Acosta R, Shergill AR, *et al.* Modifications in endoscopic practice for pediatric patients. *Gastrointest Endosc* 2014, **79**(5), 699–710.

Mahajan L, Wyllei R, Steffen R, *et al.* The effects of psychological preparation program on anxiety in children and adolescents undergoing gastrointestinal endoscopy. *J Pediatr Gastroenterol Nutr* 1998, **27**(2), 161–165.

Nanduri VR, Kelly K, Malone MM, *et al.* Colon involvement in colon Langerhans' cell histiocytosis. *J Pediatr Gastroenterol Nutr* 1999, **29**(4), 462–466.

Nieuwenhuis MH, Matus-Vliegen LM, Slors FJ, *et al.* Genotype-phenotype correlations as a guide in management of familial adenomatous polyposis. *Clin Gastroenterol Hepatol* 2007, **5**, 374–378.

Pall H, Zacur GM, Kramer RE, *et al.* Bowel preparation for pediatric colonoscopy: report of the NASPGHAN Endoscopy and Procedures Committee. *J Pediatr Gastroenterol Nutr* 2014, **59**(3), 409–416.

Pashankar DS, Uc A, Bishop WB. Polyethylene glycol 3350 without electrolytes: a new safe, effective and palatable bowel preparation for colonoscopy in children. *J Pediatr* 2004, **144**, 358–362.

Radhakrishnan CN, Bruce J. Colorectal cancer in children without any predisposing factors. A report of eight cases and review of the literature. *Eur J Pediatr Surg* 2003, **13**, 66–68.

Ravelli A, Villanacci V, Chiappa S, *et al.* Dietary protein-induced proctocolitis in childhood. *Am J Gastroenterol* 2008, **103**, 2605–2612.

Riddhiputra P, Ukarapol N. Effect of systematic psychological preparation using visual illustration prior to gastrointestinal endoscopy on the anxiety of both pediatric patients and parents. *J Med Assoc Thai* 2006, **89**(2), 231–235.

Safder S, Demintieva Y, Rewalt M, *et al.* Stool consistency and stool frequency are excellent clinical markers for adequate colon preparation after polyethylene glycol 3350 cleaning protocol: a prospective clinical study in children. *Gastrointest Endosc* 2008, **68**, 1131–1135.

Saoul R, Wolff R, Seligman H, *et al.* Symptoms of hyperphosphotemia, hypocalcemia, and hypomagnesemia in an adolescent after the oral administration of sodium phosphate in preparation for a colonoscopy. *Gastrointest Endosc* 2001, **53**, 650–652.

Singh HK, Withers GD, Ee LC. Quality indicators in pediatric colonoscopy: an Australian tertiary center experience. *Scand J Gastroenterol* 2017, **52**(12), 1453–1456.

Snyder J, Bratton B. Antimicrobial prophylaxis for gastrointestinal procedures: current practice in North American academic pediatric programs. *J Pediatr Gastroenterol Nutr* 2002, **35**, 564–569.

Snyder WH. The embryology of alimentary tract with special emphasis on the colon and rectum. In: Turell R (ed.). *Diseases of Colon and Anorectum*, vol **1**, 2nd edn. WB Saunders, Philadelphia, PA, 1969, pp. 3–19.

Tanaka K, Oikawa N, Terao R, *et al.* Evaluations of psychological preparation for children undergoing endoscopy. *J Pediatr Gastroenterol Nutr* 2011, **52**, 227–229.

Thakkar K, Holub JL, Gilger MA, et al. Quality indicators for pediatric colonoscopy: results from a multicenter consortium. *Gastrointest Endosc* 2016, **83**(3), 533–541.

Thomson M, Murphy MS. In: Winter HS, Murphy MS, Mougenot JF, *et al.* (eds). *Pediatric Gastrointestinal Endoscopy*. BC Decker, Hamilton, Ontario, 2006, pp. 81–91.

Troncone R, Descepolo V. Colon and food allergy. *J Pediatr Gastroenterol Nutr* 2009, **48**(Suppl 2), s89–s91.

Turner D, Levin A, Weiss B, *et al.* Evidence-based recommendations for bowel cleansing before colonoscopy in children: a report from a national working group. *Endoscopy* 2010, **42**, 1063–1070.

Valentin J (ed.). Alimentary system. In: *Annals of the ICRP: Basic Anatomical and Physiological Data for Use in Radiological Protection, Reference Values*. Pergamon, Oxford, 2003, pp. 109–117.

Vastyan AM, Walker J, Pinter AB, *et al.* Colorectal carcinoma in children and adolescents – a report of seven cases. *Eur J Surg* 2001, **11**, 338–341.

Vasudevan SA, Patel JC, Wesson DE, *et al.* Severe dysplasia in children with familial adenomatous polyposis: rare or simply overlooked? *J Pediatr Surg* 2006, **41**, 658–661.

Vejzovic V, Wennick A, Idvall E, *et al.* Polyethylene glycol- or sodium picosulphate-based laxatives before colonoscopy in children. *J Pediatr Gastroenterol Nutr* 2016, **62**, 414–419.

Weaver LT. Anatomy and embryology. In: Walker WA, Durie PB, Hamilton JR, *et al.* (eds). *Pediatric Gastrointestinal Disease: Pathophysiology, Diagnosis, and Management*. Mosby, St Louis, MO, 1992, pp. 195–216.

Williams C, Nicholls S. Endoscopic features of chronic inflammatory bowel disease in childhood. *Baillière's Clin Gastroenterol* 1994, **8**, 121–131.

Xanthakov SA, Schwimmer JB, Melin-Aldana H, *et al.* Prevalence and outcome of allergic colitis in healthy infants with rectal bleeding: a prospective cohort study. *J Pediatr Gastroenterol Nutr* 2005, **41**, 16–22.

Yoshioka S, Takedatsu H, Fukunaga S, *et al.* Study to determine guidelines for pediatric colonoscopy. *World J Gastroenterol* 2017, **23**(31), 5773–5779.

Zuckerman MJ, Shen B, Edwyn Harrison III M, *et al.* Informed consent for GI endoscopy. *Gastrointest Endosc* 2007, **66**(2), 213–218.

13

Handling of specimens and orientation of biopsies

Marta C. Cohen and Paul Arnold

 KEY POINTS

- Careful handling of specimens is important in the endoscopy unit.
- Orientation of small intestinal biopsies on a mesh or card is helpful immediately after they have been taken before being placed in formalin.

- Accurate labeling of specimens and good communication between endoscopist and histopathologist are key.
- Occasionally, specimens will be placed in other media, e.g., saline for disaccharidase activity analysis, glutaraldehyde for electronmicroscopy or viral culture medium.

Introduction

Biopsies are frequently obtained during endoscopic investigation of esophageal and gastrointestinal (GIT) lesions and inflammatory conditions [1]. The histopathology laboratory will receive numerous small biopsies from multiple sites of each individual patient. Precise interpretation of endoscopic esophageal and gastrointestinal biopsies requires proper handling and processing of the specimens. In addition, a requirement for any valid histological interpretation is good communication between the endoscopist and the pathologist [2].

Specimen handling in the endoscopy unit

The appropriate handling of the specimen starts in the endoscopy unit, as the endoscopist should handle the tissue with care, gently removing it from the biopsy forceps [3]. In some institutions, the specimen is orientated before being placed flat on a supportive mesh, such as filter paper [3]. Whether the specimen is orientated or not, the biopsy should be fixed in 10% buffered formalin or equivalent fixative method. Buffered formalin achieves excellent tissue fixation, allowing for good-quality staining with routine histological methods (e.g., hematoxylin and eosin, immunohistochemistry, Gram, Giemsa, etc.) as well as achieving good results in molecular tests (such as fluorescence in situ hybridization [FISH] or polymerase chain reaction [PCR]). The container should have the appropriate volume of fixative to minimize tissue desiccation and preserve tissue architecture [4].

It is of paramount importance to accurately label each specimen with the patient identification data and the site of the biopsy. The

---

Practical Pediatric Gastrointestinal Endoscopy, Third Edition. Edited by George Gershman and Mike Thomson.
© 2021 John Wiley & Sons Ltd. Published 2021 by John Wiley & Sons Ltd.
Companion website: www.wiley.com/go/gershman3e

endoscopist should ensure that a separate container is used for biopsies taken from different sites so that the precise location of each biopsy can be properly identified [5]. In addition, a pathology request form containing any pertinent clinical information should be supplied with the samples [6].

In some cases, the suspected clinical diagnosis will require confirmation with electron microscopy. As the processing of these specimens is different from that of routine histology, in these circumstances a tissue sample should be fixed in glutaraldehyde and submitted to the pathology laboratory, highlighting the specific request for electron microscopy.

Specimen handling in the histopathology laboratory

Once the specimens are received in the histopathology laboratory, the case is registered and provided with a unique identification number.

Macroscopic description

The description of each sample should include the number of tissue fragments received, the color (white, tan, yellow or red) and a three-dimensional measurement of each fragment. All samples are transferred directly into cassettes (single or multiwelled) for processing [5]. Each cassette is labeled with the corresponding pathology identifying number and suffix.

To prevent tissue loss during processing, specimens should be placed in small, mini-biopsy cassettes or alternatively wrapped in biowrap paper.

Processing, embedding, and microtomy

Unfixed specimens cannot be directly infiltrated with paraffin. First, the water from the tissues must be removed by dehydration using increasing concentrations of alcohol.

The endoscopic biopsies may be processed and embedded either as individual samples or, more usually, combined into one multicassette. The use of a multicassette is not only cost-effective but it also speeds up reporting time by the consultants (Figure 13.1).

All tissues should be orientated and embedded in a way that will facilitate optimal microtomy. GIT biopsies should be embedded on edge so that the mucosal surface is on one side (Figure 13.2).

(a)

(b)

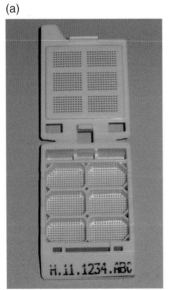
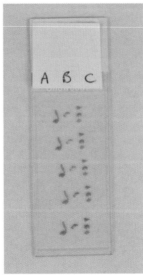

Figure 13.1 (a) GIT biopsies embedded in multicassettes (e.g., ABC). The macroscopic description should indicate which sample corresponds to which suffix. (b) Once mounted on the slide, the sample with the earliest suffix is located on the left-hand side of the slide when the frosted end is uppermost.

(a) (b)

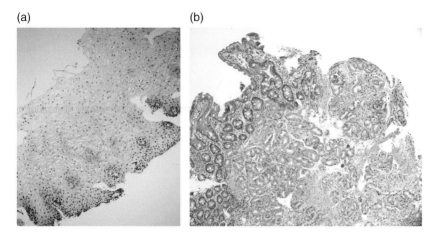

Figure 13.2 (a) Gastrointestinal sample embedded on edge, rendering a good view of the esophageal mucosa (H&E ×10). (b) Distorted short villi in D1 due to tangential orientation of the sample (H&E ×10).

If the endoscopy is described as "normal" on the accompanying request form, all blocks are trimmed to full face and a single slide of five serial 4μ sections produced per block. If the endoscopy is described as "abnormal" a specific approach is taken. For example, if clinical details suggest celiac disease, 50 serial sections are cut from all biopsy samples taken from the duodenum. These sections are picked up across 10 slides. Slides 1, 5, and10 are stained and the rest stored as unstained spares. If there is any doubt, the biomedical scientist (histotechnician) should seek advice from the pathologist.

The mucosa must be sectioned perpendicular to its long axis [3]. As the specimen will naturally curl, some tangential section during microtomy can be expected. This may be especially relevant in samples from the small bowel, as the villi can artefactually appear short and broad, with a multilayered surface epithelium and an expanded lamina propria [3] (Figure 13.2b).

The adequate handling and processing of endoscopic biopsies for histological assessment depend on the necessary steps being taken by the endoscopist, pathologists, and

Table 13.1 Artefacts related to biopsy trauma and specimen processing in endoscopic samples [3,7]

Biopsy trauma during sampling	Specimen handling in the laboratory
Tissue fragmentation	Pale staining due to poor fixation
Crushing artefact with condensation of lymphoplasmacytic cells	Tangential (oblique) orientation of the mucosa
Denudation of epithelium	Tissue curling during microtomy
Separation of surface epithelium from the underlying lamina propria	Multilayered surface and/or glandular epithelium
Hemorrhage in lamina propria	Air bubbles between the tissue and the coverslip
Edema of lamina propria	Contaminants ("floaters") from another biopsy specimen
	Shrinkage during fixation
	Formalin pigment in the section

biomedical scientists for reducing tissue trauma and processing artefacts. These artefacts may not produce any clinically significant harm, but they can create potential diagnostic problems for the pathologist during histopathological examination. Conversely, the resulting artefacts may indeed interfere with diagnosis and lead to an error with clinical consequences [7]. Artefacts related to biopsy trauma and specimen handling are listed in Table 13.1.

 • See companion website for videos relating to this chapter topic: www.wiley.com/go/gershman3e

REFERENCES

1 Lester SC. Small biopsies. In: *Manual of Surgical Pathology*. Saunders Elsevier, Philadelphia, PA, 2010, pp. 243–245.

2 Guinee DG Jr, Lee RG. Laboratory methods for processing and interpretation of endoscopic gastrointestinal biopsies. *Lab Med* 1990, **21**, 13–16.

3 Mills SE. Section VII: Alimentary Tract. In: *Histology for Pathologists*, 3rd edn. Lippincott Williams & Wilkins. Philadelphia, PA, 2007, pp. 563–760.

4 American Society for Gastrointestinal Endoscopy. Endoscopic mucosal tissue sampling. *Gastrointest Endosc* 2013, **78**, 216–224.

5 Ibrahin NB. Guidelines for handling oesophageal biopsies and resection specimens and their reporting. *J Clin Pathol* 2000, **53**, 89–94.

6 Royal College of Pathologists of Australasia. Gastrointestinal endoscopic biopsy. Macroscopic cut up manual. www.rcpa. edu.au/

7 Rastogi V, Puri N, Arora S, *et al*. Artefacts: a diagnostic dilemma – a review. *J Clin Diagn Res* 2013, **7**, 2408–2413.

14

Enteroscopy

Mike Thomson and Arun Urs

 KEY POINTS

- The techniques of Sonde or push enteroscopy have now been superseded.
- Enteroscopy complements wireless capsule endoscopy and both should be available in any unit with pretensions towards becoming a small bowel investigation center.
- Single-balloon enteroscopy does not allow the operator to advance as far beyond the pylorus or in the retrograde maneuver proximal to the ileocecal valve as double-balloon enteroscopy (DBE).
- DBE is the procedure of choice, is safe with CO_2 insufflation, and has occurred many times in children to date with no adverse events reported, and allows endotherapeutic proce-
dures of any nature to occur throughout the small bowel.
- Tattooing lesions, or tattooing the most distal part of the small bowel reached in an antegrade fashion, allows subsequent identification of the lesion by a surgeon at laparoscopy, or identification of full small bowel visualization when the retrograde transanal procedure is performed, respectively.
- Spiral enteroscopy is an emerging technology that may be helpful in enteroscopy up to 150 cm beyond the pylorus and has the advantage of allowing the operator a static platform in the small bowel from which to perform endotherapeutic procedures.

Introduction

The advent of flexible fiberoptic endoscopes transformed the diagnosis and management of gastrointestinal disorders in adults and children, allowing direct visualization with targeted mucosal biopsies. Furthermore, endotherapeutic procedures are now possible throughout the upper GI tract and ileocolon. However, the small bowel, distal to the ligament of Trietz and proximal to the terminal ileum, has to date been inaccessible to conventional GI endoscopes.

The Sonde type enteroscope, developed in the 1970s, involved the introduction of a long thin fiberoscope, with an inflatable balloon attached to its distal tip, through the nose into the stomach. The fiberoscope was guided into the duodenum by a gastroscope and the balloon attached to the tip of the fiberoscope was inflated. Normal peristalsis ensured the movement of the fiberoscope down the small bowel and theoretical visualization of the entire small bowel. However, the procedure itself was cumbersome and limited by lack of therapeutic potential.

Practical Pediatric Gastrointestinal Endoscopy, Third Edition. Edited by George Gershman and Mike Thomson.
© 2021 John Wiley & Sons Ltd. Published 2021 by John Wiley & Sons Ltd.
Companion website: www.wiley.com/go/gershman3e

Push enteroscopy, introduced in the 1990s, allowed access to the proximal small bowel beyond the ligament of Trietz. This was improvised by the addition of a semirigid overtube which made it possible to reach up to 70–100 cm of small bowel beyond the pylorus. In addition to diagnosis, endotherapy became achievable with push enteroscopy, although limited to the jejunum. The indications in adults for push enteroscopy included overt and occult GI bleeding, iron deficiency anemia abdominal pain, Crohn's disease, percutaneous endoscopic jejunostomy (PEJ) placement, and ERCP (Billroth type II). Push enteroscopy has been evaluated extensively in adults with a diagnostic yield of 41–75%. There is one report of its use in children.

Nevertheless, the diagnosis of small bowel disease beyond the proximal jejunum still remained a challenge, never mind proximal to the distal ileum. Intraoperative enteroscopy technique was developed needing an operative colotomy or enterotomy through which the endoscope was passed to visualize the small bowel. This had a very good diagnostic yield but carried a high complication rate. This technique was further refined by performing an initial upper GI endoscopy and a subsequent colonoscopy, and the surgeon manually threaded the small bowel over the tip of the endoscope, thus avoiding an enterotomy, with the advent of laparoscopic assistance. Intraoperative laparoscopy-assisted push enteroscopy offers an advantage in that the whole of the small bowel may be examined endoluminally. However, of course, this involves handling of the bowel, and the need for both a surgeon and an endoscopist.

Wireless capsule endoscopy (WCE) was the next major advance in the diagnostic assessment of the mid-small bowel. WCE made it possible to visualize the entire small bowel. The main advantage has been the relative noninvasiveness of this procedure with good diagnostic yield. WCE has been found to be superior to push enteroscopy in the diagnosis of obscure GI bleeding in adults.

However, the major limitations of WCE have been the inability to perform air insufflations, rinsing of tissue, taking biopsies or undertaking endotherapeutic procedures, and thus its major utility is limited to diagnostic input alone, at least so far. Complications, although rare, do exist and are mainly in the form of capsule retention that requires surgical intervention; however, the need for removal is extraordinarily rare.

In 2001, Yamamoto *et al.* reported a new method where two balloons were used, one at the tip and the other at the distal end of an overtube, to perform total enteroscopy without the need for laparotomy. Double-balloon enteroscopy (DBE) was thus born. DBE enables high-resolution endoscopic imaging of the entire small bowel, with the advantage over WCE of potential for mucosal biopsies and interventional endotherapy (e.g., nonvariceal hemostasis, snare polypectomy, and pneumatic balloon stricture dilation).

Double-balloon enteroscopy technique

The pediatric DBE system (Fujinon Inc., Japan) (Figure 14.1) consists of a high-resolution video enteroscope (EN-450P5/20) with a flexible overtube (TS-12140). The video enteroscope has a working length of 200 cm and an

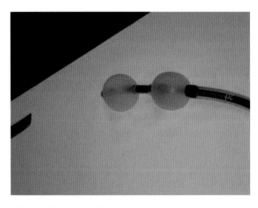

Figure 14.1 Double-balloon enteroscope system configuration.

outer diameter of 8.5 mm while the flexible overtube has a length of 140 cm and outer diameter of 12 mm. The enteroscopes either have a 2.2 mm ("P" scope) or a 2.8 mm ("T" scope) forceps channel that enables routine biopsy, and the latter allows other common therapeutic interventions. The enteroscope and the overtube are fitted with a balloon each at the tip. The overtube and balloons are disposable. The balloons can be inflated and deflated with air from a pressure-controlled pump system with maximum inflatable pressure of 60 mmHg. Since the inflation of balloons is pressure-controlled, they can be used safely, regardless of the diameter of the small bowel. The balloons help to anchor the scope and/or the overtube and stabilize the intestinal wall. This enables the further advance of the scope. The overtube prevents bending or looping of the intestine.

Both balloons are deflated at the start of the procedure. On reaching the distal duodenum or preferably jejunum, the overtube balloon is inflated to fix and stabilize the overtube within the lumen. Subsequently, the enteroscope is advanced as far as possible. Then the enteroscope tip balloon is inflated and the overtube balloon is deflated. The overtube is now advanced to reach the enteroscope tip. The overtube is again inflated and both enteroscope and overtube are gently withdrawn together in order to "concertina" the small bowel over both. The whole procedure is repeated and each set of maneuvers (or "passes") can allow up to 40–60 cm of small bowel to be examined, until the terminal ileum (TI) is reached (Figure 14.2). If the TI is not reached then the most distal region reached is "tattooed" in the submucosal plane with an endo-needle, using a bleb of normal saline then injected with methylene blue or indigo carmine (Figure 14.3). Alternatively 1 in 10 dyes in saline can be injected directly into the bowel wall, but there is a theoretical risk of intraperitoneal leak with this one-step technique.

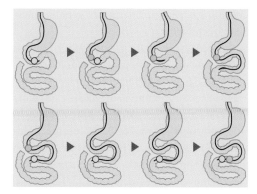

Figure 14.2 DBE technique.

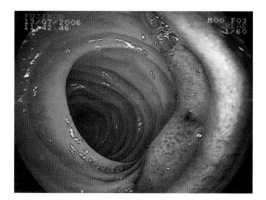

Figure 14.3 Double-balloon tattoo.

An approximate distance of postpylorus small bowel negotiation can be calculated if one assumes that 5 cm of overtube insertion equates to approximately 40 cm of small bowel. The DBE can then be repeated via the transanal route and retrograde movement from the TI proximally up the ileum, allowing full examination of the whole small bowel. Colon negotiation can be facilitated with the overtube balloon in the colon itself. Simultaneous fluoroscopy has not been found to allow further advancement of the DBE in recent studies.

On withdrawal in either procedure, close examination of the mucosal surface occurs as with standard endoscopy, but lesions are dealt with as soon as they are found, whether this is on intubation or withdrawal. Bowel preparation is as for standard ileocolonoscopy. The procedure is carried out under general anesthetic in children.

As noted above, there are two other Fujinon double-balloon enteroscopes used in adults: the EN450T5, with a diameter of 9.4 mm and a larger accessory channel of 2.8 mm allowing for therapeutic enteroscopy, and the EN450B15 with a working length of 152 cm useful in difficult colonoscopies and ERCP in patients with Roux-en-Y anastomosis. These scopes allow endotherapy as opposed to the smaller pediatric endodiagnostic scope which we previously reserved for children under 3 years or 15 kg in weight. However, as experience has been gained it is clear that the more flexible smaller enteroscope has a greater chance of full small bowel examination than the stiffer "adult" enteroscope. We have attained full small bowel examination with the smaller scope. A newer smaller diameter enteroscope with a larger 2.8 mm working channel allowing more therapeutic procedures has been produced and is promising.

Indications for DBE

Obscure GI bleeding, polyps, and evaluation of Crohn's disease are by far the most common indications for DBE in adults. DBE is also useful in the assessment of polyposis syndromes, ERCP in patients with Roux-en-Y anastomosis and suspected small intestinal tumors. A postliver transplant child has benefited from DBE to identify and treat a bilioenteric anastomotic stricture. DBE finds applications in the further evaluation of abnormal findings following WCE. Therapeutic roles include hemostasis, polypectomy, balloon dilation of strictures, and retrieval of foreign bodies. A summary of indications is listed in Table 14.1.

Pediatric experience

Limited DBE experience exists in the pediatric literature. Nishimura *et al.* performed 92 procedures in 48 patients using four different double-balloon enteroscopes including a prototype.

Table 14.1 Diagnostic and therapeutic indications for enteroscopy

Diagnostic	Therapeutic
Obscure GI bleeding	Hemostasis
Evaluation of celiac disease	Polypectomy
Malabsorption	Treatment of stenoses
Crohn's disease	Retrieval of foreign bodies
Hereditary polyposis syndromes	ERCP in patients with Billroth type II stomach or Roux-en Y anastomosis
ERCP in patients with altered surgical anatomy	Gastrostomy placement in abnormal bowel anatomy
Suspected tumors	Treatment of early postoperative small bowel obstruction

The mean duration of procedures was 96 minutes (range 30–220 minutes). The most common indication was stricture of biliary anastomosis following living donor liver transplantation (23 patients). Other indications included obscure GI bleeding (10 patients), surveillance and treatment of hereditary polyposis syndromes (five patients), abdominal pain (four patients), and inflammatory bowel disease (two patients). The overall diagnostic yield was 65%. Therapeutic interventions were performed in 40% of patients including balloon dilation, biliary stenting, or removal of stones in 13 patients, polypectomy in five patients and argon plasma coagulation in one patient. Complications reported included self-limiting abdominal pain in 10 patients, mucosal injury of the small bowel in one patient, and postpolypectomy bleeding in one patient.

Liu *et al.* reported a retrospective case series of 31 patients. Oral approach was used in 18 patients and anal approach in 11 patients. Two patients underwent both oral and anal approaches and the entire small bowel was visualized. The procedure time ranged from 40 to 70 minutes. Twenty seven of these patients were investigated for obscure GI bleeding.

A source for the bleeding was found in 21 patients, giving a diagnostic yield of 77%. Angiomata and Crohn's disease were the most common causes for bleeding. Four patients were investigated for chronic diarrhea; two were found to have lymphangiectasia, and one each had a diagnosis of IBD and celiac disease. The overall diagnostic yield was 80%.

In our own experience, initial description n = 14 (now n = 40), we have examined 40 patients: eight for Peutz–Jeghers syndrome (PJS), 24 for obscure or occult GI bleeding, two for recurrent abdominal pain, one patient with Cowden's syndrome and persistent GI bleeding, and five for suspected but unproven (by conventional endoscopy) Crohn's disease. The median time was 118 minutes (range 95–195 minutes) for the whole procedure. The entire small bowel was examined in six patients and a length of 200–320 cm distal to pylorus in the remaining. Sixteen patients had only an oral approach; the remainder had oral and anal approaches. Polyps were detected and successfully removed (Figure 14.4) in all eight patients with PJS, in one patient with tubulovillous adenoma of the duodenum, in one patient with significant anemia and occult bleeding, and in a patient with Cowden's syndrome. A diagnosis was made in a patient with multiple angiomata (Figure 14.5) not amenable to endotherapy, and in one with a discrete angioma which was treated with argon plasma coagulation. The source of bleeding was identified in a further patient with varices. DBE was normal

or revealed minor mucosal friability in the remaining patients. Hence, a diagnostic yield in the majority was achieved with therapeutic success in all but one in whom lesions required intervention. Incidentally, a Meckel's diverticulum was found in one patient (Figure 14.6).

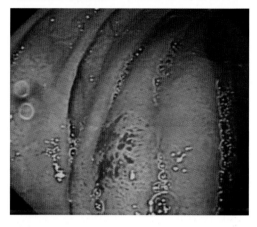

Figure 14.5 Multiple angiomas in small bowel.

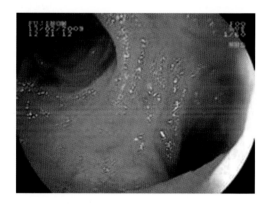

Figure 14.6 Meckel's diverticulum.

(a)　　　　　　　　　　(b)

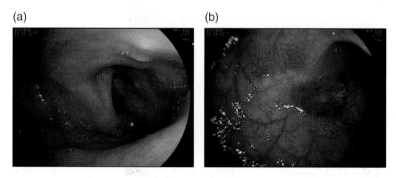

Figure 14.4 Polyp detected (a) and removed (b).

Two patients with blue rubber bleb nevus syndrome had successful ablation of the lesions with argon plasma coagulation with no complications (Figure 14.7).

No complications were encountered. All patients underwent general anesthesia and were allowed home on the same day. Part of the ability to perform the procedure as a day case was due to the use of carbon dioxide insufflation – a much more rapid absorption led to a greater depth of intubation as the peritoneal cavity was thus less encumbered by gas-filled small bowel loops preventing advancement, and once woken the patients experienced minimal or no abdominal distension-related pain. Interestingly, the end expired CO_2 recorded during anesthesia rose, but not to any level that was considered compromising, nor higher than observed during CO_2-assisted laparoscopy. ERCP via a balloon enteroscope is now well established in adult endoscopy, and is particularly useful when a Roux-en-Y loop is present.

Complications

From the three pediatric case series reported involving 107 children undergoing 186 procedures when oral and anal approaches are included, no major complications have been reported. Minor complications included abdominal pain, sore throat, minor aspiration, and bleeding following polypectomy. The lack of any significant complications reported reflects the small number of patients involved and the different indications for DBE in comparison to adults. In the adult literature, acute pancreatitis, perforation, and bleeding are known significant complications. Minor complications include pain, fever, and vomiting. Single case reports of intraperitoneal bleeding and paralytic ileus have also been published.

Several mechanisms have been proposed for the occurrence of acute pancreatitis. These include sphincter injury from direct compression by the balloons, duodenal pancreatic reflux, and direct pancreatic injury secondary to endoscopic compression of the pancreas against the spine.

In one large international survey, 40 complications occurred from 2362 procedures (1.7%). The incidences of acute pancreatitis and perforations were similar at 0.3% each. Twelve bleeding complications were reported from 364 polypectomies, none of which were a major bleed. In another large pooled data study from the German national register involving 3894 procedures, a complication rate of 1.2% was reported. Rates of acute pancreatitis were similar while perforations were higher at 3.4%. There were also six major bleeding episodes. Similar complication rates were reported in data from nine US centers.

Training issues and learning curve

In view of the small number of cases requiring DBE in children, training remains an issue. In

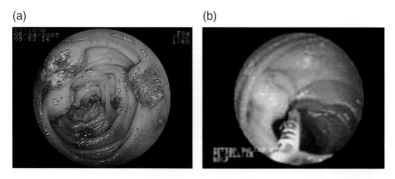

(a)   (b)

Figure 14.7 (a) Blue rubber bleb nevus syndrome lesions. (b) Blue rubber bleb nevus syndrome lesions after argon plasma coagulation

adults a step-by-step approach has been found to be useful. The first step is to be familiar with the pathological conditions in the small gut as well as the technique of DBE. The second step involves observation of live procedures in patients conducted by experienced endoscopists as well as hands-on training using a fresh ex vivo model, and finally one-to-one training with an experienced DBE endoscopist. Mehdizadeh *et al.* found a significant decrease in the overall procedural time after the initial 10 DBE cases in a study involving 188 patients and 237 DBE procedures from six US centers. The mean duration decreased from 109 minutes for the first 10 cases to 92 minutes for subsequent cases. Close coordination with the adult GI units performing DBE may be beneficial. Further, with the low case volume requiring DBE in children, it may be practical and cost-effective to limit the use of DBE to specialized pediatric GI endoscopic units.

Single-balloon enteroscopy

Using an Olympus platform and standard push enteroscope or pediatric-size colonoscope, this technique has its followers (Figure 14.8). It has the advantage of using existing equipment, but suffers from certain disadvantages that preclude deep small bowel intubation – this is

identifed by most users. Hence, it is useful for proximal small bowel lesions, but rarely is full small bowel traverse acquired. As there is only one balloon, it relies (during withdrawal to concertina the bowel over the scope, once the balloon has been deflated to facilitate this part of the enteroscopy) on the operator trying to hook the tip of the scope over one of the valvulae coneventes in the small bowel. However, inevitably during withdrawal, there is retrograde slippage, and a seesaw motion occurs during intubation and withdrawal, after only a few "passes." For deep small bowel intubation it is therefore not the procedure of choice, although it seems to be safe. Only one small series of seven patients exists in the pediatric literature to date. It has been used successfully in case reports in children, for example, for the treatment of small bowel varices with a child having a hepaticojejunostomy.

Spiral enteroscopy

This is an exciting recent development which arose from the application of novel thinking to an enduring problem – how to insert a flexible tube through a flexible tube. Thus, instead of pushing, this principle is the screw and advance concept, thus pulling the enteroscope through the small bowel. A mathematical relationship exists between the rotational force/movement, the acuteness of the spiral, and the resultant forward progression of the tip of the scope.

A disposable overtube with an outer spiral is placed transorally over an endoscope (Figure 14.9) – typically, a Fujinon enteroscope

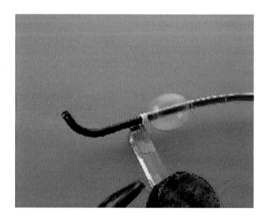

Figure 14.8 Single-balloon enteroscopy.

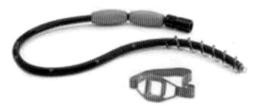

Figure 14.9 Spiral enteroscopy outside the patient.

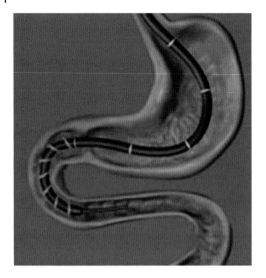

Figure 14.10 Spiral enteroscope advancing intraluminally.

at present – and after the pylorus is negotiated, the operator simply rotates the handles of the overtube which remain outside the patient in a clockwise direction to produce forward movement (Figure 14.10). Remarkable forward movement with simultaneous "concertina"-ing of the small bowel over the instrument occurs. When this motion is stopped, then stable nonmovement of the tip of the scope can be observed. Simple reversal (counterclockwise) results in removal of the tip of the scope through the small bowel. With this degree of control, lesions can be targeted accurately for endotherapy without the distraction of intestinal peristalsis. Recent large adult studies have been published, although some groups identify that the diagnostic yield may be less than that of DBE, although insertion depth seems to be greater than SBE.

Intraoperative or laparoscopy-assisted enteroscopy

It has to be said that this is an inferior technique to nonoperative enteroscopy. Intraoperative or laparoscope-assisted enteroscopy starts with conventional enteroscopic jejunal intubation followed by surgical assistance. The endoscopist's role is relatively passive, deflecting the tip of the instrument while the surgeon, either with hands or laparoscopic instruments, concertinas examined parts of the small bowel over the enteroscope. Both the mucosal and serosal surfaces can be examined. Very little air is insufflated into the bowel to avoid hindering the surgeon. Dimmed lights in the operating field also help to identify the position of the tip of the instrument. In experienced hands, all the small bowel is examined in 60% of cases, taking up to 2–3 hours (Figure 14.11). An enterotomy may be used to insert a sterilized enteroscope in some situations. Lesions can be marked by injection of ink or placement of a suture.

Intraoperative or laparoscopy-assisted enteroscopy is the most successful technique for identifying sites of obscure gastrointestinal bleeding with diagnostic yields of between 83% and 100%. Laser or bipolar coagulation can be used, and resection of lesions is recommended if intraoperative. This technique has demonstrable advantages in assessment of the extent

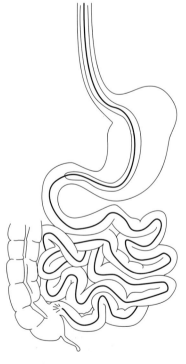

Figure 14.11 Extent of laparoscopic-assisted enteroscopy.

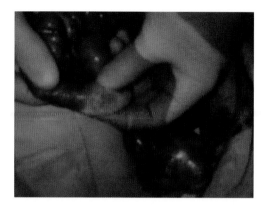

Figure 14.12 Intraoperative enteroscopy and transillumination of a discrete area of intestinal lymphangiectasia.

of polyposis syndromes. "On-table" enteroscopy has a better pick-up rate for polyps at laparotomy than external transillumination and palpation. It can be helpful to view both serosal and mucosal surfaces simultaneously, especially with transillumination, when trying to identify small isolated lesions such as isolated pockets of intestinal lymphangiectasia (Figure 14.12). When attempted in Crohn's disease, up to 65% of patients have had lesions not previously identified in the small bowel by other investigations, including direct vision of the serosal surface of the bowel. As previously mentioned, occult Crohn's disease can be identified in children using enteroscopy. Partial intestinal obstruction and Meckel's diverticulum have also been identified at intraoperative enteroscopy. Small bowel neoplasia must not be forgotten as the second most common cause of obscure gastrointestinal bleeding in younger patients, accounting for 5–10% of cases in young adults. Exploratory laparoscopy and enteroscopy are important in preventing missed diagnoses.

In essence, intraoperative enteroscopy is likely to give way to DBE in the very near future.

General complications

Complications are not often encountered with simple push enteroscopy, but when the overtube is employed, significant patient discomfort has been described. Other, rare complications of the overtube include pharyngeal tear, Mallory–Weiss tear, gastric mucosal stripping, pancreatitis, and duodenal perforation. DBE may be associated with pancreatitis in some cases, especially if the overtube balloon is first inflated too proximally, i.e., this needs to occur past the ligament of Treitz. Intraoperative enteroscopy has a 5% incidence of perforation and, in one series, a 50% incidence of mucosal laceration. Prolonged ileus has been occasionally described.

None of these rare complications have been reported in the limited studies investigating children.

Conclusion

Flexible GI endoscopy is sufficient for diagnostic and therapeutic procedures in the vast majority of pediatric cases, and in adult patients with obscure gastrointestinal bleeding is known to determine the source in up to 90%. However, in the small number of cases when the pathology is confined to the small bowel beyond the reach of conventional endoscopy, WCE and DBE have a role. DBE allows examination of the entire small bowel, making it possible to diagnose small bowel Crohn's disease, obscure GI bleeding and tumors otherwise not attainable by conventional GI endoscopy, and also to perform endotherapeutic procedures such as hemostasis, polypectomy, balloon dilation of strictures, and retrieval of foreign bodies. DBE has a high diagnostic and therapeutic yield and a low risk of complications in 1–2% of cases. DBE is feasible and safe in children.

 • See companion website for videos relating to this chapter topic: www.wiley.com/go/gershman3e

FURTHER READING

Apelgren KN, Vargish T, Al-Kawas F. (1988) Principles for use of intraoperative enteroscopy for hemorrhage from the small bowel. *Am J Surg*, **54**, 85–88.

Appleyard M, Fireman Z, Glukhovsky A, *et al.* (2000) A randomized trial comparing wireless capsule endoscopy with push enteroscopy for the detection of small-bowel lesions. *Gastroenterology*, **119**, 1431–1438.

Attar A, Maissiat E, Sebbagh V, *et al.* (2005) First case of paralytic intestinal ileus after double balloon enteroscopy. *Gut*, **54**, 1823–1824.

Barkin J, Lewis B, Reiner D, *et al.* (1996) Diagnostic and therapeutic jejunoscopy with a new, longer enteroscope. *Gastrointest Endosc*, **38**, 55–58.

Barth BA, Channabasappa N. (2010) Single-balloon enteroscopy in children: initial experience at a pediatric center. *J Pediatr Gastroenterol Nutr*, **51**(5)**,** 680–684.

Bowden TA Jr, Hooks VH IIIrd, Teeslink CR, *et al.* (1980) Occult gastrointestinal bleeding: locating the cause. *Am J Surg*, **46**, 80–87.

Chak A, Koehler MK, Sundaram SN, *et al.* (1998) Diagnostic and therapeutic impact of push enteroscopy: analysis of factors associated with positive findings. *Gastrointest Endosc*, **47**, 18–22.

Cheng DW, Han NJ, Mehdizadeh S, *et al.* Intraperitoneal bleeding after oral double-balloon enteroscopy: a case report and review of the literature. *Gastrointest Endosc*, **66**, 627–629.

Chong J, Tagle M, Barkin J, *et al.* (1994) Small bowel push-type fiberoptic enteroscopy for patients with occult gastrointestinal bleeding or suspected small bowel pathology. *Am J Gastroenterol*, **89**, 2143–2146.

Curcio G, Sciveres M, Mocciaro F, *et al.* (2012) Out-of-reach obscure bleeding: single-balloon enteroscopy to diagnose and treat varices in hepaticojejunostomy after pediatric liver transplant. *Pediatr Transplant*, **16**, E78–80.

Darbari A, Kalloo AN, Cuffari C. (2006) Diagnostic yield, safety, and efficacy of push

enteroscopy in pediatrics. *Gastrointest Endosc*, **64**, 224–228.

Di Caro S, May A, Heine DGN, *et al.* (2005) The European experience with double-balloon enteroscopy: indications, methodology, safety, and clinical impact. *Gastrointest Endosc*, **62**, 545–550.

Douard R, Wind P, Panis Y, *et al.* (2000) Intraoperative enteroscopy for diagnosis and management of unexplained gastrointestinal bleeding. *Am J Surg*, **180**, 181–184.

Duggan C, Shamberger R, Antonioli D, *et al.* (1995) Intraoperative enteroscopy in the diagnosis of partial intestinal enteroscopy in infancy. *Dig Dis Sci*, **40**, 236–238.

Frieling T, Heise J, Sassenrath W, *et al.* (2010) Prospective comparison between double-balloon enteroscopy and spiral enteroscopy. *Endoscopy*, **42**(11)**,** 885–888.

Foutch PG, Sawyer R, Sanowski RA. (1990) Push-enteroscopy for diagnosis of patients with gastrointestinal bleeding of obscure origin. *Gastrointest Endosc*, **36**, 337–341.

Gerson LB, Flodin JT, Miyabayashi K. (2008) Balloon-assisted enteroscopy: technology and troubleshooting. *Gastrointest Endosc*, **68**, 1158–1167.

Gerson LB, Tokar J, Chiorean M, *et al.* (2009) Complications associated with double balloon enteroscopy at nine US centers. *Clin Gastroenterol Hepatol*, **7**, 1177–1182, 1182, e1171–e1173.

Gong F, Swain P, Mills T. (2000) Wireless endoscopy. *Gastrointest Endosc*, **51**, 725–729.

Heine GD, Hadithi M, Groenen MJ, *et al.* (2006) Double-balloon enteroscopy: indications, diagnostic yield, and complications in a series of 275 patients with suspected small-bowel disease. *Endoscopy*, **38**, 42–48.

Hopkins H, Kapany YS. (1954). A flexible fiberoscope using static scanning. *Nature*, **173**, 39.

Hyer W, Neale K, Fell J, *et al.* (2000) At what age should routine screening start in children at risk of familial adenomatous polyposis? *J Pediatr Gastroenterol Nutr*, **405**, 417.

Khashab MA, Lennon AM, Dunbar KB, *et al.* (2010) A comparative evaluation of single-balloon enteroscopy and spiral enteroscopy for patients with mid-gut disorders. *Gastrointest Endosc*, **72**(4), 766–772.

Landi B, Cellier C, Fayemendy L, *et al.* (1996) Duodenal perforation occurring during push enteroscopy. *Gastrointest Endosc*, **43**, 631.

Lau WY. (1990) Intraoperative enteroscopy – indications and limitations. *Gastrointest Endosc*, **36**, 268–271.

Lewis B, Kornbluth A, Waye J. (1991) Small bowel tumors: the yield of enteroscopy. *Gut*, **32**, 763–765.

Lewis B, Wenger J, Waye J. (1991) Intraoperative enteroscopy versus small bowel enteroscopy in patients with obscure GI bleeding. *Am J Gastroenterol*, **86**, 171–174.

Lescut D, Vanco D, Bonniere P, *et al.* (1993) Peri-operative endoscopy of the whole small bowel in Crohn's disease. *Gut*, **34**, 3647–3649.

Li XB, Dai J, Chen HM, *et al.* (2010) A novel modality for the estimation of the enteroscope insertion depth during double-balloon enteroscopy. *Gastrointest Endosc*, **72**(5), 999–1005.

Liu W, Xu C, Zhong J. (2009) The diagnostic value of double-balloon enteroscopy in children with small bowel disease: report of 31 cases. *Can J Gastroenterol*, **23**, 635–636.

Linder J, Cheruvattath R, Truss C, *et al.* (2002) Diagnostic yield and clinical implications of push enteroscopy: results from a nonspecialized center. *J Clin Gastroenterol*, **35**, 383–386.

Lo SK, Simpson PW. (2007) Pancreatitis associated with double-balloon enteroscopy: how common is it? *Gastrointest Endosc*, **66**, 1139–1141.

Manner H, May A, Pohl J, *et al.* (2010) Impact of fluoroscopy on oral double-balloon enteroscopy: results of a randomized trial in 156 patients. *Endoscopy*, **42**(10), 820–826.

Manno M, Barbera C, Dabizzi E, *et al.* (2010) Safety of single-balloon enteroscopy: our experience of 72 procedures. *Endoscopy*, **42**(9), 773, author reply, 774.

Mata A, Bordas JM, Feu F, *et al.* (2004) Wireless capsule endoscopy in patients with obscure gastrointestinal bleeding: a comparative study with push enteroscopy. *Aliment Pharmacol Therapeut*, **20**, 189–194.

Mathus-Vliegen E. (1989) Laser treatment of intestinal vascular abnormalities. *Int J Colorect Dis*, **4**, 20–25.

May A. (2008) Performing double-balloon enteroscopy: the utility of the Erlangen EndoTrainer. *Techn Gastrointest Endosc*, **10**, 54–58.

May A, Nachbar L, Wardak A, *et al.* (2003) Double-balloon enteroscopy: preliminary experience in patients with obscure gastrointestinal bleeding or chronic abdominal pain. *Endoscopy*, **35**, 985–991.

Mehdizadeh S, Ross A, Gerson L, *et al.* (2006) What is the learning curve associated with double-balloon enteroscopy? Technical details and early experience in 6 U.S. tertiary care centers. *Gastrointest Endosc*, **64**, 740–750.

Mensink PBF. (2008) Complications of double balloon enteroscopy. *Techn Gastrointest Endosc*, **10**, 66–69.

Monkemuller K, Bellutti M, Fry LC, Malfertheiner P. (2008) Enteroscopy. *Best Pract Res Clin Gastroenterol*, **22**, 789–811.

Morgan D, Upchurch B, Draganov, P *et al.* (2010) Spiral enteroscopy: prospective U.S. multicenter study in patients with small-bowel disorders. *Gastrointest Endosc*, **72**(5), 992–998.

Mylonaki M, Fritscher-Ravens A, Swain P. (2003) Wireless capsule endoscopy: a comparison with push enteroscopy in patients with gastroscopy and colonoscopy negative gastrointestinal bleeding. *Gut*, **52**, 1122–1126.

Nishimura N, Yamamoto H, Yano T, *et al.* (2009) Safety and efficacy of double-balloon enteroscopy in pediatric patients. *Gastrointest Endosc*, **71**, 287–294.

O'Mahony S, Morris AJ, Straiton M, *et al.* (1996) Push enteroscopy in the investigation of small-intestinal disease. *Q J Med*, **89**, 685.

Pennazio M, Arrigoni A, Risio M, *et al.* (1995) Clinical evaluation of push-type enteroscopy. *Endoscopy*, **27**, 164–170.

Sanada Y, Mizuta K, Yano T, *et al.* (1995) Double-balloon enteroscopy for bilioenteric anastomotic stricture after pediatric living donor liver transplantation. *Transplant Int*, **24**(1), 85–90.

Schnoll-Sussman F, Kulkarni K. (2008) Risks of capsule endoscopy. *Techn Gastrointest Endosc*, **10**, 25–30.

Shimizu S, Tada M, Kawai K. (1987) Development of a new insertion technique in push-type enteroscopy. *Am J Gastroenterol*, **82**, 844–847.

Sunada K, Yamamoto H. (2008) Double balloon enterosocopy: techniques. *Techn Gastrointest Endosc*, **10**, 46–53.

Tada M, Akasaka Y, Misaki F, *et al.* (1977) Clinical evaluation of a sonde-type small intestinal fiberscope. *Endoscopy*, **9**, 33–38.

Thomson M, Venkatesh K, Elmalik K, *et al.* (2010) Double balloon enteroscopy in children: diagnosis, treatment and safety. *World J Gastroenterol*, **16**, 56–62.

Turck D, Bonnevalle M, Gottrand F, *et al.* (1990) Intraoperative endoscopic diagnosis of heterotopic gastric mucosa in the ileum causing recurrent acute intussusception. *J Pediatr Gastroenterol Nutr*, **11**, 275–278.

Whelan R, Buls J, Goldberg S, *et al.* (1989) Intraoperative enteroscopy: University of Minnesota experience. *Am J Surg*, **55**, 281–286.

Yamamoto H, Sekine Y, Sato Y, *et al.* (2001) Total enteroscopy with a nonsurgical steerable double-balloon method. *Gastrointest Endosc*, **53**, 216–220.

Yamamoto H, Kita H, Sunada K, *et al.* (2004) Clinical outcomes of double-balloon endoscopy for the diagnosis and treatment of small-intestinal diseases. *Clin Gastroenterol Hepatol*, **2**, 1010–1016.

Yang R, Laine L. (1995) Mucosal stripping: a complication of push enteroscopy. *Gastrointest Endosc*, **41**, 156–158.

Zaman A, Katon RM. (1998) Push enteroscopy for obscure gastrointestinal bleeding yields a high incidence of proximal lesions within reach of a standard endoscope. *Gastrointest Endosc*, **47**, 372–376.

15

Wireless capsule endoscopy

Mike Thomson

 KEY POINTS

- Wireless capsule endoscopy (WCE) can reveal small bowel pathologies which cannot be evaluated by standard endoscopy (except enteroscopy) and can be missed by radiological means.
- Most children over 8 years can swallow the capsule with appropriate training.
- Younger children need the capsule to be introduced into the duodenum by endoscopic delivery devices.
- WCE is safe and feasible in children as young as 6 months and with a weight of 8 kg.

- Pathologies such as obscure GI bleeding, small bowel IBD, polyp syndromes, and intestinal lymphangiectasia are particularly amenable to this technology.
- Advances include a magnetically controlled capsule which can be maneuvered from outside the patient.
- Esophageal-specific and colon-specific capsules are now available but their indications/applications in children are relatively limited.

Introduction

Wireless capsule video-endoscopy (WCE or VCE) has been used in pediatric small bowel investigation for over 20 years and is a standard tool for the investigation of pathologies such as occult/obscure GI bleeding (see Chapter 31) (Figure 15.1), polyp syndromes (see Chapter 43) (Figure 15.2), small bowel Crohn's (see Chapter 25) (Figure 15.3), and less common pathologies such as diaphragm disease (also known as chronic mucosal ulcerating and stenosing enteropathy, CMUSE) and tumors (Figures 15.4 and 15.5). It is now preferred by most as the tool for investigating a Meckel's diverticulum (Figure 15.6) and has

become standard in IBD staging complementing magnetic resonance enteroclysis (MRE) and standard endoscopy (see Figure 15.3). Possible NSAID enteropathy can be excluded (Figure 15.7), which includes Crohn's-like lesions and ulcerating stenoses (Figure 15.8), and the patchy nature of celiac disease can be identified (Figure 15.9). Ideally, it is accompanied by a sister therapeutic technique such as double-balloon enteroscopy (DBE) (see Chapter 14) or occasionally intraoperative enteroscopy (IOE).

This chapter will deal with the practicalities of WCE in children and is not meant as an atlas – there are already very good texts that cover this area in more detail than space allows here.

Practical Pediatric Gastrointestinal Endoscopy, Third Edition. Edited by George Gershman and Mike Thomson.
© 2021 John Wiley & Sons Ltd. Published 2021 by John Wiley & Sons Ltd.
Companion website: www.wiley.com/go/gershman3e

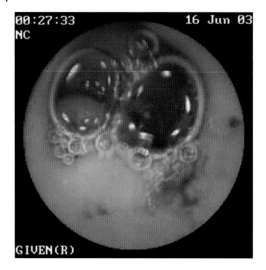

Figure 15.1 Occult bleeding from an angiodysplasia.

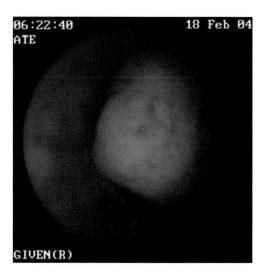

Figure 15.2 Jejunal Peutz–Jeghers polyp.

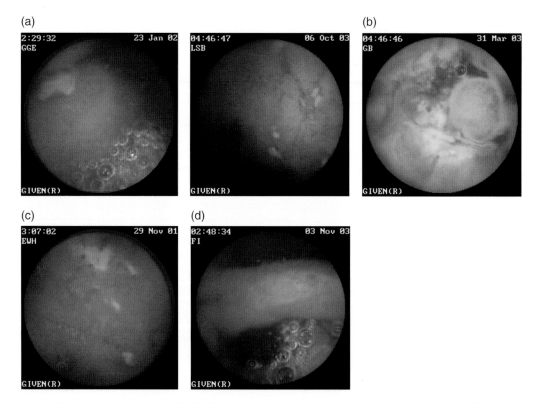

Figure 15.3 (a) Crohn's disease. (b) A follow-up study in a 16-year-old male treated for Crohn's disease shows inflammatory pseudopolyps in the ileum. (c) Small bowel Crohn's disease. (d) Flat Crohn's-like lesion in jejunum.

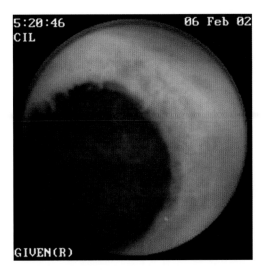

Figure 15.4 CMUSE or diaphragm disease.

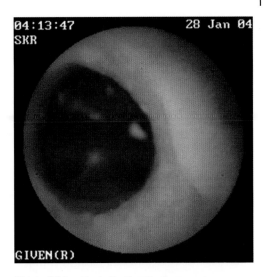

Figure 15.6 Meckel's diverticulum.

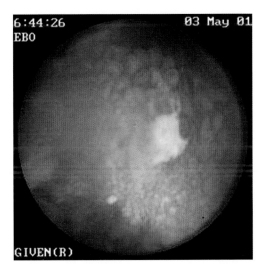

Figure 15.5 Lymphoma.

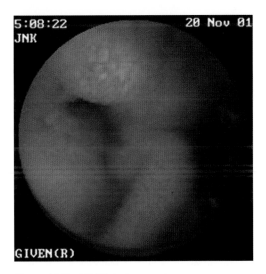

Figure 15.7 NSAID lesions.

Practical approach

Bowel preparation and starving/oral intake instructions are those which are standard for the unit's ileocolonoscopy (see Chapter 12). Often a detergent such as simethicone can be given 1–2 hours before the procedure to decrease bubbles and alalow better mucosal visualization – 10 mL under 5 years, 20 mL 5–10 years and 40 mL over 10 years. A propulsion agent may be employed such as metoclopramide or domperidone but this is not usually necessary unless profound dysmotility is previously identified – and unfortunately is rarely beneficial anyway. Children under 12 but over 8 can be taught to swallow the capsule by a number of weeks of tutoring to swallow jelly beans whole – it is very patient-specific in terms of whether or not they will swallow a capsule and generally we would have a back-up plan of placing the child first on the

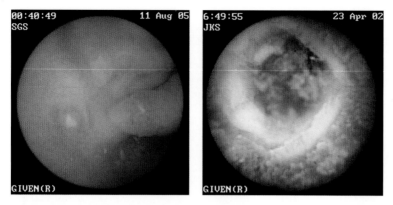

Figure 15.8 Crohn's aphthoid ulcers and stricture.

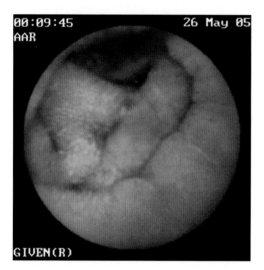

Figure 15.9 Celiac disease.

afternoon endoscopy list and starved in order to place the capsule endoscopically if swallowing fails, thereby avoiding the waste of a capsule. In this approach gastro nurses are invaluable in persuasion.

Introduction of the capsule endoscopically into the small bowel in children who will not swallow it is well described and used to involve a Roth net but this caused too much mucosal trauma – we now have a capsule delivery device (Acorn®, US Endoscopy) which is "front-loaded" onto the endoscope and introduced with a normal endoscopic approach (Figure 15.10). This can occur down to 6 months

of age. In practice, the flashing end of the capsule is loaded towards the endoscope – this allows the endoscopist to identify when the capsule is deployed; if they can no longer see the flashing of the capsule, then the capsule has left the device. Once the endoscope has entered the stomach, the capsule and delivery device can be protruded away from the end of the endoscope (prior to which the endoscopist's view is somewhat obscured in the esophagus by the capsule) and a better view towards the pylorus may be allowed.

On insertion of the capsule and delivery device through the pylorus in older children with a more spacious duodenal bulb, negotiation into the more distal part of the duodenum may be possible. However, in younger children and infants, deployment in the first part of the duodenum may be necessary. In this scenario it is important to avoid deployment against the distal wall of the duodenum which will result in the capsule being "half-deployed" and kept in the delivery device. A trick to avoid this is to give a small IV dose of buscopan (hyoscine) to relax the duodenum and to have only the first third of the capsule protruding into the duodenum.

When one is trying to detect occult/obscure GI bleeding lesions, it is recommended to avoid taking duodenal biopsies which will bleed and the blood will often travel down the small intestine with the capsule, causing visual confusion.

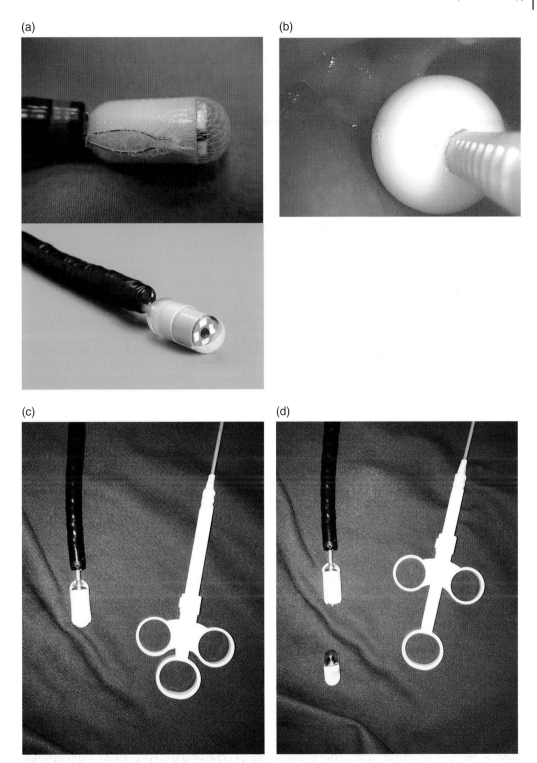

Figure 15.10 Methods of "front-loading" the PillCam™ onto a gastroscope. (a) Using a Roth net. (b) Endoscopic insertion of a PillCam with the capsule delivery device. (c,d) Illustration of how the US Endoscopy device deploys the capsule.

One must be aware of the technology of the receiving module, ensuring that it is kept close to the patient at all times. Otherwise if no signal is detected, it will cease to record after a period of time and not reinitialize. Of course, the battery must be fully charged and the patient details input into the base station. A number of models are now available from different companies; there is little to choose between the alternatives and price may differ. Most give a recording life on one battery of up to 15 hours which is more than sufficient to traverse the small bowel in all children, barring the presence of strictures.

The question of whether or not to use a dissolvable practice capsule in case of strictures has been debated. It is common in adults but in children it is not generally useful. This is because of two considerations: first, to place such a capsule in young children would need a separate GA for endoscopic insertion and second, a video capsule can stay in the small bowel for months if not years in reported experience without causing any problems at all. In any event, if the capsule did cause obstructive symptoms then it would highlight an area that would require surgery anyway. If really necessary, it is possible to remove a capsule from the mid-small bowel by DBE. If it is arrested due to an inflammatory pathology, it is our experience that with antiinflammatories such as steroids which diminish the inflammatory component of such a stricture/stenosis, the capsule will often pass uneventfully. If obstructive symptoms occur then it is likely that the stricture would have needed surgery in any case.

Pediatric experience and pathologies

Small bowel IBD and inflammatory pathologies

Although nonsteroidal antiinflammatory drugs are less commonly employed in children, they commonly cause mucosal injury, including ulcerations that mimic Crohn's disease. The drug-induced lesions may include mucosal breaks, focal ulcerations (see Figure 15.7) and circumferential, ulcerated strictures – so-called diaphragm disease or CMUSE. However, in children this is more usually a congenital condition of prostaglandin receptor abnormal function (see Figure 15.4). Histological confirmation of specific diagnoses suggested by capsule endoscopy should thus always be considered, where feasible – this can be provided reliably by balloon enteroscopy. Crohn's disease may be identified occurring only in the small bowel by WCE and may be missed by MRE (see Figures 15.3 and 15.8).

Polyposis syndromes and other intestinal tumors

Among adult patients, capsule endoscopy has been shown to be highly efficient in detecting small bowel tumors that were missed by conventional endoscopic and imaging methods, including push enteroscopy. Although small bowel malignancies are rare in children, inherited gastrointestinal polyposis disorders such as Peutz–Jeghers syndrome are not uncommonly seen by pediatric gastroenterologists and surgeons. Complications of these tumors include small bowel intussusception, bleeding and less commonly malignancy (see Figure 15.2). Polyp syndrome surveillance recommendations are published as guidelines by ESPGHAN for children. Polyps less than 15 mm are better detected with capsule endoscopy than MRE or other imaging studies. The available data thus suggest that capsule endoscopy should replace barium X-rays, MRI, and push enteroscopy for the identification of small bowel polyps in the pediatric age group. The localization software is not useful for guiding the clinician to the possibility of reaching a polyp for removal endoscopically, but calculation of the time from pylorus to polyp divided by total small bowel transit time can give a percentage of the length of the small bowel which the polyp might be located at enteroscopy.

Occult or obscure intestinal bleeding

Obscure/occult bleeding is defined as bleeding of unknown origin that persists or recurs (recurrent or persistent visible bleeding, iron-deficiency anemia with positive fecal occult blood testing) after a negative initial or primary endoscopy (upper and/or lower endoscopy). The source of bleeding is frequently located in the small bowel and may result from a number of conditions, including vascular lesions and inflammatory lesions, or tumors (see Figures 15.1, 15.5 and 15.6).

Imaging techniques for evaluation of the small bowel are relatively insensitive for intestinal bleeding lesions that are flat, small, infiltrative, or inflammatory. Angiography and radioisotope bleeding scans are insensitive in the absence of brisk active bleeding but CT angiography is occasionally helpful, as is a plain CT scan for lesions such as gastric duplication cysts, etc. As noted above, intraoperative enteroscopy is the most thorough but also the most invasive means to visualize the small bowel. Double-balloon enteroscopy is the best method that offers the possibility of achieving complete small bowel enteroscopy and providing therapy without the need for laparoscopy/laparotomy.

Capsule endoscopy is a useful tool for diagnosing and monitoring the effects of therapy in patients with blue rubber bleb nevus syndrome. Bleeding from small bowel varices in pediatric cases with portal hypertension is also described, allowing banding by enteroscopy if in the proximal small bowel (see Figure 15.7). WCE may be considered the diagnostic modality of choice for lesions such as angiodyplasia of the small bowel including Diuelafoy's and Meckel's diverticulum (see Figure 15.6), in which isotope scanning is notoriously unreliable. NSAID lesions are also sources of jejunal bleeding (see Figure 15.8).

For celiac disease, histological diagnosis remains the gold standard although recent guidelines suggest that with a tissue transglutaminase 10 times the upper limit of normal in a symptomatic child, a biopsy may not be necessary. WCE can show typical features macroscopically with scalloping or a mosaic appearance but it is unlikely to replace formal upper GI endoscopy (see Figure 15.9).

Other indications

In addition to the more common indications that have been discussed above, capsule endoscopy is likely to prove clinically useful for a variety of other potential disorders of the small bowel in the pediatric age group (see Table 15.1). The identification of abnormal but undiagnosed findings on small bowel imaging is a worthwhile indication for capsule study. Pathologies that have been uncovered include

Table 15.1 Potential indications for capsule endoscopy in pediatric patients

---

Small bowel inflammatory disorders

Crohn's disease; celiac disease; food allergic or eosinophilic enteropathies; intestinal vasculitis/angiodysplasia; Henoch–Schönlein purpura; drug-induced mucosal injury (nonsteroidal antiinflammatory or chemotherapy); radiation enteropathy; graft-versus-host disease; intestinal transplantation

Small bowel polyps and tumors

Peutz–Jeghers syndrome; other familial and nonfamilial polyposes; lymphoma, leiomyoma, carcinoid and other tumors

Occult or obscure intestinal bleeding

Including vascular malformations, portal hypertension, and small bowel varices

Abnormal findings on small bowel imaging

Unexplained malabsorption and protein-losing enteropathies

Intestinal lymphangiectasia, allergic or congestive enteropathies, etc.

Chronic abdominal pain with high suspicion of small bowel pathology

Motility disorders – not an ideal modality but may give an impression

Esophageal disorders

Esophagitis, Barrett's esophagus, esophageal varices

---

small bowel lymphomas (see Figure 15.5), intestinal lymphangiectasia (Figure 15.11), chronic intermittent intussusception and ischemic bowel disease as causes of recurrent abdominal pain by capsule endoscopy in adolescent patients (Figure 15.12). Capsule endoscopy can also be useful to ascertain the intestinal manifestations of immunodeficiency disorders and graft-versus-host disease, but in essence these remain histology-dependent diagnoses.

Recent developments

An esophageal capsule with a video camera at each end has been developed but its utility in children is somewhat limited as it is mainly aimed at esophageal cancer and varices in adults (Figure 15.13). Hence it has not drawn advocates in pediatric GI circles. Equally, the colon capsule has not caught on in children (Figure 15.14), possibly because this WCE device, with a delayed onset of imaging in order to focus on the colon, requires extremely good bowel prep. In addition, the difference in the pediatric GI world is that we require tissue diagnosis generally with biopsies.

One interesting recent evolution is that of the magnetically controlled capsule that can be maneuvered in the upper GI tract by a strong external magnet (Figure 15.15). This may be helpful in acute GI bleeding scenarios; the disadvantage is that it requires the stomach to be filled with fluid for good 100% mucosal visualization and once into the duodenum, it can pass rapidly, precluding decent images of the duodenal cap. Once in the duodenum, the magnet is no longer strong enough to coax it back into the first part of the duodenum or stomach.

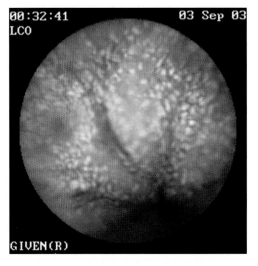

Figure 15.11 Intestinal lymphangiectasia.

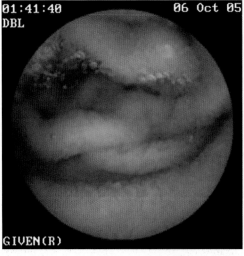
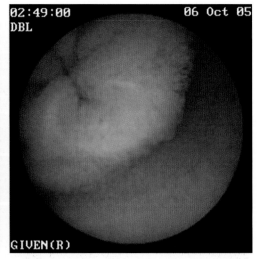

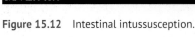

Figure 15.12 Intestinal intussusception.

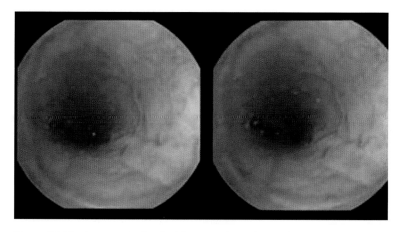

Figure 15.13 Images obtained with an esophageal capsule.

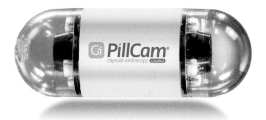

Figure 15.14 Colon capsule.

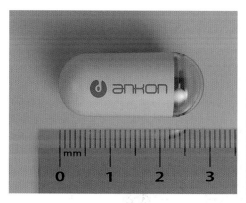
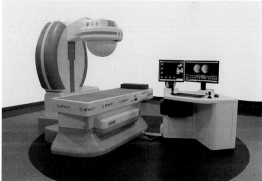

Figure 15.15 Mechanism for magnetic capsule propulsion.

Conclusion

Wireless capsule endoscopy represents an extraordinary technical innovation in diagnostic gastrointestinal endoscopy. As in adult patients, it opens new horizons that permit an accurate and noninvasive approach to identify occult lesions in the small bowel in children and adolescents. It can be successful even in infants as young as 6 months old.

 • See companion website for videos relating to this chapter topic: www.wiley.com/go/gershman3e

REFERENCES

1 Arguelles-Arias F, Caunedo A, Romero J, *et al.* The value of capsule endoscopy in pediatric patients with a suspicion of Crohn's disease. *Endoscopy* 2004, **36**, 869–873.

2 Barkay O, Moshkowitz M, Reif S. Crohn's disease diagnosed by wireless capsule endoscopy in adolescents with abdominal pain, protein-losing enteropathy, anemia and negative endoscopic and radiologic findings. *Isr Med Assoc J* 2005, **7**, 262–263.

3 Barth BA, Donovan K, Fox VL. Endoscopic placement of the capsule endoscope in children. *Gastrointest Endosc* 2004, **60**, 818–821.

4 Caspari R, von Falkenhausen M, Krautmacher C, Schild H, Heller J, Sauerbruch T. Comparison of capsule endoscopy and magnetic resonance imaging for the detection of polyps of the small intestine in patients with familial adenomatous polyposis or with Peutz–Jeghers' syndrome. *Endoscopy* 2004, **36**, 1054–1059.

5 Cellier C, Green PH, Collin P, Murray J. ICCE consensus for celiac disease. *Endoscopy* 2005, **37**, 1055–1059.

6 Costamagna G, Shah SK, Riccioni ME, *et al.* A prospective trial comparing small bowel radiographs and video capsule endoscopy for suspected small bowel disease. *Gastroenterology* 2002, **123**, 999–1005.

7 De Bona M, Bellumat A, de Boni M. Capsule endoscopy for the diagnosis and follow-up of blue rubber bleb nevus syndrome. *Dig Liver Dis* 2005, **37**, 451–453.

8 de Mascarenhas-Saraiva MN, da Silva Araujo Lopes LM. Small-bowel tumors diagnosed by wireless capsule endoscopy: report of five cases. *Endoscopy* 2003, **35**, 865–868.

9 Ell C, Remke S, May A, Helou L, Henrich R, Mayer G. The first prospective controlled trial comparing wireless capsule endoscopy with push enteroscopy in chronic gastrointestinal bleeding. *Endoscopy* 2002, **34**, 685–689.

10 Goldstein JL, Eisen GM, Lewis B, *et al.* Video capsule endoscopy to prospectively assess small bowel injury with celecoxib, naproxen plus omeprazole, and placebo. *Clin Gastroenterol Hepatol* 2005, **3**, 133–141.

11 Iddan G, Meron G, Glukhovsky A, Swain P. Wireless capsule endoscopy. *Nature* 2000, **405**, 417.

12 MacKenzie JF. Push enteroscopy. *Gastrointest Endosc Clin North Am* 1999, **9**, 29–36.

13 Maiden L, Thjodleifsson B, Theodors A, Gonzalez J, Bjarnason I. A quantitative analysis of NSAID-induced small bowel pathology by capsule enteroscopy. *Gastroenterology* 2005, **128**, 1172–1178.

14 Mata A, Bordas JM, Feu F, *et al.* Wireless capsule endoscopy in patients with obscure gastrointestinal bleeding: a comparative study with push enteroscopy. *Aliment Pharmacol Therapeut* 2004, **20**, 189–194.

15 Mihaly F, Nemeth A, Zagoni T, *et al.* Gastrointestinal manifestations of common variable immunodeficiency diagnosed by video- and capsule endoscopy. *Endoscopy* 2005, **37**, 603–604.

16 Murray JA, Brogan D, van Dyke C, Knipshield MA, Gostout CJ. Mapping the extent of untreated celiac disease with capsule enteroscopy. *Gastrointest Endosc* 2004, **59**, AB101.

17 Pennazio M, Eisen G, Goldfarb N. ICCE consensus for obscure intestinal bleeding. *Endoscopy* 2005, **37**, 1046–1050.

18 Pennazio M, Santucci R, Rondonotti E, *et al.* Outcome of patients with obscure gastrointestinal bleeding after capsule endoscopy: report of 100 consecutive cases. *Gastroenterology* 2004, **126**, 643–653.

19 Peretti N, Sant'Anna AMGA, Dirks MH, Seidman EG. Capsule endoscopy detects lymphangiectasia missed by other means. 4th International Conference on Capsule Endoscopy, Miami, FL, **7–8** March 2005, p. 189.

20 Petroniene R, Dubenco E, Baker JP, *et al.* Given capsule endoscopy in celiac disease: evaluation of diagnostic accuracy and interobserver variation. *Am J Gastroenterol* 2005, **100**, 685–694.

21 Sant'Anna AMGA, Seidman EG. Wireless capsule endoscopy: comparison study in pediatric and adult patients. *J Pediatr Gastroenterol Nutr* 2003, **37**, 332.

22 Sant'Anna AMGA, Dubois J, Miron MJ, Seidman EG. Wireless capsule endoscopy for obscure small bowel disorders: final results of the first pediatric controlled trial. *Clin Gastroenterol Hepatol* 2005, **3**, 264–270.

23 Schulmann K, Hollerbach S, Kraus K, *et al.* Feasibility and diagnostic utility of video capsule endoscopy for the detection of small bowel polyps in patients with hereditary polyposis syndromes. *Am J Gastroenterol* 2005, **100**, 27–37.

24 Seidman EG, Sant'Anna AMGA, Dirks MH. Potential applications of wireless capsule endoscopy in the pediatric age group. *Gastrointest Endosc Clin North Am* 2004, **14**, 207–218.

25 Soares J, Lopes L, Vilas Boas G, Pinho C. Wireless capsule endoscopy for evaluation of phenotypic expression of small-bowel polyps in patients with Peutz–Jeghers syndrome and in symptomatic first-degree relatives. *Endoscopy* 2004, **36**, 1060–1066.

26 Thomson M, Tringali A, Landi R, *et al.* ESPGHAN/ESGE Pediatric Endoscopy Guidelines. *J Pediatr Gastroenterol Nutr* 2017, **64**(1), 133–153.

27 Triester SL, Leighton JA, Gurudu SR, *et al.* A meta-analysis of capsule endoscopy (CE) compared to other modalities in patients with non-stricturing small bowel Crohn disease (NSCD). *Am J Gastroenterol* 2004, **99**, S271–S272.

28 Waye JD. Small-bowel endoscopy. *Endoscopy* 2003, **35**, 15–21.

29 Yakoub-Agha I, Maunoury V, Wacrenier A, *et al.* Impact of small bowel exploration using video-capsule endoscopy in the management of acute gastrointestinal graft-versus-host disease. *Transplantation* 2005, **79**, 1767.

30 Yamamoto H, Kita H, Sunada K, *et al.* Clinical outcomes of double-balloon endoscopy for the diagnosis and treatment of small-intestinal diseases. *Clin Gastroenterol Hepatol* 2004, **2**, 1010–1016.

16

Endoscopic ultrasonography

Simona Faraci, Luigi Dall'Oglio, Paola de Angelis, and Douglas S. Fishman

---

 KEY POINTS

- Radial (diagnostic) and linear (therapeutic) endoscopic ultrasound (EUS) allow transmural and extraluminal examination to take place.
- Extent of lesions can be accurately determined allowing targeted biopsies and endotherapy to be conducted.
- Fine needle aspiration (FNA) of lesions such as mediastinal lymph nodes can obtain tissue

which previously would have required operations such as thoracoscopy/thoracotomy or laparoscopy/laparotomy.
- In children, esophageal and pancreatobiliary congenital anomalies make up a higher percentage of indications for EUS than in adults.

Introduction

Endoscopic ultrasound (EUS) is a minimally invasive method that combines the advantages of ultrasound and endoscopy [1]. The main advantage of EUS compared to conventional gastrointestinal endoscopy is its unique capacity for detailed cross-sectional examination of the walls of the esophagus, stomach, duodenum, and rectum and detection of extraluminal lesions or structures within the surrounding compartments (e.g., the mediastinum) and acquisition of biological material through EUS-guided fine needle aspiration (EUS-FNA) [2–4]. The wall of the digestive tract on EUS appears as several hyperechoic and hypoechoic layers. The distortion of one or more of these layers will reflect the depth, size, and nature of the lesions.

Instruments and technique

Application of EUS falls into two main categories: diagnostic and interventional/therapeutic endosonography. The latter includes EUS-FNA and therapeutic procedures.

Over the last decade, innovations in EUS technology have significantly expanded utilization of EUS. Most EUS devices require an echo-transmitting physical medium (water), interposed between the probe and the anatomical structures being studied. In linear EUS, a latex balloon should be attached to the distal end of the scope and filled with water. A similar approach applies for examination of the esophagus with front-loading radial ultrasound probes. For the study of gastric lesions, water instead is injected directly into the stomach. For investigation of the duodenum

---

Practical Pediatric Gastrointestinal Endoscopy, Third Edition. Edited by George Gershman and Mike Thomson.
© 2021 John Wiley & Sons Ltd. Published 2021 by John Wiley & Sons Ltd.
Companion website: www.wiley.com/go/gershman3e

and rectum, it is useful to combine the two techniques [5]. The ultrasound transducer may have a frequency ranging from a minimum of 5 MHz to a maximum of 20 MHz and the scan can be radial or sectoral (Table 16.1).

Reported experience with standard EUS scopes and miniprobes in children is limited to a small series [6–8]. Only a few articles including approximately 50 cases are reported [9], partly because commercially available echo-endoscopes have a distal end diameter of 11–14 mm for radial probes and 14 mm for linear probes, which cannot traverse easily and without trauma from the first to the second portion of the duodenum in small children. The use of adult echo-endoscopes has been described in children >3 years with weight >15 kg [6]. In children less than 15 kg, the endobronchial ultrasound (EBUS) endoscope or miniprobes are a good and useful alternative. A recent multicenter study described the efficacy and safety of EBUS with transbronchial needle aspiration and endoscopic ultrasound with an echo-bronchoscope-guided FNA in children with mediastinal lymphadenopathy of undefined etiology [10].

Miniprobes can be used with standard endoscopes in small children when standard EUS scopes cannot be maneuvered through the narrowed esophageal or intestinal lumen [7,11–14].

Ultrasound catheter probe (radial EUS)

The high-frequency (12–25 MHz) ultrasound catheter probes (Figure 16.1) are designed to pass through the working channel of standard endoscopes, which is exceptionally important for EUS in small children and patients with luminal narrowing, making application of the linear echo-endoscope with a rigid 5–12 mm tip questionable or impossible [15,16]. These devices provide excellent recognition of structures within 5–20 mm from

Table 16.1 Commercially available echo-endoscopes and miniprobes

Manufacturer	Type	Product	Max diameter (mm)	Insertion tube diameter (mm)	Channel size (mm)
Pentax	Radial	EG-3670URK	n/a	12.1	2.4
	Linear	EG-3270UK	11.5	10.8	2.8
	Linear	EG-3870UTK	n/a	12.8	3.8
	EBUS (Linear)	EB-1970UK	6.3	n/a	2.0
Olympus	Mini-probe	UM2R/3R	2.5	n/a	n/a
	Radial	GF-UE160-AL5	13.8	11.8	2.2
	Linear	GF-UCT180	14.6	12.6	3.7
	Linear	GF-UC140P-AL5	14.2	11.8	2.8
	Linear	GF-UC140-AL5	14.6	12.6	3.7
	Linear	TGF-UC180J	14.6	12.6	3.7
	EBUS	BF-UC180F	n/a	6.2	2.2
Fujinon	Radial	EG-580UR	n/a	11.4	2.8
	Radial	EG-530UR2	11.4	11.5	2.2
	Linear	EG-580UT	13.9	n/a	3.8
	Linear	EG-530UT2	13.9	12.1	3.8
	EBUS	EB-530US	6.7	6.3	2.0

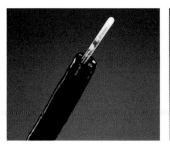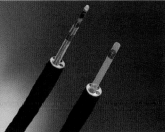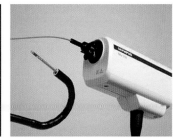

Figure 16.1   Ultrasound catheter probe.

the transducer and are very useful for examining the layers of the gastrointestinal wall.

Front-loading ultrasound probe

The diagnostic potential of a standard high-frequency ultrasound catheter probe is quite limited when the lesions are large or broad-based. To insure high-quality EUS scanning of large lesions with deep penetration into and/or beyond the wall of the GI tract, a low-frequency 7.5 MHz front-loading probe was developed [15,17] (Figure 16.2).

Radial endoscopic ultrasonography

Radial endoscopic ultrasonography allows complete examination of large areas of the gastrointestinal tract and adjacent organs with simple and rapid visualization of these structures. The direction of scanning is perpendicular to the longitudinal axis of the device, producing a full 360° field of view. The

available high-frequency miniaturized probes can be used with standard endoscopes for evaluation of stenotic areas or small superficial lesions.

Balloon contact method

This method requires filling of the balloon at the tip of the echo-endoscope with 1–7 mL of deaerated water and direct contact between the balloon and the wall of the GI tract. It is used primarily for evaluation of the esophagus and pancreatobiliary system and adjacent lesions.

Water-filling method

In this method, the deaerated water is pumped into the GI tract through the working channel of the echo-endoscope until the lumen is adequately distended. The volume of water varies between 100 and 500 mL. This method is useful to evaluate the penetration depth of GI lesions, for example for cancer staging.

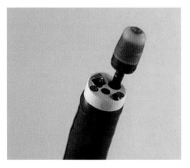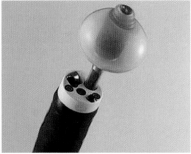

Figure 16.2   Front-loading ultrasound probe.

Balloon contact plus water-filling method

This is a combination of the two methods and is useful for GI tract lesions and lesions of the papilla of Vater [18] (Figure 16.3).

Linear endoscopic ultrasonography

The linear echo-endoscope has a curved laterally oriented transducer providing a 120° sector scanning ultrasound view (Figure 16.4).

Although linear EUS is designed for one-sided sectoral scanning, a complete 360° image can be achieved by clockwise and/or counterclockwise torques of the scope in small incremental steps.

The working channel opens just above the transducer (Figure 16.5) which is ideal for safe and effective use of FNA procedures because the needle and the target lesion are within the same ultrasound view (Figure 16.6).

The parallel orientation of the ultrasonic beam to the longitudinal axis of the instrument allows precise navigation of the FNA needle to the target lesion for cytological sampling or therapeutic manipulations (Figure 16.7).

This technique is particularly important for the diagnosis and treatment of conditions including pancreatobiliary tumors, mediastinal lymph node in patients with suspected TB or sarcoidosis, and other pathology. The wide (3.8 mm) instrumental channel of some lineal echo-endoscopes allows passage of accessories up to 10 Fr in diameter. The instruments with an electronic transducer have color Doppler and power Doppler signals.

Needles for FNA are equipped with a handle connected to the operator channel of the echo-endoscope. The needle flows inside a metal or plastic protective sheath, which simplifies

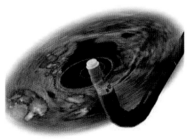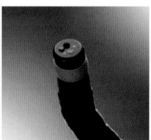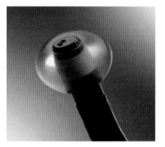

Figure 16.3 Radial scan ultrasound. Distal tip of echo-endoscope with balloon inflation.

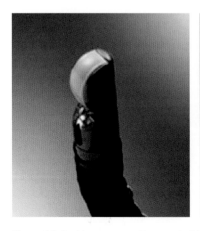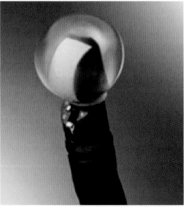

Figure 16.4 Linear scan ultrasound video endoscope. Distal tip of echo-endoscope with balloon inflation.

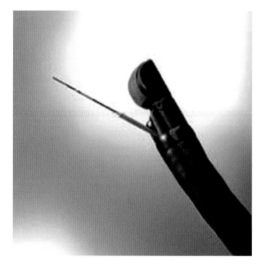

Figure 16.5 The linear probe with advanced aspiration/biopsy needle.

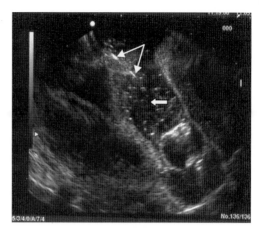

Figure 16.6 EUS of the needle (*double arrow*) advanced into a pancreatic pseudocyst (*solid arrow*).

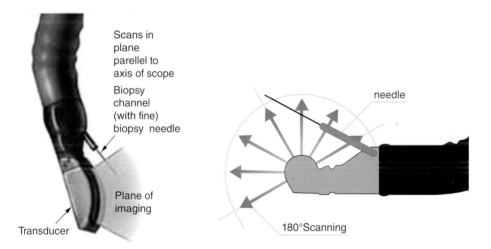

Figure 16.7 Orientation of a FNA needle advanced through the operative channel under direct EUS control.

manipulations. The needles are available in three sizes: 19, 22, and 25 G. The aspiration system consists of a negative pressure syringe connected to a tap, which is opened after having engaged the needle system [19,20]. An application of the color Doppler modality of the linear EUS scope with electronic transducer substantially reduces an accidental puncture of neighboring vessels.

Once the needle has been advanced into the lesion safely, changing the penetration angle and rapid withdrawal of the needle are helpful for better tissue sampling. The collected specimen is placed in fixative solution for histology and other histochemical and cytogenetic studies.

Appearance of the gastrointestinal wall on EUS images

Under low-frequency (7.5 MHz) EUS scanning, the walls of the esophagus, stomach, and rectum appear as five concentric layers that alternate according to the echogenicity. From the inside out, the first two hyper- and hypoechoic layers correspond to the mucosa and muscularis mucosa; the third hyperechoic layer is associated with the submucosa; the fourth hypoechoic layer represents muscularis propria; and the fifth hyperechoic layer is related to the serosa (Figure 16.8).

Due to the relatively thin wall of the esophagus, it is not easy to distinguish mucosa and submucosa. In the stomach, the fourth layer (muscularis propria) may consist of two sublayers (inner circular muscle and outer longitudinal muscle) divided by a hyperechoic line.

High-frequency (20 MHz) probes provide a better resolution of the wall architecture (up to nine layers) at the expense of depth of scanning of the surrounding structures. In contrast, many vital structures are within the reach of a low-frequency EUS. From the esophagus it is possible to study the posterior mediastinum: thoracic aorta, azygos vein,

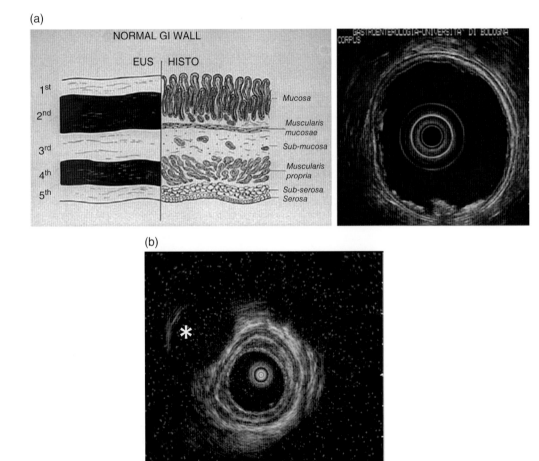

Figure 16.8 (a) Esophagus wall; the first inner hyperechoic (bright) layer is mucosa followed by hypoechoic (dark) muscularis mucosa, hyperechoic (bright) submucosa, hypoechoic (dark) muscularis propria, and hyperechoic (bright) serosa. An arrow points to the folded mucosa. (b) The extramural structure is marked by a star.

pulmonary arteries, and lymph nodes. EUS from the stomach provides access to the spleen, left adrenal gland, celiac tripod/axis, body and tail of pancreas, splenic vessels up to the portal vein, left lobe of liver and gallbladder. From the duodenum, the head of the pancreas, extrahepatic biliary ducts, major duodenal papilla, and right lobe of the liver can be visualized [21].

Indications in children

Endoscopic ultrasonography is a useful imaging technique that has applications for the pediatric population. In 2017, ESPGHAN-ESGE released their guidelines for pediatric gastrointestinal endoscopy. The panel of experts emphasized that proposed recommendations for EUS in children have been made based on low quality of evidence [22]. Pancreaticobiliary and duodenal indications include differentiation between autoimmune pancreatitis and neoplasm [23]; assessment of anatomy of the pancreas in pancreatitis [24] and biliary anatomical abnormalities [25]; pancreatic pseudocyst drainage and duodenal duplication cyst assessment [26,27].

ESPGHAN-ESGE suggested the following.

- The use of radial EUS with miniprobes to diagnose congenital esophageal strictures (tracheobronchial remnants vs fibromuscular stenosis subtypes).
- EUS for diagnosis of pancreatobiliary diseases in children in whom noninvasive imaging modalities (US, MRCP) are inconclusive.
- EUS-guided drainage of pancreatic pseudocyst in children should be performed in a large EUS center with specific expertise. Therapeutic EUS with drainage of pancreatic pseudocysts can be performed with the same technique described in adult patients or utilizing a miniprobe [6,8,28,29].

Indications for EUS in children are summarized in Table 16.2.

Table 16.2 Indications for EUS in children

Esophagus	• Esophageal stenosis (congenital, postcorrosive, postsurgical, etc.) • Eosinophilic esophagitis • Esophageal duplication • Vascular disease • Achalasia
Stomach	• Gastric duplication • Gastric varices • Masses, lymphoma • Hypertrophy of gastric folds
Duodenum	• Duodenal duplication • Duodenal web • Vascular disease • Submucosal tumor
Pancreatobiliary	• Choledocholithiasis and microlithiasis and other causes of biliary obstruction • Pancreatic pseudocysts (diagnosis and treatment), • Recurrent and chronic pancreatitis, autoimmune pancreatitis • Ampullary adenoma • Pancreatic trauma • Congenital anomalies (e.g., pancreas divisum) • Diagnosis, evaluation, and staging of mass lesions of the pancreas, tumors of the bile ducts, gallbladder and liver • Evaluation of retroperitoneal masses and lymphadenopathy • Evaluation of chronic intractable upper abdominal pain of suspected biliary-pancreatic etiology

In children, esophageal and pancreatobiliary congenital anomalies comprise a higher percentage of indications for EUS than in adults.

As mentioned above, successful application of EUS and EUS-guided FNA has been reported in children with pancreatobiliary diseases [23–25], in whom noninvasive imaging modalities (i.e., US, MRCP, CT, etc.) were inconclusive.

EUS features in pediatric diseases

Esophageal strictures

Esophageal strictures in children are predominantly benign and associated with many conditions including reflux and eosinophilic esophagitis, caustic ingestion, tuberculosis, post surgical (anastomotic), IgG4-related esophagitis, radiation and drug-induced esophageal injuries (Figures 16.9 and 16.10).

In children with congenital esophageal stenosis, miniprobe EUS can distinguish between tracheobronchial remnants (TBR) and fibromuscular stenosis (FMS). In congenital esophageal stenosis with TBR, there are multiple echogenic regions in the muscle layer that represent aberrant cartilaginous remnants. Patients with TBR often require surgical resection because of the increased risk of perforation during dilation. In contrast, patients with FMS or membranous stenosis can be treated safely with esophageal dilation [12,23]. EUS is

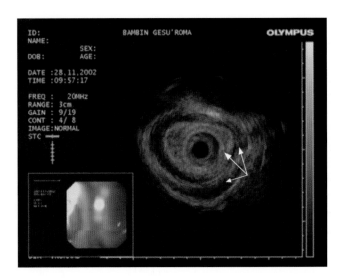

Figure 16.9 Esophageal anastomotic stenosis: thickening of concentric layers marked by arrows.

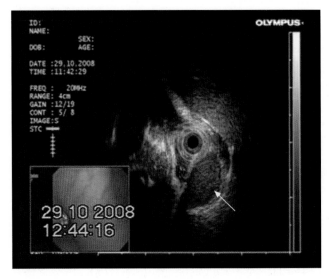

Figure 16.10 Esophageal duplication marked by arrow.

the best diagnostic test to distinguish between these conditions. High correlation between EUS miniprobe evidence of TBR and surgical findings has been documented [7]. Both high-frequency miniprobe and three-dimensional EUS have been used for preoperative evaluation of congenital esophageal stenosis in children [14]. After a pediatric endoscope is positioned just above the narrowed esophagus, the probe is inserted through the instrument channel and negotiated across the stricture. The miniprobe EUS procedure is performed using the direct contact method (Figure 16.11).

Other structural abnormalities of the esophageal wall and submucosal lesions such as esophageal duplications, malignant lesions, and lymphomas are generally well defined by EUS [30–33]. EUS is considered the primary diagnostic tool in preoperative staging of esophageal carcinoma.

Endoscopic treatment by mucosal EUS-guided resection is used effectively to treat Barrett's esophagus in adults. Barrett's esophagus has no specific EUS characteristics but only a slight thickening of the mucosa. However, if complicated by severe dysplasia, it shows infiltration of the underlying layers and lymphadenopathy [34]. To study Barrett's esophagus and other infiltrating lesions of the esophagus, it is necessary to utilize EUS at high frequency (e.g., 20 MHz).

EUS features of esophageal lesions are listed in Table 16.3.

Stomach

Many studies have shown that EUS is superior to CT in the staging of gastric tumors and associated lymph nodes. The information from EUS helps to indicate the surgical intervention, type of surgery, and any adjuvant chemotherapy. EUS assesses the degree of infiltration of the neoplasm in early and advanced stages. In pediatric patients it is very useful both in the rare cases of mass and of lymphoma.

Both the radial instrument and the miniprobe can be used in relation to age. Bowel or balloon filling is necessary for the study. Neoplastic lesions can infiltrate deeply into the gastric wall with complete disappearance of stratification [33] (Figures 16.12–16.14).

Congenital anomalies are common in children, for example duodenal duplication (Figure 16.15). In congenital duodenal duplications, EUS may identify anomalous pancreatobiliary ducts that may not be as well defined

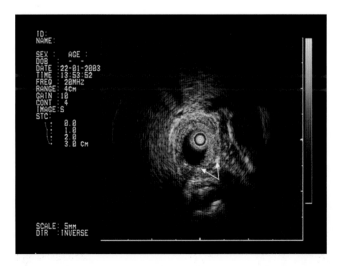

Figure 16.11 Congenital stenosis with aberrant cartilaginous remnants (*white dots*) indicated by arrows; thickening of layers consistent with congenital stenosis.

Table 16.3 EUS features in esophageal diseases

Disease	Layer	Feature
Caustic stenosis	Mucosa/muscularis mucosa	Subversion and dissection of the layers
Congenital stenosis	Mucosa/muscularis mucosa	Thickening of the layers
Eosinophilic esophagitis	Mucosa	Thin wall, variable thickness
Achalasia	Muscularis mucosa	Thickening of the layers
Varices	Mucosa/submucosa	Anechoic, tortuous, color Doppler
Duplication cyst	Variable	Hypoechoic, roundish, variable inside
Barrett's/esophageal cancer	Mucosa/submucosa/muscularis mucosa	Parietal thickening of esophagus with fusion of layers that involves the wall including muscle layers

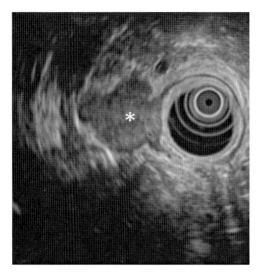

Figure 16.12 Gastrointestinal stromal tumor (GIST) (arising from submucosal layer; mass marked by asterisk).

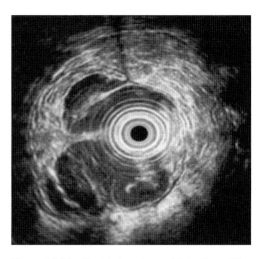

Figure 16.14 Gastric lymphoma (distortion of the gastric wall and enlarged lymph nodes).

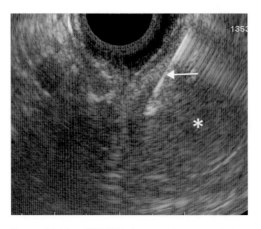

Figure 16.13 GIST-FNA. Arrow points toward the FNA within the labeled mass (asterisk).

by CT scan or MRCP [26,27]. This information is essential for choosing between surgical and endoscopic therapy.

The plicate hypertrophy of the stomach is amenable to study by EUS for differential diagnosis with lymphomas (Figure 16.16).

In case of duodenal web, it is important to perform EUS before endoscopic dilation or dissection to evaluate the thickness of the web and the outlet of the biliary tract [33–35] (Figure 16.17).

EUS features of the main lesions of the stomach are detailed in Table 16.4.

Pancreatobiliary ducts

Given its high accuracy and sensitivity, EUS is particularly effective in evaluating pancreatobiliary

Figure 16.15 Duodenal duplication.

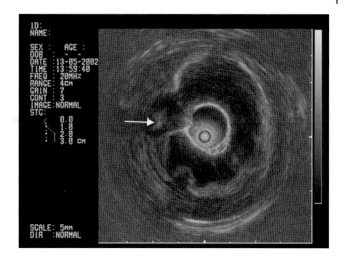

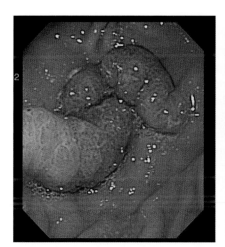

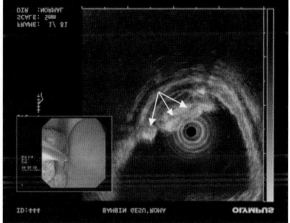

Figure 16.16 Plicate hypertrophy of the stomach related to *Helicobacter pylori*.

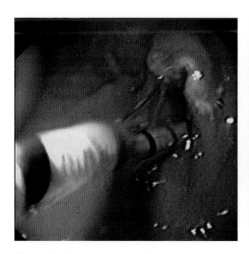

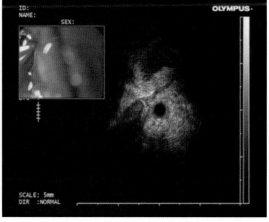

Figure 16.17 Duodenal web.

Table 16.4 EUS features in gastric pathology

Disease	Layer	Feature
Leiomyoma	Mucosa/muscularis mucosa	Hypoechogenic, roundish, net margins
Lipoma	Submucosa	Echogenic, smooth margins
Cyst	Variable	Hypoechogenic, roundish
Aberrant pancreas	Submucosa/muscularis mucosa	Hypoechoic, mixed, bile ducts?
Varices	Mucosa/submucosa	Size, depth, tortuousity, color Doppler
Gastrointestinal stromal tumor	Muscularis mucosa	<3 cm hypoechoic, net margins; >3 cm cystic weakness, irregular margins
Lynphoma	Mucosa/submucosae/ muscularis mucosa	Hypoechogenic

diseases. One of the important benefits of EUS is a reduction of unnecessary diagnostic ERCP [10,29,30]. The diagnosis of lithiasis or microlithiasis of the common bile duct by EUS is superior to conventional ultrasound technique (Figure 16.18).

In children with chronic pancreatitis, EUS is more sensitive than CT scan, especially in the early stage of the disease, and helps to depict the focal or diffuse changes of the pancreatic parenchyma such as echogenic foci, interlobular septa, small cystic cavities, lobulated glandular margins, parenchymal heterogeneity, and pancreatic ducts/ectasia of collateral branches (Figure 16.19).

In children with pancreatic pseudocysts, it is often necessary to perform an internal drainage through the stomach (Figure 16.20). For a detailed description of pancreatic cystogastrostomy see Chapter 38. Complications related to

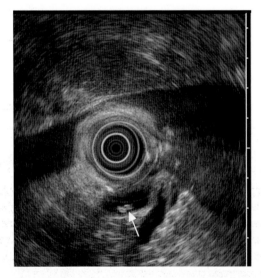

Figure 16.18 Choledocholithiasis: two stones (*arrow*) in the dilated common bile duct. Solid arrow points toward the dilated main pancreatic duct.

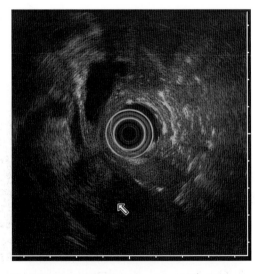

Figure 16.19 Autoimmune pancreatitis (white arrow pointing at fullness in pancreatic head).

(a)

(b)

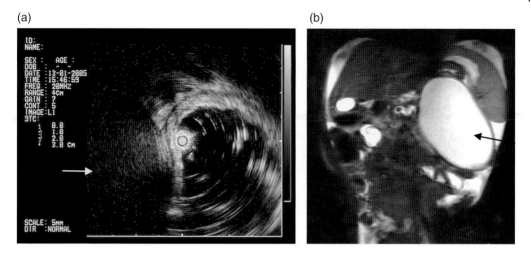

Figure 16.20 Pancreatic pseudocyst. (a) Hypoechoic/anechoic cyst (*white arrow*). (b) MRI view of pseudocyst (*black arrow*).

Table 16.5 EUS features of the cystic and mass lesions of the pancreas and biliary ducts

Disease	Features
Neuroendocrine tumors	Tiny, discrete, encapsulated, hypoechoic mass lesions, often along the anterior/posterior surface of pancreas. High vascularity on color Doppler. Large tumors show cystic and necrotic areas
Pseudocysts	Large and hypoechogenic. Well-formed fibrous wall
Pancreatitis	Variable, heterogeneous with hypo- and hyperechogenic areas
Lithiasis of the common bile	Hyperechogenic lesions evident in the common bile duct
Portal hypertension	Use of Doppler

this intervention (perforation or bleeding) can be prevented by EUS.

EUS with FNA allows precise histological analysis and differential diagnosis of cystic lesions/tumors of the pancreas and biliary ducts (Table 16.5).

Overall, current data support a high diagnostic value of EUS in many pancreatobiliary conditions including cholelithiasis, recurrent, chronic and autoimmune pancreatitis, idiopathic fibrosing pancreatitis, pancreas divisum, congenital anomalies, microlithiasis, pancreatic pseudocysts, and pancreatic mass lesions [19,35–43]. Therapeutic EUS with pancreatic fluid collection in children appears promising, although larger prospective studies

will be needed for conclusion [44]. EUS and EUS-guided interventions could alter clinical management in pediatric patients and should be considered in some challenging cases of pancreatobiliary disorders [45].

EUS is shown to be a safe and cost-effective modality with both diagnostic and therapeutic capabilities in the pediatric population. It is now increasingly being recognized as a standard of care when evaluating pancreatobiliary conditions in children [40].

 • See companion website for videos relating to this chapter topic: www.wiley.com/go/gershman3e

REFERENCES

1 Fusaroli P, Vallar R, Caletti G, *et al*. Scientific publications in endoscopic ultrasonography: a 20-year global survey of the literature. *Endoscopy* 2002, **34**(6), 451–456.

2 Fusaroli P, Caletti G. Endoscopic ultrasonography. *Endoscopy* 2003, **35**(2), 127–135.

3 Williams DB, Sahai AV, Aabakken L, *et al*. Endoscopic ultrasound guided fine needle aspiration biopsy: a large single centre experience. *Gut* 1999, **44**, 720–726.

4 Mortensen MB, Pless T, Durup J *et al*. Clinical impact of endoscopic ultrasound-guided fine-needle aspiration biopsy in patients with upper gastrointestinal tract malignancies: a prospective study. *Endoscopy* 2001, **33**, 478–483.

5 Akahoshi K, Tanaka T, Matsui N *et al*. Newly developed all in one EUS system: one cart system, forward-viewing optics type 360° electronic radial array echoendoscope and obliqueviewing type convex array echoendoscope. *Fukuoka Acta Med* 2007, **98**, 82–89.

6 Sheers I, Ergun MA, Aouattah T, *et al*. Diagnostic and therapeutic roles of endoscopic ultrasound in pediatric pancreatobiliary disorders. *J Pediatr Gastroenterol Nutr* 2015, **61**, 238–247.

7 Romeo E, Foschia F, de Angelis P, *et al*. Endoscopic management of congenital esophageal stenosis. *J Pediatr Surg* 2011, **46**(5), 838–841.

8 Jazrawi SF, Barth BA, Sreenarasimhaiah J. Efficacy of endoscopic ultrasound guided drainage of pancreatic pseudocyst in a pediatric population. *Dig Dis Sci* 2011, **56**, 902–908.

9 Al Rashdam A, LeBlanc J, Sherman S, *et al*. Role of endoscopic ultrasound for evaluating gastrointestinal tract disorders in pediatrics: a tertiary care center experience. *J Pediatr Gastroenterol Nutr* 2010, **51**, 718–722.

10 Dhooria S, Madan K, Pattabhiraman V, *et al*. A multicenter study on the utility and safety of EBUS-TBNA and EUS-B-FNA in children. *Pediatr Pulmonol* 2016, **51**(10), 1031–1039.

11 Usui N, Kamata S, Kawahara H, *et al*. Uses of endoscopic ultrasonography in the diagnosis of congenital esophageal stenosis. *J Pediatr Surg* 2002, **37**, 1744–1746.

12 Quiros JA, Hirose S, Patino M, *et al*. Esophageal tracheobronchial remnant, EUS diagnosis and minimally invasive surgical management. *J Pediatr Gastroenterol Nutr* 2013, **56**(30), e14.

13 Takamizawa S,Tsugawa C, Mouri N, *et al*. Congenital esophageal stenosis: therapeutic strategy based on aetiology. *J Pediatr Surg* 2002, **37**, 197–201.

14 Bocus P, Realdon S, Eloubeidi MA, *et al*. High-frequency miniprobes and 3-dimensional EUS for preoperative evaluation of the etiology of congenital esophageal stenosis in children (with video). *Gastrointest Endosc* 2011, **74**(1), 204–207.

15 Hocke M. Basic of radial endoscopic ultrasound. In: Dietrich CF (ed.). Endoscopic Ultrasound: An Introductory Manual and Atlas. Thieme, Stuttgart, 2006, p. 1.

16 Menzel J, Domschke W. Gastrointestinal miniprobe sonography: the current status. *Am J Gastroenterol* 2000, **95**, 605–616.

17 Chak A, Canto M, Stevens PD, *et al*. Clinical applications of a new through-the-scope ultrasound probe: prospective comparison with an ultrasound endoscope. *Gastrointest Endosc* 1997, **45**(3), 291–295.

18 LeBlanc JK. An overview of endoscopic ultrasound equipment. *Minerva Gastroenterol Dietol* 2008, **54**(2), 177–187.

19 Iwashita T, Nakai Y, Lee JG, *et al*. Newly-developed, forward-viewing echoendoscope: a comparative pilot study to the standard echoendoscope in the imaging of abdominal organs and feasibility of endoscopic ultrasound-guided interventions. *J Gastroenterol Hepatol* 2012, **27**(2), 362–367.

20 Irisawa A, Imaizumi H, Hikichi T, *et al*. Feasibility of interventional endoscopic ultrasound using forward-viewing and curved linear-array echoendoscope: a

literature review. *Dig Endosc* 2010, **22** Suppl 1, S128–131.

21 Tio TL, Tytgat GN. Endoscopic ultrasonography of normal and pathologic upper gastrointestinal wall structure. Comparison of studies in vivo and in vitro with histology. *Scand J Gastroenterol* 1986, **123**, 27–33.

22 Thomson M, Tringali A, Dumonceau JM, *et al*. Pediatric gastrointestinal endoscopy: European Society for Pediatric Gastroenterology Hepatology and Nutrition and European Society of Gastrointestinal Endoscopy guidelines. *J Pediatr Gastroenterol Nutr* 2017, **64**(1), 133–163.

23 Friedlander J, Quiros JA, Morgan T, *et al*. Diagnosis of autoimmune pancreatitis vs neoplasms in children with pancreatic mass and biliary obstruction. *Clin Gastroenterol Hepatol* 2012, **10**(9), 1051–1055.

24 Attila T, Adler DG, Hilden K, *et al*. EUS in pediatric patients. *Gastrointest Endosc* 2009, **70**(5), 892–898.

25 Varadarajulu S, Wilcox CM, Eloubeidi MA. Impact of EUS in the evaluation of pancreaticobiliary disorders in children. *Gastrointest Endosc* 2005, **62**(2), 239–244.

26 Romeo E, Torroni F, Foschia F, *et al*. Surgery or endoscopy to treat duodenal duplications in children. *J Pediatr Surg* 2011, **46**(5), 874–878.

27 Stelling T, von Rooij WJ,Tio TL, *et al*. Pancreatitis associated with congenital duodenal duplication cyst in an adult. *Endoscopy* 1987, **19**, 171–173.

28 Ramesh J, Bang JY, Trevino J, *et al*. Endoscopic ultrasound-guided drainage of pancreatic fluid collections in children. *J Pediatr Gastroenterol Nutr* 2013, **56**, 30–35.

29 De Angelis P, Romeo E, Rea F, *et al*. Miniprobe EUS in management of pancreatic pseudocyst. *World J Gastrointest Endosc* 2013, **5**, 255–260.

30 Brand B, Oesterhelweg L, Binmoeller KF, *et al*. Impact of endoscopic ultrasound for evaluation of submucosal lesions in gastrointestinal tract. *Dig Liver Dis* 2002, **34**, 290–297.

31 Zhu X, Zhang XQ, Li BM, *et al*. Esophageal mesenchymal tumors: endoscopy, pathology and immunohistochemistry. *World J Gastroenterol* 2007, **13**(5), 768–773.

32 Turhan N, Aydog G, Ozin Y, *et al*. Endoscopic ultrasonography-guided fine-needle aspiration for diagnosing upper gastrointestinal submucosal lesions: a prospective study of 50 cases. *Diagn Cytopathol* 2011, **39**(11), 808–817.

33 Lugering N, Menzel J, Kucharzik T, *et al*. Impact of miniprobes compared to conventional endosonography in the staging of low-grade gastric MALT lymphoma. *Endoscopy* 2001, **33**, 832–837.

34 Scotiniotis IA,Kochman ML, Lewis JD, *et al*. Accuracy of EUS in the evaluation of Barrett's esophagus and high grade dysplasia or intramucosal carcinoma. *Gastrointest Endosc* 2001, **54**, 689–686.

35 Menzel J, Domschke W. Intraductal ultrasound in the biliary tract. *Curr Gastroenterol Rep* 2001, **3**, 141–146.

36 Frossard JL, Sosa-Valencia L, Amouyal G, *et al*. Usefulness of endoscopic ultrasonography in patients with "idiopathic" acute pancreatitis. *Am J Med* 2000, **109**, 1196–2000.

37 Bhutani MS, Hoffman BJ, Hawes RH. Diagnosis of pancreas divisum by endoscopic ultrasonography. *Endoscopy* 1999, **31**, 167–169.

38 Nadler EP, Novikov A, Landzberg BR, *et al*. The use of endoscopic ultrasound in the diagnosis of solid pseudopapillary tumors of the pancreas in children. *J Pediatr Surg* 2002, **37**, 1370–1373.

39 Buxbaum JL, Eloubeidi MA, Varadarajulu S. Utility of EUS-guided FNA in the management of children with idiopathic fibrosing pancreatitis. *J Pediatr Gastroenterol Nutr* 2011, **52**(4), 482–484.

40 Patel S, Marshak J, Daum F, Iqbal S. The emerging role of endoscopic ultrasound for pancreaticobiliary diseases in the pediatric population. *World J Pediatr* 2017, **13**(4), 300–306.

41 Singh SK, Srivastava A, Rai P, Yachha SK, Poddar U. Yield of endoscopic ultrasound in children and adolescent with acute recurrent pancreatitis. *J Pediatr Gastroenterol Nutr* 2018, **66**(3), 461–465.

42 Fugazza A, Bizzarri B, Gaiani F, *et al.* The role of endoscopic ultrasound in children with pancreatobiliary and gastrointestinal disorders: a single center series and review of the literature. *BMC Pediatr* 2017, **17**(1), 203.

43 Fujii LL, Chari ST, El-Youssef M, *et al.* Pediatric pancreatic EUS-guided trucut biopsy for evaluation of autoimmune pancreatitis. *Gastrointest Endosc* 2013, **77**(5), 824–828.

44 Nabi Z, Talukdar R, Reddy DN. Endoscopic management of pancreatic fluid collections in children. *Gut Liver* 2017, **11**(4), 474–480.

45 Gordon K, Conway J, Evans J, Petty J, Fortunato JE, Mishra G. EUS and EUS-guided interventions alter clinical management in children with digestive diseases. *J Pediatr Gastroenterol Nutr* 2016, **63**(2), 242–246.

17

Chromoendoscopy

Mike Thomson and Paul Hurlstone

 KEY POINTS

- Chromoendoscopy facilitates optimal mucosal sampling, for example, in children with Barrett's esophagus, celiac sprue, polyposis syndromes, and long history of inflammatory bowel disease.

- The technique of mucosal staining is simple and adds only a few minutes to a routine endoscopic procedure.
- It is an essential part of enhanced magnification endoscopy or magnification chromoendoscopy.

Indications

Esophageal disorders

One potential indication of chromoendoscopy in the pediatric esophagus is intestinal metaplasia, i.e., Barrett's esophagus. If this condition is suspected, the main aim of chromoendoscopy is to help increase the diagnostic yield of endoscopic biopsies. Positive staining with methylene blue could also be used to identify endoscopically invisible intestinal metaplasia of the cardia region which may exist in patients with GERD. However, it is questionable if methylene blue staining should be applied to all patients with long-standing GERD who undergo upper endoscopy, since intestinal metaplasia can also be found in asymptomatic individuals and the advantage of methylene blue staining over random biopsy is controversial. In adult patients with short-segment Barrett's esophagus, the sensitivity of methylene blue staining for the detection of

intestinal metaplasia varies from 60% to 98%, but is generally higher than that of random biopsies. Abnormal methylene blue staining can also be helpful in delineating dysplastic or malignant areas for endoscopic treatment such as mucosal resection or photodynamic therapy. If mucosectomy is planned, a minimum amount of methylene blue injected with saline into the underlying submucosa which stain it blue, thereby facilitating an accurate removal of the mucosal lesion.

In patients who have undergone mucosal ablation, chromoendoscopy could also help distinguish the regenerating squamous epithelium from residual Barrett's mucosa. Lugol's solution has also been used in follow-up endoscopic examination of young patients who have been treated for Barrett's esophagus or dysplasia, in order to promptly detect remnants of unstained Barrett's epithelium.

Studies in adults have shown that chromoendoscopy with Lugol's solution is superior to conventional endoscopy for the detection of

Practical Pediatric Gastrointestinal Endoscopy, Third Edition. Edited by George Gershman and Mike Thomson.
© 2021 John Wiley & Sons Ltd. Published 2021 by John Wiley & Sons Ltd.
Companion website: www.wiley.com/go/gershman3e

severe dysplasia and early squamous cell carcinoma of the esophagus. In a Chinese population with a high esophageal cancer rate, chromoendoscopy with Lugol's solution showed a sensitivity of 62–96% and specificity of 63%. However, esophageal dysplasia and cancer are extremely uncommon in pediatric patients and it should be kept in mind that Lugol's solution can also stain an inflamed esophageal mucosa, namely reflux esophagitis.

Other staining techniques such as indigo carmine and acetic acid have been proposed in association with magnification endoscopy to detect Barrett's esophagus and dysplasia. Staining with toluidine blue has been reported to have a very high (98%) sensitivity for Barrett's esophagus, but cannot distinguish between gastric and intestinal metaplasia.

Although studies in adults have shown promising results, so far there are insufficient data supporting routine use of chromoendoscopy for detecting Barrett's esophagus and dysplasia in children.

Helicobacter pylori infection and related disorders

To date, there are no clear-cut indications for the use of chromoendoscopy to detect specific gastric disorders in clinical practice. At least two reactive dyes, however, deserve attention and may prove useful in the near future. Congo red stains acid-secreting mucosa and has been used in adult patients to detect gastric atrophy, which appears as an area of negative staining on the dark blue/black background of the normal mucosa of the gastric fundus and body. Phenol red turns from yellow to red in the presence of alkaline pH, such as that related to the hydrolysis of urea by urease-producing *H. pylori*, and has been used to map the extent of *H. pylori* colonization in the stomach. Both these staining techniques could, therefore, find an application in pediatric patients with long-standing or refractory *H. pylori* infection.

Celiac disease

Gluten-sensitive enteropathy (celiac disease) usually result in endoscopically visible changes of the duodenal mucosa, including a "mosaic" pattern, loss or indentation (scalloping) of Kerckring's folds, and a visible vascular pattern. Chromoendoscopy with methylene blue emphasizes the mosaic pattern, although it does not seem to increase the diagnostic yield of endoscopy, at least when performed by experienced gastroenterologists. In one study, indigo carmine scattering combined with magnification endoscopy proved superior to standard endoscopy for the detection of small bowel enteropathy, mainly because it was able to distinguish between total and partial villous atrophy. However, since the diagnosis of celiac disease is established by histology and not by endoscopy, duodenal biopsies should be taken whenever celiac disease is suspected, irrespective of the endoscopic appearance of the duodenal mucosa. Therefore, the major contribution of chromoendoscopy in celiac disease is to allow for better targeting – and consequently some sparing – of duodenal biopsies.

Polyposis syndromes

Chromoendoscopy may be very useful to detect smaller lesions in the duodenum of patients with familial adenomatous polyposis (FAP). Small flat duodenal adenomas may, in fact, go unnoticed during standard endoscopy and even capsule endoscopy, but can be identified as negative-staining lesions when an absorptive dye such as methylene blue is sprayed onto the mucosa. In *colonic polyposis*, the main aim of chromoendoscopy is the same as in the duodenum, i.e., to increase the detection rate by facilitating the identification of small flat polyps, especially adenomas. The preferred dye for the detection of colonic polyps is indigo carmine, a contrast stain that pools in areas of mucosal irregularity and often gives a three-dimensional effect, which is particularly useful for the detection of small protruding lesions. Needless to say, magnification endoscopy and high-resolution endoscopy can add to the accuracy of the technique. In adult studies, left-sided or total colonic indigo carmine staining significantly increased the detection rate of small flat or depressed adenomas. Chromoendoscopy can also help distinguish between hyperplastic and adenomatous polyps, as they produce different staining patterns. In a recent multicenter study, more than 90% of colonic polyps were correctly classified according to the staining pattern, and for adenomatous polyposis, the sensitivity and specificity were 82% and the negative predictive value was 88%.

Inflammatory bowel disease

In inflammatory bowel disease (IBD), the greatest potential for chromoendoscopy is the ability to detect dysplasia or cancer early in patients with long-standing ulcerative colitis. Colonic dysplasia and colitis-related colon cancer may also, occasionally, be a problem in pediatric patients, as in the case of ulcerative colitis presenting before 10 years of age, especially if associated with sclerosing cholangitis. In a randomized controlled trial on 174 patients with long-standing ulcerative colitis, total colonic methylene blue staining was clearly superior to conventional surveillance endoscopy with biopsy for the detection of early neoplasia (32 versus 10 overall intraepithelial lesions; 24 versus 8 low-grade and 24 versus 10 in flat mucosa).

Other indications

In the duodenal bulb, methylene blue spray can help identify areas of gastric metaplasia, which is a marker of inflammation such as that related to *H. pylori* infection. Methylene blue was also used to identify the minor papilla in patients with pancreas divisum.

Application technique

Equipment

Special reusable spray catheters such as those used for ERCP (e.g., Olympus PW-5L1) are

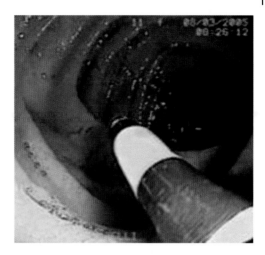

Figure 17.1 The tip of a pediatric ERCP catheter pushed through the biopsy channel is seen in the distal duodenum, prior to dye spraying.

preferable. The biopsy channel of all modern pediatric video-endoscopes allows the passage of such catheters (Figure 17.1). It is also convenient to use a new biopsy channel cap in order to minimize the leakage of dye. Endoscopists and support staff with less experience in chromoendoscopy should be particularly careful, as most dyes can produce a fairly persistent staining of skin and clothing. Depending on the specific indication and need, different types of stains can be used, such as stains that are absorbed by the mucosa (vital stains), stains that produce contrast (reactive stains), and stains for tattooing of the mucosa (Table 17.1).

Methylene blue

Methylene blue is actively absorbed by the intestinal epithelium and does not stain nonabsorptive tissues such as the normal esophageal or gastric mucosa. Optimal staining requires washing of the mucosa with a mucolytic agent such as N-acetylcysteine prior to spraying a 0.25–0.5% solution of the dye, and subsequent washing with water. The absorptive intestinal epithelium – including metaplastic epithelium as in Barrett's esophagus – is stained blue, whereas the nonabsorptive

Table 17.1 Types of staining

Dye (%)	Staining mechanism	Color	Main clinical application(s)
Methylene blue (0.5%)	Absorption into intestinal epithelial cells	Blue	Intestinal metaplasia in esophagus (Barrett's)
			Intestinal metaplasia in stomach
			Gastric metaplasia in duodenum (*negative staining*)
			Celiac disease
Lugol's solution (1–5%)	Binding to glycogen-containing cells	Dark green/brown or black	Squamous esophageal cancer (*negative staining*)
			Residual postablation Barrett's (*negative staining*)
			Esophagitis (*negative staining*)
Toluidine blue (1%)	Binding to nuclear DNA of malignant cells	Blue	Squamous esophageal cancer
Indigo carmine (0.1–0.5%)	Pools in mucosal crevices and pits	Indigo (blue-violet)	Small, flat or superficial polyps Barrett's esophagus
			Dysplasia or cancer in ulcerative colitis
Congo red (0.3–0.5%)	Stains acid-producing mucosa (pH <3)	Turns red to dark blue/black	Mapping of acid-secreting mucosa
			Gastric cancer, gastric atrophy and intestinal metaplasia (*negative staining*)
Phenol red (0.1%)	Stains alkalinized mucosa	Turns yellow to red	Mapping of *H. pylori*-infected mucosa
			Gastric metaplasia (*negative staining*)
India ink (1%)	Staining of mucosa at site of injection	Black (permanent)	Site of endoscopically removed polyp

Source: Reproduced with permission from Kiesslich R, Neurath MF. Surveillance colonoscopy in ulcerative colitis: magnifying chromoendoscopy in the spotlight. *Gut* 2004, **53**, 165–167.

epithelium – such as ectopic gastric metaplasia – is delineated as an area of negative staining against a blue-stained background. The presence of dysplasia or early malignancy within Barrett's epithelium results in inhomogeneous staining, as a consequence of the differential absorption of methylene blue from cells that are depleted of goblet cells and have less cytoplasm.

Methylene blue is generally considered to be safe. However, it has been reported that, once photosensitized by white light, methylene blue may induce oxidative damage of the DNA and although it does not usually stain the dysplastic intestinal epithelium, there is concern that it may increase the risk of carcinogenesis in patients with Barrett's esophagus. The parents of patients in whom methylene blue staining is being used should be warned that their child's urine and stool might temporarily acquire a green-bluish color.

Lugol's solution

Lugol's solution contains iodine, which has a special affinity for the glycogen contained in squamous epithelia. For this reason, it is most commonly used in the esophagus, where the normal squamous epithelium is stained green/brown to dark brown or black. Malignancy, dysplasia, metaplasia or even simple inflammation is associated with glycogen depletion and the affected mucosa will thus appear as an unstained area on a dark stained background. Severe allergic reactions to iodine have been reported, so allergy to iodine should be carefully excluded in patients who are undergoing chromoendoscopy with Lugol's solution.

Toluidine blue

Toluidine blue is a basic dye that binds to the nuclear DNA of epithelial cells, and can, therefore, be used to identify tissues with an increased DNA synthesis such as malignancy. Toluidine blue staining has mainly been used in endoscopic screening for malignant gastric ulcers and early squamous esophageal cancers in at-risk populations, such as heavy alcohol drinkers and smokers.

Indigo carmine

Indigo carmine is the most widely used contrast stain, and is especially useful to identify and define the margins of neoplastic lesions. Indigo carmine, in fact, typically pools in areas of mucosal irregularity, which are stained indigo (blue/violet) color. After washing, pits, grooves and edges of the lesion are highlighted and this may produce a three-dimensional effect, which is particularly useful for the detection of small superficial lesions. Indigo carmine at a concentration of 0.1–0.5% is usually sprayed onto the gut mucosa, but may also be given orally in a capsule. Although mostly utilized to identify small superficial polyps, indigo carmine has been applied in several other conditions such as Barrett's esophagus, gastric cancer, sprue, and ulcerative colitis.

Congo red

Congo red reacts to an acidic pH by changing from red to dark blue or black. Its major application is the identification and mapping of nonsecretory gastric mucosa such as that of gastric atrophy, intestinal metaplasia and gastric cancer, which will appear red in contrast to blue/black secretory areas. A stimulation of acid production with pentagastrin is therefore necessary before staining.

Phenol red

Phenol red is also a reactive dye, but unlike Congo red it reacts to an alkaline pH by changing from yellow to red. Patients should undergo pretreatment with a proton pump inhibitor and an anticholinergic, plus the local application of a mucolytic. Once 0.1% phenol red and 5% urea have been sprayed onto the gastric mucosa of *H. pylori*-infected individuals, the alkalinized mucosa is stained red whereas areas of intestinal metaplasia in the stomach will stain negative.

Acetic acid

Acetic acid is a newcomer to GI chromoendoscopy. Preliminary studies suggest that acetic acid stain may help identify Barrett's esophagus as well as duodenal atrophy in celiac disease, by delineating the features of the metaplastic or atrophic intestinal epithelium.

India ink

When injected into the mucosa, 1% India ink produces a permanent black staining. India ink can be injected superficially into the mucosa to mark the site where a worrisome polyp has been endoscopically removed, or it can be injected deeper to mark a lesion that has to be removed surgically.

Patient sedation

As the main aim of chromoendoscopy is to allow for the visualization of small and fine features of the gut mucosa, the whole procedure can be rendered completely useless if the patient is restless or agitated. Therefore, unless the patient is fully cooperative – which is the exception rather than the rule in pediatric endoscopy – adequate sedation is mandatory to maintain the patient still throughout the procedure. Conscious sedation with midazolam 0.05–0.01 mg/kg IV may not be sufficient in infants or very anxious children, where deep sedation with propofol or a brief general anesthesia may be necessary.

Preparation of the mucosa

There is no doubt that chromoendoscopy gives better results when the gut mucosa to be examined is cleared of mucus (and blood, bile or food debris, if present). So, whenever possible, the mucosa should be washed prior to staining. A better washing is obtained if forceful pressure is applied with a syringe either through the spray catheter or directly into the biopsy channel. If absorptive dyes such as methylene blue or Lugol's solution are to be used, the mucosa should be washed with a few mL of 10% N-acetylcysteine to adequately remove mucus. Once the tissue has been stained, a wash with water or saline can remove the excess, nonabsorbed dye. If the vision is disturbed by bubbles or foam, a small volume of an antifoam preparation (e.g., simethicone 10–20 drops) can be added to the wash. A spasmolytic drug such as hyoscine N-butylbromide can be administered IV to reduce peristalsis or smooth muscle spasm and maximize visualization of the mucosal area of interest. As mentioned above, when a pH-sensitive dye is used, acid secretion should be either stimulated or suppressed, depending on the dye being used.

Staining technique

The technique for staining is fairly simple. Once the gut area of interest has been reached and adequately washed (see above), the endoscope and the tip of the catheter should be directed towards the mucosa with a combination of clockwise and counterclockwise rotation movements, and the dye should be sprayed onto the mucosa while the tip of the endoscope is gently and slowly withdrawn. The only exception is

India ink staining which is, in fact, a permanent tattoo of the mucosa and as such requires injection into the mucosa or submucosa. Once satisfactory images are obtained, it is always advisable to take photographs of the stained mucosa, in order to compare staining features with the histological abnormalities, to assess interobserver variability and also to monitor the improvement of the staining technique over time. Recently, guidelines have been proposed for optimal chromoendoscopy in ulcerative colitis (Table 17.2), but most of these guidelines do apply to chromoendoscopy in general.

Table 17.2 "Surface" guidelines for chromoendoscopy in ulcerative colitis

---

1) Strict patient selection

Patients with histologically proven ulcerative colitis and at least 8 years' duration in clinical remission; avoid patients with active disease

2) Unmask the mucosal surface

Excellent bowel preparation; remove mucus and remaining fluid in the colon when necessary

3) Reduce peristaltic waves

When drawing back the endoscope, a spasmolytic agent should be used if necessary

4) Full-length staining of the colon

In ulcerative colitis, perform panchromoendoscopy rather than local staining

5) Augmented detection with dyes

Vital staining with 0.4% indigo carmine or 0.1% methylene blue should be used to unmask flat lesions more frequently than with conventional colonoscopy

6) Crypt architecture analysis

Using magnification endoscopy, all lesions should be analyzed according to the pit pattern classification; whereas pit pattern types I–II suggest the presence of nonmalignant lesions, staining patterns III–IV suggest the presence of intraepithelial neoplasias and carcinomas

7) Endoscopic targeted biopsies

Perform targeted biopsies of all mucosal alterations, particularly of circumscribed lesions with staining patterns indicative of intraepithelial neoplasias and carcinomas, i.e., pit patterns III–IV.

Source: Reproduced with permission from Kiesslich R, Neurath MF. Surveillance colonoscopy in ulcerative colitis: magnifying chromoendoscopy in the spotlight. *Gut* 2004, **53**, 165–167.

Recognition of lesions

Barrett's esophagus and related disorders

Methylene blue is absorbed by the intestinal epithelium, so it has been used for the endoscopic detection of the intestinal metaplasia typical of Barrett's esophagus, especially when the diagnosis is uncertain, as it may be in short-segment Barrett's. The staining is usually homogeneous but in short-segment Barrett's it may be somewhat patchy due to the presence of nonintestinal columnar cells. More importantly, in Barrett's esophagus, the pattern of methylene blue staining is irregular and heterogeneous if dysplasia or cancer is present (Figure 17.2). Heterogeneously stained or light blue/unstained areas should be biopsied with particular care in search of high-grade dysplasia

and early adenocarcinoma. If Lugol's solution is used, Barrett's epithelium, dysplasia or carcinoma will appear as areas of negative staining on the dark green/brown stained background of the normal squamous epithelium.

Helicobacter pylori infection and related disorders

In patients with long-lasting *H. pylori* infection, chromoendoscopy with Congo red will demonstrate gastric atrophy as an area of negative staining on the dark blue/black background of the normal mucosa of the gastric fundus and body. Chromoendoscopy with phenol red will define the extent of *H. pylori* colonization in the stomach by producing a yellow staining throughout the affected gastric mucosa, which is alkalinized by urease.

(a) (b)

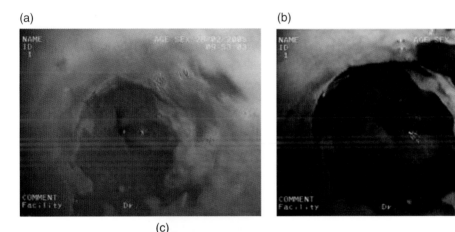

(c)

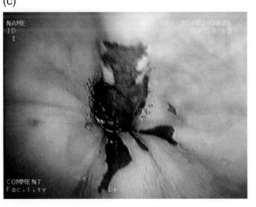

Figure 17.2 Endoscopic view of Barrett's esophagus: (a) plain close view; (b) close view after 0.1% methylene blue staining; (c) with the endoscope slightly withdrawn, a small area of negative staining can be seen in the uppermost part of the lesion (*top*); biopsy of this area showed moderate-grade dysplasia.

Celiac disease

Staining with methylene blue, even without preparation of the duodenal mucosa, makes the typical mosaic pattern more prominent and crisp, emphasizing the coarse, "cobblestone" appearance of the celiac mucosa that may not be evident at standard endoscopy (Figure 17.3). Immersion chromoendoscopy – that is, 1% methylene blue spray combined with magnification obtained by immersion of the endoscope tip – can amplify the difference between the mosaic pattern due to villous atrophy and the normal duodenal mucosa where villi can be clearly seen along the duodenal folds (Figure 17.4).

Polyposis syndromes

In patients with familial adenomatous polyposis (FAP), small flat duodenal adenomas will be easily identified as negative-staining plaques following methylene blue spray (Figure 17.5). In colonic polyposis, indigo carmine staining can help identify small

(a) (b)

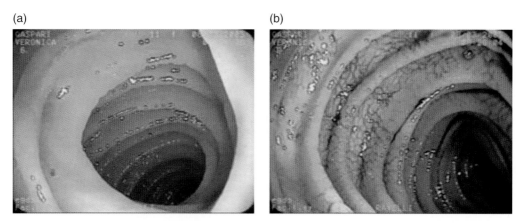

Figure 17.3 Endoscopic view of the distal duodenum in a patient with celiac disease and total villous atrophy. (a) A very mild scalloping of Kerckring's folds can be seen, but there is no clear evidence of mucosal atrophy. (b) Even without preparation of the mucosa, the mosaic pattern typical of gluten-sensitive enteropathy is clearly seen following methylene blue spray.

(a) (b)

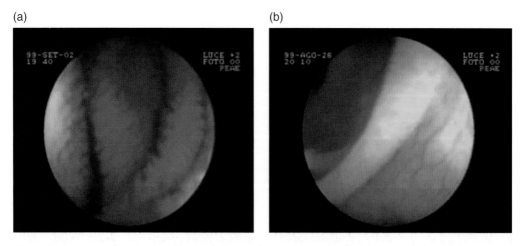

Figure 17.4 Immersion chromoendoscopy after methylene blue spray, without preparation of the mucosa. Unlike the normal duodenum, where villi are clearly seen along the mucosal folds (a), in patients with celiac disease and total villous atrophy duodenal folds appear flat and "denudated" and the typical cobblestone or mosaic pattern of the mucosa is highlighted (b).

superficial lesions such as flat or depressed adenomas. Indigo carmine and methylene blue can also differentiate hyperplastic (i.e., nonneoplastic) polyps from adenomatous (i.e., neoplastic) polyps, as the former are characterized by a regular pitted pattern (see Figure 17.5), whereas a grooved or sulcus pattern is typical of adenomatous polyps (Figure 17.6).

(a)   (b)

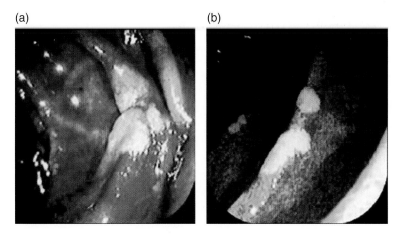

Figure 17.5 In a patient with familial adenomatous polyposis coli, flat (a) or minimally raised (b) duodenal adenomas stand out as small areas of negative staining following methylene blue spray. *Source:* Reproduced with permission from Weinstein W. Tissue sampling, specimen handling, and chromoendoscopy. In: Ginsberg GG, Kochman ML, Norton ID, Gostout CJ (eds). *Clinical Gastrointestinal Endoscopy.* Elsevier Science, Philadelphia, PA, 2005, pp. 59–75.

(a)

(b)

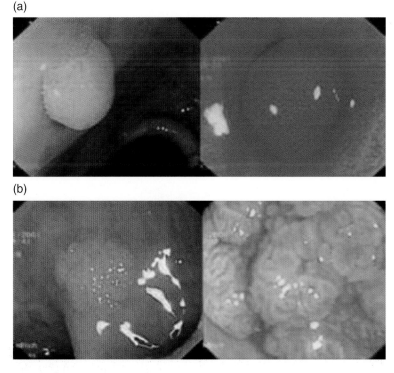

Figure 17.6 Colonic polyps before and after chromoendoscopy. (a) Hyperplastic polyp showing a regular pitted pattern. (b) Neoplastic polyp showing a sulciform pattern. *Source:* Reproduced with permission from Kiesslich R, Neurath MF. Surveillance colonoscopy in ulcerative colitis: magnifying chromoendoscopy in the spotlight. *Gut* 2004, **53**, 165–167.

Inflammatory bowel disease

In patients with long-standing ulcerative colitis, colonic dysplasia will appear as an area of negative-staining following methylene blue spray. If an early cancer is present within a metaplastic area, the staining will appear inhomogeneous and subsequent carmine red staining could be helpful to outline the margins of the lesion. As in colonic polyposis syndromes, methylene blue and indigo carmine staining can help discriminate between hyperplastic and neoplastic lesions (see Figure 17.6).

 • See companion website for videos relating to this chapter topic: www.wiley.com/go/gershman3e

 FURTHER READING

Acosta MM, Boyce HW Jr. Chromoendoscopy: where is it useful? *J Clin Gastroenterol* 1998, **27**, 13–20.

Bernstein CN. The color of dysplasia in ulcerative colitis. *Gastroenterology* 1999, **124**, 1135–1138.

Canto MI. Staining in gastrointestinal endoscopy: the basics. *Endoscopy* 1999, **31**, 479–486.

Canto MI, Yoshida T, Gossner L. Chromoscopy of intestinal metaplasia in Barrett's esophagus. *Endoscopy* 2002, **34**, 330–336.

Da Costa R, Wilson BC, Marcon NE. Photodiagnostic techniques for the endoscopic detection of premalignant gastrointestinal lesions. *Diagn Endosc* 2003, **15**, 153–173.

Eisen GM, Kim CY, Fleischer DE, *et al*. High-resolution chromoendoscopy for classifying colonic polyps: a multicenter study. *Gastrointest Endosc* 2002, **55**, 687–694.

Kiesslich R, Neurath MF. Surveillance colonoscopy in ulcerative colitis: magnifying chromoendoscopy in the spotlight. *Gut* 2004, **53**, 165–167.

Kiesslich R, Mergener K, Naumann C, *et al*. (Value of chromoendoscopy and magnification endoscopy in the evaluation of duodenal abnormalities: a prospective, randomized comparison. *Endoscopy* 2003, **35**, 559–563.

Siegel LM, Stevens PD, Lightdale CJ, *et al*. Combined magnification endoscopy with chromoendoscopy in the evaluation of patients with suspected malabsorption. *Gastrointest Endosc* 1997, **46**, 226–230.

Weinstein W. Tissue sampling, specimen handling, and chromoendoscopy. In: Ginsberg GG, Kochman ML, Norton ID, Gostout CJ (eds). *Clinical Gastrointestinal Endoscopy*. Elsevier Science, Philadelphia, PA, 2005, pp. 59–75.

18

Confocal laser endomicroscopy in the diagnosis of pediatric gastrointestinal disorders

Mike Thomson and Krishnappa Venkatesh

 KEY POINTS

- Confocal laser endomicroscopy (CLE) is feasible and safe in children as young as 18 months.
- Avoidance of biopsies in certain conditions such as graft-versus-host disease is desirable and CLE allows this.
- Targeting of biopsies is facilitated by CLE, affording greater histological efficiency.
- Consequent cost savings on conventional histology are potentially large and a viable business case can be drawn around this

- premise for purchase and use of CLE in the pediatric setting.
- *In vivo* histology using CLE has revealed interesting new findings in situations such as celiac disease, which are lost in conventional histology due to fixing of tissue and associated artefact.
- CLE may prove particularly useful in situations such as the detection of polyp syndrome-associated dysplasia.

Modern endoscopy has recently seen the development of technological advances with the aim of increasing and optimizing diagnostic yield from the procedure. These have included video and magnification endoscopes. Greater surface definition has been achieved with chromoendoscopy and recently, narrow-band imaging has allowed greater definition of vascular architecture. However, in vivo subsurface pathology remained obscure to the endoscopist until the advent of confocal endomicroscopy which affords magnification up to 1000×, and with sequentially deeper images from the epithelial surface to approximately 250 µm below the surface, producing histological assessment of the in vivo gastrointestinal (GI) mucosal structure at the cellular and subcellular levels. In addition, this technique avoids crush artefact from the grasp

biopsy forceps and changes from histopathological processing.

The diagnosis of upper GI disorders in children depends, to a great extent, on endoscopy and subsequent histology of biopsy specimens. Pathologies such as gastroesophageal reflux disease (GERD), eosinophilic esophagitis (EE), *Helicobacter pylori* gastritis, and celiac disease (CD), in conjunction with various other investigative modalities, have histological confirmation as pivotal to their diagnosis. Similarly, pediatric ileocolonic conditions such as inflammatory bowel disease (IBD), familial adenomatous polyposis (FAP), graft-versus-host disease (GVHD), and allergic colitis necessitate a tissue diagnosis.

Confocal laser endomicroscopy involves the use of a highly miniaturized confocal microscope which has been incorporated into the

Practical Pediatric Gastrointestinal Endoscopy, Third Edition. Edited by George Gershman and Mike Thomson.
© 2021 John Wiley & Sons Ltd. Published 2021 by John Wiley & Sons Ltd.
Companion website: www.wiley.com/go/gershman3e

distal tip of a flexible endoscope to allow *in vivo* microscopic examination of the gut mucosa. The confocal microscope uses a single optical fiber to deliver 488 nm laser light to the distal tip of the endoscope where it is focused to a single diffraction limited point within the tissue. The laser light excites fluorescent molecules within the tissue. Fluorescent light emanating from the specific point of focus is collected into the same optical fiber of the confocal microscope and delivered to the photodetector. Light emanating from outside the focally illuminated spot is not focused into the optical fiber and is therefore rejected from detection. The focused point of laser light is scanned in a raster pattern across the field of view, and the intensity of the fluorescent signal returning to the detector from successive points is measured (12-bit digitization) to produce two-dimensional images that are *en face* to the tissue surface. By moving the microscope optics within the confocal microscope, the operator can dynamically adjust the imaging depth to allow microscopic imaging at and below the surface of the mucosa; hence, each image is an optical section representing one focal plane within the specimen, and collection of multiple optical sections at successive depths results in true volumetric sampling of the tissue. As a three-dimensional volume is thus sampled, this can be thought of as a "virtual biopsy."

The Pentax EC3870CILK endoscope has a 5 mm diameter miniaturized confocal microscope integrated into the distal tip of the endoscope (Figure 18.1). The diameter of the distal tip and insertion tube of the endoscope is 12.8 mm. In addition to the integrated confocal microscope, the distal tip also contains a colour CCD camera which enables simultaneous confocal microscopy with standard videoendoscopy, air and water jet nozzles, two light guides, a 2.8 mm working channel and an auxiliary water jet channel. During CLE, the laser delivers an excitation wavelength of 488 nm at a maximum laser output of 1 mW to the tissue (typically 300–700 W). Confocal images can

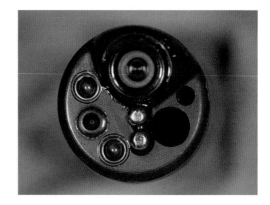

Figure 18.1 Confocal laser endomicroscope (Pentax).

then be collected at either 1024 × 1024 pixels (0.8 frames/second) or 1024 × 512 pixels (1.6 frames second). The optical sections have a 475 × 475 µm field of view, with a lateral resolution of 0.7 µm, axial resolution of 7.0 µm, and the imaging depth (z-axis) range of 0–250 µm below the tissue surface in 4 µm steps. The imaging depth below the tissue surface can be dynamically controlled by the operator. CLE magnifies images 1000-fold and they are visualized in real time on a monitor. A library of images is then collected and analyzed subsequently or contemporaneously.

Contrast agents

Fluorescein sodium (FS) 10% and acriflavine hydrochloride (AH) 0.05% are used as contrast agents. FS is highly water soluble and, on intravenous administration, rapidly diffuses in seconds from the capillaries into the extravascular tissue. FS, when exposed to light of wavelength 465– 490 nm (blue), emits light at longer wavelengths (520–65 nm, with peak emission in the 520–530 nm green-yellow region). This enables visualization of microvessels, cells, and connective tissue. However, FS is not enriched in the nuclei of intestinal epithelial cells and hence the nuclei are not readily visible in the confocal images. To circumvent this limitation, AH (0.05%) is used topically to enrich the superficial nuclei and to a lesser extent the cytoplasm.

To limit peristaltic artefacts, 10–20 mg Buscopan (hyoscine-N-butyl-bromide, Boehringer, Ingelheim, Germany) can be given intravenously. Following duodenal or ileal intubation, 0.05 0.1 mL/kg of 10% fluorescein sodium is administered intravenously and flushed adequately with normal saline. AH (0.05%) is applied to the mucosa using a spray catheter at all sites undergoing confocal imaging.

Confocal laser endomicroscopy image acquisition is performed by placing the tip of the colonoscope in direct contact with the target tissue site. Using gentle suction to stabilize the mucosa, image acquisition and focal plane z-axis scanning depth is actuated using two discrete handpiece control buttons. Confocal images are sequentially obtained from third-part duodenum, gastric antrum and body, distal and proximal esophagus in the upper GI tract, and ileum, cecum, ascending, transverse, descending, and sigmoid colon, and rectum in the ileocolon. Confocal images are acquired simultaneously with ongoing video-endoscopic imaging. Same-site mucosal specimens are obtained using standard biopsy forceps. The biopsy specimens are fixed in buffered formalin solution, embedded in paraffin wax, serial section obtained and stained with hematoxylin and eosin (H&E). The histological specimens from each site are compared with same-site confocal images jointly by the endoscopists and experienced pediatric and GI histopathologists, who are often in the endoscopy room. It is notable that the CLE images are cross-sectional in parallel with the mucosal surface, which is in contrast to standard histology in which a vertical section is made. Once this adjustment in perception is made by the observer, it is relatively easy to compare CLE images in vivo and postfixed tissue sections by histology. Of course, no artefact due to fixing and staining occurs in the CLE images.

Recently in our center, CLE occurred in 57 children intubating the duodenum at upper GI endoscopy, and the terminal ileum at ileocolonoscopy. In all those in whom this occurred, the pylorus at upper GI CLE and the terminal ileum at lower GI CLE were intubated in all patients except one – the exception being a patient who weighed 10 kg and who was 8 months old in whom the pylorus and ileocecal valve were both too narrow to accept the confocal endomicroscope. The youngest and smallest patient to have full successful examinations up to third-part duodenum and terminal ileum was 18 months old and 11 kg. The procedure time for upper GI endoscopy ranged from 7 to 25 minutes (median 16.4 minutes), and for ileocolonoscopy 15–45 minutes (median 27.9 minutes). A total of 132 pinch biopsies were taken from the upper GI tract from 33 procedures and 184 from the ileocolon from 30 procedures, i.e., not all patients had both upper and lower GI CLE.

No complications or adverse effects occurred except on one occasion when precipitation was observed in the peripheral venous line when fluorescein was injected immediately after neostigmine, but no patient morbidity occurred as the precipitant did not enter the patient.

Upper GI tract

In our unit, 33 patients underwent upper GI CLE, and the duodenum was intubated in all but one. A total of 4368 confocal images was obtained which included 1835 from the duodenum, 1451 from the stomach and 1082 from the esophagus, which were compared with 44 biopsies from each site.

The esophagus is lined by nonkeratinized squamous epithelium with polygonal epithelial cells. The nuclei of the epithelial cells are highlighted clearly following topical administration of acriflavine. Further, the capillary loops in the papillae are visible in deeper planes following subsurface optical sectioning, and surface to capillary distance can be measured as each level is deeper by 4 μm. This allows assessment of GERD-like histopathology given that papillary height is increased and epithelial surface to papillary tip (i.e., where capillary loops appear on confocal endomicroscopy) distance is thereby shorter. Recent in vivo data indicate that the epithelium is thinner in GERD versus normal versus EE and this is a very interesting phenomenon as it may allow real-time differentiation of esophageal pathologies.

The gastric pits or foveolae appear as invaginations on the surface epithelium. Each confocal image shows several evenly spaced such pits lined by columnar epithelium. The centers of the pits appear dark.

On confocal imaging, the duodenal villi have a long, slender and finger-like appearance similar to histological specimens. The single layer of brush border columnar epithelial cells interspersed with intraepithelial lymphocytes and goblet cells is well visualized. Crypts are not usually visible except in the presence of villous atrophy.

Celiac disease is particularly amenable to diagnosis by CLE. Comparative histological and CLE images are shown in Figure 18.2. On confocal imaging, in CD with subtotal villous atrophy (Marsh type 3a/b) (Figure 18.2a), the duodenal villi are broad with loss of the hexagonal pattern of the surface epithelium and a decrease in goblet cells. A characteristic feature observed was linking between adjacent villi giving an appearance of the villi being "sticky" (Figure 18.2b). Furthermore, the villi appear to be folded onto themselves. In contrast, in CD with total villous atrophy (Marsh type 3c on histology) (Figure 18.2c), on confocal imaging, villi are absent and crypts are visible with dense cellular infiltration in the surrounding stroma (Figure 18.2d), similar to histology.

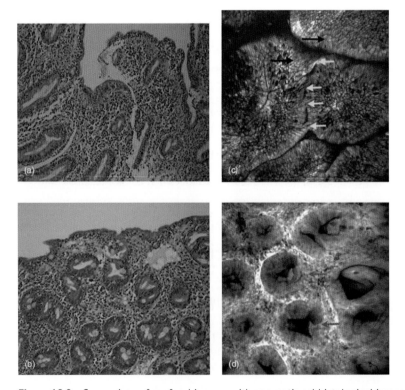

Figure 18.2 Comparison of confocal images with conventional histological images in celiac disease. (a) Histological image showing marked villous atrophy with increased intraepithelial lymphocytes and crypt hyperplasia. (b) Comparative confocal image. (c) Histological image showing total villous atrophy of the duodenum. (d) Comparative confocal image.

Lower GI tract

The typical features of the colonic crypt pattern can be seen in Figure 18.3 with a polygonal appearance. Goblet cells show up as dark cells, whilst enterocytes are light gray.

Technological innovations have led to the development of chromoendoscopy in which dyes such as methylene blue and indigo carmine have been used to aid localization of lesions, and magnifying endoscopy has enabled visualization of surface structures at approximately 100-fold magnification. In adults, several studies have validated these techniques in differentiating neoplastic from nonneoplastic lesions, diagnosis of neoplastic lesions in flat and depressed lesions in the colorectum, and in cancer surveillance in patients with long-standing ulcerative colitis. Differentiation of types of colitis is feasible although specificities such as presence of eosinophils are not observable. Typical features of ulcerative colitis are demonstrable, and CLE allows targeting of biopsy taking in order to allow such issues as dysplasia to be identified.

The following features are seen in inflammatory bowel disease on histology and on CLE (Figure 18.4).

- Goblet cell depletion
- Bifid crypt pattern

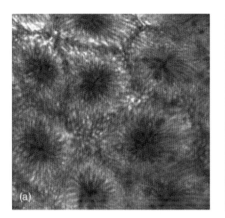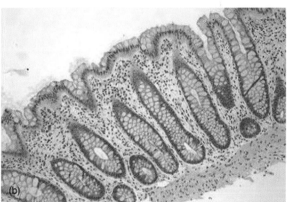

Figure 18.3 Comparison of confocal images with conventional histological images of the lower GI tract. (a) Confocal image of normal colonic mucosa showing regularly spaced crypts with numerous goblet cells. (b) Comparative histological image – note different plane.

(a)   (b)

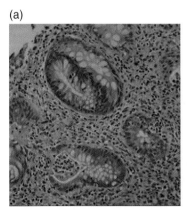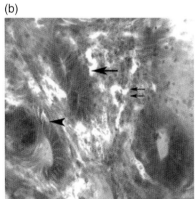

Figure 18.4 (a) Inflammatory bowel disease showing bifid crypt pattern, crypt distortion/destruction/abscess and cryptitis, goblet cell depletion, inflammatory cell infiltration prominence. (b) Comparative confocal image showing similar features plus tortuous vessel architecture suggesting inflammatory activity.

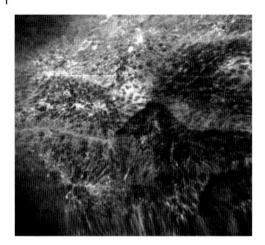

Figure 18.5 CLE of GVHD showing nuclear debris representing apoptotic bodies and obviating the need for taking of actual biopsies for histological confirmation.

- Crypt distortion
- Crypt abscess/cryptitis
- Crypt destruction
- Tortuous vessels

Granulomata cannot reliably be distinguished as yet, in our experience, but ileal inflammatory features can be, and therefore distinction between ulcerative colitis and Crohn's disease is further aided. Other pathologies such as collagenous colitis are noted easily with the typical increase in the thickness of the basement membrane. Graft-versus-host disease (GVHD) may also be identified with nuclear debris representing apoptotic bodies in the rectal mucosa (Figure 18.5), and this would potentially negate the need for biopsy which, in immunocom-promised children who may be at increased risk of mucosal infection and hemorrhage associated with biopsies being obtained, offers a cogent clinical benefit over standard endoscopy and biopsy.

Conclusion

The technology of CLE offers an insight into in vivo histology and allows targeting of biopsies which not only allow more accurate diagnostics but may help in diminishing the number of biopsies and concurrent costs to an endoscopy service. Smaller endoscopes may be useful but we have shown this technology to be applicable practically in children as young as 18 months of age. The tantalizing prospect of targeted biopsies or even a biopsy-free endoscopic procedure in the diagnosis of childhood GI disorders arises with obvious potential benefits in terms of avoidance of biopsy-associated complications and diminution of the considerable histological burden that this patient cohort places on already overstretched histopathological services with the prospect of considerable associated cost savings.

 • See companion website for videos relating to this chapter topic: www.wiley.com/go/gershman3e

 FURTHER READING

Carvalho R, Hyams JS. Diagnosis and management of inflammatory bowel disease in children. *Semin Pediatr Surg* 2007, **16**, 164–171.

Delaney P, Harris M. Fiber-optics in scanning optical microscopy. In: Pawley JB (ed.). *Handbook of Biological Confocal Microscopy*, 3rd edn. Springer, New York, pp. 501–515.

Fefferman DS, Farrell RJ. Endoscopy in inflammatory bowel disease: indications, surveillance, and use in clinical practice. *Clin Gastroenterol Hepatol* 2005, **3**, 11–24.

Gono K, Obi T, Yamaguchi M, *et al.* Appearance of enhanced tissue features in narrow band endoscopic imaging. *J Biomed Optics* 2004, **9**, 568–577.

Hoffman A, Goetz M, Vieth M, *et al.* Confocal laser endomicroscopy: technical status and current indications. *Endoscopy* 2006, **38**, 1275–1283.

Jung M, Kiesslich R. Chromoendoscopy and intravital staining techniques. *Best Pract Res Clin Gastroenterol* 1999, **13**, 11–19.

Kiesslich R, Fritsch J, Holtman M, *et al.* Methylene blue-aided chromoendoscopy for the detection of intraepithelial neoplasia and colon cancer in ulcerative colitis. *Gastroenterology* 2003, **124**, 880–888.

Kiesslich R, Burg J, Vieth M, *et al.* Confocal laser endoscopy for diagnosing intraepithelial neoplasias and colorectal cancer in vivo. *Gastroenterology* 2004, **127**, 706–713.

Lipson BK, Yannuzzi L. Complications of intravenous fluorescein injections. *Int Ophthalmol Clin* 2006, **29**, 200–205.

Polglase AL, McLaran WJ, Skinner SA, *et al.* A fluorescence confocal endomicroscope for in vivo microscopy of the upper- and the lower-GI tract. *Gastrointest Endosc Clin North Am* 2005, **62**, 686–695.

Thomson M. The pediatric esophagus comes of age. *J Pediatr Gastroenterol Nutr* 2002, **34**(S1), 40–45.

Tung, SY, Wu CS, Su MY. Magnifying colonoscopy in differentiating neoplastic from non-neoplastic colorectal lesions. *Am J Gastroenterol* 2001, **96**, 2628–2632.

Venkatesh K, Cohen M, Evans C, *et al.* Feasibility of confocal endomicroscopy in the diagnosis of paediatric gastrointestinal disorders. *World J Gastroenterol* 2009, **15**(18), 2214–2219.

Venkatesh K, Abou-Taleb A, Cohen M, *et al.* Role of confocal endomicroscopy in the diagnosis of celiac disease. *J Pediatr Gastroenterol Nutr* 2010, **51**, 274–279.

19

High-risk pediatric endoscopy

Jenifer R. Lightdale, Mike Thomson, and Douglas S. Fishman

 KEY POINTS

- Children who are particularly at risk fall into two main categories: those at risk from the cardiopulmonary anesthesia-related problems and those at risk from the procedure itself.
- Specific examples of patients at high risk for sedation complications include infants <1 year of age, infants and children with

congenital heart disease, pulmonary hypertension, cystic fibrosis, muscular dystrophy, and obesity.
- Endoscopy-related at-risk patients include those with predisposition to increased bleeding tendency, infection likelihood, and perforation risk.

Introduction

Adverse events associated with pediatric endoscopy are rare, but do occur. Published data from the Pediatric Clinical Outcomes Research Initiative (PEDS-CORI) suggest the overall rate of complications during pediatric endoscopy is 2.3%, including a specific risk of hypoxia (1.5%) and bleeding (0.3%) [1]. Generally speaking, endoscopy complications can be categorized as involving cardiopulmonary compromise, bleeding, perforation, and infection. Children at high risk for adverse events during pediatric endoscopy are often those with underlying disorders that put them at increased risk for events that fall into these four categories.

Patients at high risk for cardiopulmonary and sedation-related events

Cardiopulmonary events that occur during pediatric endoscopy are typically related to procedural sedation and anesthesia, which accounts for ~60% of all complications related to endoscopic procedures in children [1–3]. Cardiopulmonary events during pediatric endoscopy can range from minor to major complications, and include transient oxygen desaturation, aspiration, respiratory arrest, shock, and myocardial infarction [4]. Patients at high risk for cardiopulmonary events include those with compromised cardiopulmonary function, including decreased forced expiratory volumes

Practical Pediatric Gastrointestinal Endoscopy, Third Edition. Edited by George Gershman and Mike Thomson.
© 2021 John Wiley & Sons Ltd. Published 2021 by John Wiley & Sons Ltd.
Companion website: www.wiley.com/go/gershman3e

(as measured by FEV$_1$) [5]. Specific examples of patients at high risk for sedation complications include infants <1 year of age, infants and children with congenital heart disease, pulmonary hypertension, cystic fibrosis, muscular dystrophy, and obesity [1–3].

In addition, all children with difficult airways should be recognized to be at risk for sedation-related complications. Pediatric populations at highest risk for having difficult airways are those with craniofacial congenital abnormalities, including a large tongue, a highly arched or narrow palate, a short, thick neck, and prominent overbite, as well as those with limited range of motion of their necks [6]. Specific patient diagnoses that should elicit concern for increased cardiopulmonary risks during endoscopy include Pierre Robin syndrome, Treacher Collins' syndrome, and patients with laryngeal atresia.

Patients with history of lung disease, including chronic aspiration or other aerodigestive disease, reactive airways, pulmonary hypertension and cystic fibrosis should be recognized to be at particular risk of ventilatory compromise during endoscopy [7]. Medications which can potentiate cardiopulmonary effects of sedation include antiseizure, psychotropic, and pain medicines [7]. Children receiving benzodiazepines or opioids on a chronic basis should be identified during preprocedure patient preparation to be at high risk for cardiopulmonary events during endoscopy [8].

Patients at high risk for bleeding

Significant bleeding is a rare adverse event of endoscopic procedures in children, and generally speaking occurs more commonly during therapeutic procedures with instrumentation [1,9,10]. Endoscopy-related bleeding can also result from endoscope manipulation or tissue sampling. In terms of the latter, the risk of bleeding during mucosal biopsy is generally related more to patient-specific risk factors (i.e., inflammation, coagulopathy, hemophilia)

than the total number of biopsies obtained [11–13]. When bleeding is associated with endoscopy in children, it may be intraluminal or intramural. The former is typically noted during the procedure, whereas the latter may present in a delayed fashion, often after a patient has been discharged.

Bleeding can also occur with endoscope advancement, especially around blind or angulated turns, due to mucosal shearing or tearing, and is more common in certain anatomical areas. For example, the sigmoid colon may be at particular risk of intraluminal bleeding or intramural hematoma during colonoscopic advancement and loop reduction [14]. In addition, the duodenum may also be particularly vulnerable to intramural hematomas post EGD with mucosal biopsy. The incidence of EGD with biopsy-related duodenal hematoma in children has been reported to be 1 in 1922 procedures [15]. Cases typically present as abdominal pain and/or vomiting within 72 hours post procedure [15].

Unique features of the third portion of the duodenum have been hypothesized to account for this anatomical location being particularly vulnerable to hematoma, including a relatively fixed retroperitoneal position, adjacency to the lumbar spine, a lack of well-developed retroperitoneal serosal layer, and a rich submucosal vascular plexus susceptible to shearing forces during biopsy acquisition [16,17]. As such, it has been theorized that one may be able to decrease the risk of a duodenal hematoma by avoiding extension of the biopsy forceps more than 2–3 cm beyond the endoscope tip, thereby decreasing the chances of stripping of the mucosa from the immobile bowel wall behind it [18,19].

Specific patient co-morbidities that may increase the risk of duodenal hematoma include leukemia and history of hematopoetic bone marrow transplant [19–21]. Underlying coagulation disorders may also predispose to intramural duodenal hematoma [22]. Once a hematoma occurs, it generally requires about three weeks to resolve, unless surgical evacuation is performed.

Patient risk factors for bleeding during endoscopy also include anemia, thrombocytopenia, coagulopathy, and use of certain medications. Pediatric patient populations at increased risk of bleeding complications during endoscopic procedures include those with bone marrow failure or hematological malignancies, history of hematopoietic stem cell transplant (HSCT), end-stage liver disease, disorders of coagulation and those taking antithrombotic medications. Antithrombotic agents carry varying degrees of bleeding risks, and include anticoagulants (heparin, low molecular weight heparin, and warfarin) and antiplatelet medications (nonsteroidal antiinflammatory drugs, aspirin, clopidrogrel, ticlopidine, and glycoprotein IIb/IIIa inhibitors).

Finally, it is reasonable to assume that comorbidities of uremia, hypoalbuminemia, or a recent bleeding event may confer additional risk of bleeding in children related to platelet dysfunction [23–25].

Patients at high risk for perforation

Perforation during endoscopy can be defined as instrumental injury leading to a defect in the wall of the bowel, with evidence of air or luminal contents outside the GI tract [5]. The reported incidence of perforation during pediatric endoscopy is 0.06–0.3% [26], and perforation is generally classified as large or small.

Large perforations usually result from injury from the shaft of the endoscope. Risk factors for large perforations include large intracolonic loops, particularly when formed in the rectosigmoid region, and often involve the antimesenteric side of the bowel [27]. Presentation of large perforations is immediate, and patients will have peritoneal signs. Computed tomography (CT) scans will demonstrate extraluminal free air.

In comparison, small perforations are usually due to the endoscope tip and can occur when advancing through a turn with a "sliding by" technique [27]. Therapeutic maneuvers, such as hot snare polypectomy and sphincterotomy, can also result in small focal perforations. Presentation of small perforations can be delayed by hours to days with nonspecific abdominal pain and tenderness [27].

Generally speaking, patients with intestinal strictures may be at risk for perforation in part due to intermittent obstruction that occurs mechanically when a colonoscope traverses a stricture. With air unable to pass distally around the endoscope, it will accumulate in the proximal colon, stretching the mucosa and decreasing wall strength. In addition, patients with both primary and secondary pseudoobstruction leading to massive dilated bowel (e.g., spinal muscular atrophy, metabolic disorders) should be recognized to be at increased risk of perforation during endoscopic procedures [28]. This includes increased risk for perforation during therapeutic decompression, which should be mitigated by employing CO_2 and performing intermittent suctioning [28,29].

A number of other factors may increase a patient's risk for perforation. These include using a larger endoscope in small patients, poor or compromised endoscopic visualization, and impaired bowel wall strength [30]. It is important to recognize that performance of endoscopic procedures in small children may require larger endoscopes, with larger working channels and greater availability of endoscopic accessories [31]. For example, to control gastrointestinal bleeding in neonates and young infants, a larger gastroscope than standard neonatal scopes is needed to use bipolar electrocautery or hemostatic clips [31]. Also, to successfully perform colonoscopy in infants and small children, gastroscopes may be used, which may be stiff and relatively large for a small child's intestinal lumen [2]. Although patient–endoscope mismatch may be unavoidable, it is prudent to recognize the increased risks of perforation and proceed accordingly.

Patients with inflammatory bowel disease may be at high risk for perforation due to intestinal strictures and mucosal inflammation, which may compromise wall strength. This risk can be compounded when patients are on high-dose steroids, which can decrease bowel wall thickness and strength [32]. High-dose steroid use can also mask and delay the onset of peritoneal symptoms [33]. It is therefore important to have a high suspicion for bowel perforation in patients receiving high-dose steroids who develop persistent abdominal pain post endoscopy.

There are two additional specific conditions which may increase patient risks for endoscopic perforation: recessive dystrophic epidermolysis bullosa (RDEB) and type 4 (vascular type) Ehlers–Danlos syndrome (EDS) [34,35]. In children with severe generalized RDEB, epithelial and mucosal scarring due to even minimal manipulation or abrasion is a significant risk, and can occur with taping of the skin or with establishment of a secure airway [36,37]. Ideally, specially designed adhesives should be used exclusively, and careful decision making about airway management should occur prior to the procedure [37]. When performing upper endoscopy in children with RDEB, it is particularly important to recognize that esophageal scarring can lead to esophageal stricturing [38]. If dilation in RDEB is pursued, a conservative target of no more than three times the stricture diameter during any one procedure should be preferentially performed via endoscopic radial force balloons with fluoroscopic guidance [35].

Patients with EDS type IV (vascular type) have an extremely high risk of bowel perforation and GI bleeding during endoscopy [34]. EDS type IV accounts for 5% of EDS prevalence and has an autosomal dominant inheritance pattern. Complications associated with endoscopy, particularly colonic perforations, have higher rates in children and teenagers [34,39–41]. Therefore endoscopic procedures should be considered in type IV EDS only if necessary and performed with extreme caution.

Acquired patient risk factors for endoscopic perforation include certain types of ingestions, history of prior perforation,

prolonged procedures and hemopoietic stem cell transplant [42]. In particular, compromised mucosal wall strength may increase risks of esophageal perforation in patients with caustic ingestion, disk battery ingestion, and tracheal-esophageal atresia surgical anastomotic sites [42,43].

Warning signs associated with perforation include pain out of proportion to exam, persistent tachycardia, atypical use of pain medication, as well as fever and pain lasting beyond a few hours [42]. Initial imaging should include a KUB and left lateral decubitus (LLD) radiograph. The patient should ideally be in the LLD position for 5–10 minutes. If the imaging is normal, repeat imaging or CT scan should be considered.

Patients at high risk for endoscopy-related infections

Adverse events associated with infection are infrequent during pediatric endoscopy, but have been well described [44]. They may result from either exposing patients to infectious agents through the use of contaminated equipment (exogenous transmission) or by creating a portal of entry through which host flora may set up infection (endogenous transmission) [44,45]. Generally speaking, rates of postprocedural infectious events are dependent on the fidelity of postprocedural equipment processing, the presence of patient-specific risk factors such as a compromised immune system, and the nature of the procedure being performed.

Exogenous infection transmission

During endoscopy, the external portion of the endoscope, its channels, and the utilized accessories are inevitably contaminated with bodily fluids, organic debris, and the microorganism milieu of the patient [44,45]. The most often quoted estimated rate of transmission is 1 out of 1.8 million procedures [46,47]. It should be noted that even meticulous adherence to high-level disinfection techniques does not completely eliminate the risk of transmitting infection [48]. Nevertheless, infectious transmission is an extremely rare event in the setting of appropriately implemented endoscopy equipment processing standards.

Patient risk factors for endogenous infection transmission

Endogenous infection transmission generally involves transient bacteremia associated with endoscopy that may result from subclinical mucosal tears. Rate of transient bacteremia after diagnostic EGD or colonoscopy with biopsy in adult patients is reported to be ~4% [49] and small pediatric series suggest that transient bacteremia after routine gastrointestinal endoscopy with biopsy is similarly uncommon [50,51]. All these reports note that such rates of bacteremia are not dissimilar to rates associated with activities of daily living, such as chewing food (7–51%), flossing and tooth brushing (20–40%) [52]. Nevertheless, children with cardiovascular disease may be at higher risk for developing endocarditis after gastrointestinal endoscopy, particularly due to atypical anatomy, vascular flow or synthetic repair [53].

To date, there has been no study demonstrating that administration of antibiotic prophylaxis prevents development of infectious endocarditis associated with endoscopy [2,49]. Nevertheless, when performing endoscopy in children with cardiac conditions, it is important to have a conversation with the patient's cardiologist to consider unique patient factors that may influence decision making. Patient-specific decision making around antibiotic prophylaxis for endoscopic procedures may also be reasonable to pursue in patients who possess congenital or acquired defects in their immune response. Examples of such patients include those with a diagnosed solid or other hematological malignancy; on immunosuppressive medications; with absolute or functional neutropenia; with cirrhosis; as well as those with hyposplenism or asplenism [54–56]. The primary concern in immunocompromised patients is they may not be able to clear transient bacteremia that may occur during endoscopic procedures which could consequently result in deep seeded infections or sepsis.

Risk factors for procedure-related infections

Certain therapeutic interventions, such as stricture dilation, sclerotherapy, and esophageal banding, are associated with increased rates of bacteremia. In turn, prophylaxis during these procedures in certain high-risk patient groups (i.e., those with profound neutropenia) is recommended [49,56]. Another high-risk group of children for infectious complications is those undergoing placement of percutaneous endoscopic gastrostomy (PEG) tubes. Society guidelines currently list a grade 1A recommendation to administer parenteral cefazolin (or equivalent) 30 minutes prior to the placement of PEGs [49]. Antibiotic prophylaxis should also be provided when complete relief of biliary obstruction via endoscopic retrograde cholangiopancreatograhy (ERCP) may not be achieved, such as in the setting of patients with primary sclerosing cholangitis or hilar tumors, as well as in patients requiring biliary interventions after liver transplantation; stenting in the setting of biliary malignancy; and when a combined percutaneous-endoscopic approach is undertaken [49,57].

 • See companion website for videos relating to this chapter topic: www.wiley.com/go/gershman3e

REFERENCES

1 Thakkar K, El-Serag HB, Mattek N, Gilger MA. Complications of pediatric EGD: a 4-year experience in PEDS-CORI. *Gastrointest Endosc* 2007, **65**, 213–221.

2 ASGE Standards of Practice Committee, Lightdale JR, Acosta R, *et al.* Modifications in endoscopic practice for pediatric patients. *Gastrointest Endosc* 2014, **79**, 699–710.

3 Gilger MA, Gold BD. Pediatric endoscopy: new information from the PEDS-CORI project. *Curr Gastroenterol Rep* 2005, **7**, 234–239.

4 Cravero JP. Risk and safety of pediatric sedation/anesthesia for procedures outside the operating room. *Curr Opin Anaesthesiol* 2009, **22**, 509–513.

5 Cotton PB, Eisen GM, Aabakken L, *et al.* A lexicon for endoscopic adverse events: report of an ASGE workshop. *Gastrointest Endosc* 2010, **71**, 446–454.

6 Engelhardt T, Weiss M. A child with a difficult airway: what do I do next? *Curr Opin Anaesthesiol* 2012, **25**, 326–332.

7 Sharma VK, Nguyen CC, Crowell MD, Lieberman DA, de Garmo P, Fleischer DE. A national study of cardiopulmonary unplanned events after GI endoscopy. *Gastrointest Endosc* 2007, **66**, 27–34.

8 Nusrat S, Mahmood S, Bitar H, Tierney WM, Bielefeldt K, Madhoun MF. The impact of chronic opioid use on colonoscopy outcomes. *Dig Dis Sci* 2015, **60**, 1016–1023.

9 Enestvedt BK, Eisen GM, Holub J, Lieberman DA. Is the American Society of Anesthesiologists classification useful in risk stratification for endoscopic procedures? *Gastrointest Endosc* 2013, **77**, 464–471.

10 Enestvedt BK, Tofani C, Lee DY, *et al.* Endoscopic retrograde cholangiopancreatography in the pediatric population is safe and efficacious. *J Pediatr Gastroenterol Nutr* 2013, **57**, 649–654.

11 Cerezo Ruiz A, Parras Mejias E, Martos Becerra JM. A complication following a biopsy sample in eosinophilic esophagitis. *Rev Esp Enferm Dig* 2017, **109**, 537.

12 Yao MD, von Rosenvinge EC, Groden C, Mannon PJ. Multiple endoscopic biopsies in research subjects: safety results from a National Institutes of Health series. *Gastrointest Endosc* 2009, **69**, 906–910.

13 Yankov IV, Spasova MI, Andonov VN, Cholakova EN, Yonkov AS. Endoscopic diagnosis of intramural hematoma in the colon sigmoideum in a child with high titer inhibitory hemophilia A. *Folia Med* 2014, **56**, 126–128.

14 Katsurahara M, Horiki N, Kitade T, *et al.* Acute colonic intramural hematoma: a rare complication of colonoscopy. *Endoscopy* 2014, **46** Suppl 1 UCTN, E180–1.

15 Sahn B, Anupindi SA, Dadhania NJ, Kelsen JR, Nance ML, Mamula P. Duodenal hematoma following EGD: comparison with blunt abdominal trauma-induced duodenal hematoma. *J Pediatr Gastroenterol Nutr* 2015, **60**, 69–74.

16 Zinelis SA, Hershenson LM, Ennis MF, Boller M, Ismail-Beigi F. Intramural duodenal hematoma following upper gastrointestinal endoscopic biopsy. *Dig Dis Sci* 1989, **34**, 289–291.

17 Guzman C, Bousvaros A, Buonomo C, Nurko S. Intraduodenal hematoma complicating intestinal biopsy: case reports and review of the literature. *Am J Gastroenterol* 1998, **93**, 2547–2550.

18 Bechtel K, Moss RL, Leventhal JM, Spiro D, Abo A. Duodenal hematoma after upper endoscopy and biopsy in a 4-year-old girl. *Pediatr Emerg Care* 2006, **22**, 653–654.

19 Ramakrishna J, Treem WR. Duodenal hematoma as a complication of endoscopic biopsy in pediatric bone marrow transplant recipients. *J Pediatr Gastroenterol Nutr* 1997, **25**, 426–429.

20 Lipson SA, Perr HA, Koerper MA, Ostroff JW, Snyder JD, Goldstein RB. Intramural duodenal hematoma after endoscopic biopsy in leukemic patients. *Gastrointest Endosc* 1996, **44**, 620–623.

21 Grasshof C, Wolf A, Neuwirth F, Posovszky C. Intramural duodenal haematoma after endoscopic biopsy: case report and review of the literature. *Case Rep Gastroenterol re* 2012, **6**, 5–14.

22 Hameed S, McHugh K, Shah N, Arthurs OJ. Duodenal haematoma following endoscopy as a marker of coagulopathy. *Pediatr Radiol* 2014, **44**, 392–397.

23 Friedmann AM, Sengul H, Lehmann H, Schwartz C, Goodman S. Do basic laboratory tests or clinical observations predict bleeding in thrombocytopenic oncology patients? A reevaluation of prophylactic platelet transfusions. *Transfus Med Rev* 2002, **16**, 34–45.

24 Park YB, Lee JW, Cho BS, *et al*. Incidence and etiology of overt gastrointestinal bleeding in adult patients with aplastic anemia. *Dig Dis Sci* 2010, **55**, 73–81.

25 Li M, Wang Z, Ma T, *et al*. Enhanced platelet apoptosis in chronic uremic patients. *Renal Fail* 2014, **36**, 847–853.

26 Friedt M, Welsch S. An update on pediatric endoscopy. *Eur J Med Res* 2013, **18**, 24.

27 Anderson ML, Pasha TM, Leighton JA. Endoscopic perforation of the colon: lessons from a 10-year study. *Am J Gastroenterol* 2000, **95**, 3418–3422.

28 Saunders MD. Acute colonic pseudo-obstruction. *Best Pract Res Clin Gastroenterol* 2007, **21**, 671–687.

29 Sajid MS, Caswell J, Bhatti MI, Sains P, Baig MK, Miles WF. Carbon dioxide insufflation vs conventional air insufflation for colonoscopy: a systematic review and meta-analysis of published randomized controlled trials. *Colorect Dis* 2015, **17**, 111–123.

30 Farley DR, Bannon MP, Zietlow SP, Pemberton JH, Ilstrup DM, Larson DR. Management of colonoscopic perforations. *Mayo Clin Proc* 1997, **72**, 729–733.

31 Barth BA, Banerjee S, Bhat YM, *et al*. Equipment for pediatric endoscopy. *Gastrointest Endosc* 2012, **76**, 8–17.

32 Navaneethan U, Kochhar G, Phull H, *et al*. Severe disease on endoscopy and steroid use increase the risk for bowel perforation during colonoscopy in inflammatory bowel disease patients. *J Crohns Colitis* 2012, **6**, 470–475.

33 ReMine SG, McIlrath DC. Bowel perforation in steroid-treated patients. *Ann Surg* 1980, **192**, 581–586.

34 Stillman AE, Painter R, Hollister DW. Ehlers–Danlos syndrome type IV: diagnosis and therapy of associated bowel perforation. *Am J Gastroenterol* 1991, **86**, 360–362.

35 Okada T, Sasaki F, Shimizu H, *et al*. Effective esophageal balloon dilation for esophageal stenosis in recessive dystrophic epidermolysis bullosa. *Eur J Pediatr Surg* 2006, **16**, 115–119.

36 Gottschalk A, Venherm S, Vowinkel T, Tubergen D, Frosch M, Hahnenkamp K. Anesthesia for balloon dilatation of esophageal strictures in children with epidermolysis bullosa dystrophica: from intubation to sedation. *Curr Opin Anaesthesiol* 2010, **23**, 518–522.

37 Van Den Heuvel I, Boschin M, Langer M, *et al*. Anesthetic management in pediatric patients with epidermolysis bullosa: a single center experience. *Minerva Anestesiol* 2013, **79**, 727–732.

38 Vowinkel T, Laukoetter M, Mennigen R, *et al*. A two-step multidisciplinary approach to treat recurrent esophageal strictures in children with epidermolysis bullosa dystrophica. *Endoscopy* 2015, **47**, 541–544.

39 Allaparthi S, Verma H, Burns DL, Joyce AM. Conservative management of small bowel perforation in Ehlers–Danlos syndrome type IV. *World JGastrointest Endosc* 2013, **5**, 398–401.

40 Burcharth J, Rosenberg J. Gastrointestinal surgery and related complications in patients with Ehlers–Danlos syndrome: a systematic review. *Dig Surg* 2012, **29**, 349–357.

41 Yoneda A, Okada K, Okubo H, *et al*. Spontaneous colon perforations associated with a vascular type of Ehlers–Danlos syndrome. *Case Rep Gastroenterol* 2014, **8**, 175–181.

42 Hsu EK, Chugh P, Kronman MP, Markowitz JE, Piccoli DA, Mamula P. Incidence of perforation in pediatric GI endoscopy and colonoscopy: an 11-year experience. *Gastrointest Endosc* 2013, **77**, 960–966.

43 Jain P, Debnath PR, Jain V, Chadha R, Choudhury SR, Puri A. Multiple anastomotic complications following repair of oesophageal atresia with tracheoesophageal fistula: a report of two cases. *Afr J Paediatr Surg j* 2011, **8**, 244–248.

44 Reprocessing Guideline Task Force, Petersen BT, Cohen J, *et al*. Multisociety guideline on reprocessing flexible GI endoscopes: 2016 update. *Gastrointest Endosc* 2017; www.sgna. org/Portals/0/MS_guideline_reprocessing_ GI_endoscopes.pdf.

45 Visrodia K, Petersen BT. Echoing concerns related to endoscope reprocessing. *Gastrointest Endosc* 2017, **85**, 398–400.

46 Spach DH, Silverstein FE, Stamm WE. Transmission of infection by gastrointestinal endoscopy and bronchoscopy. *Ann Intern Med* 1993, **118**, 117–128.

47 Petersen BT, Chennat J, Cohen J, *et al*. Multisociety guideline on reprocessing flexible GI endoscopes: 2011. *Infect Control Hosp Epidemiol* 2011, **32**, 527–537.

48 Epstein L, Hunter JC, Arwady MA, *et al*. New Delhi metallo-beta-lactamase-producing carbapenem-resistant Escherichia coli associated with exposure to duodenoscopes. *JAMA* 2014, **312**, 1447–1455.

49 ASGE Standards of Practice Committee, Khashab MA, Chithadi KV, *et al*. Antibiotic prophylaxis for GI endoscopy. *Gastrointest Endosc* 2015, **81**, 81–89.

50 el-Baba M, Tolia V, Lin CH, Dajani A. Absence of bacteremia after gastrointestinal procedures in children. *Gastrointest Endosc* 1996, **44**, 378–381.

51 Byrne WJ, Euler AR, Campbell M, Eisenach KD. Bacteremia in children following upper gastrointestinal endoscopy or colonoscopy. *J Pediatr Gastroenterol Nutr* 1982, **1**, 551–553.

52 Wilson W, Taubert KA, Gewitz M, *et al*. Prevention of infective endocarditis: guidelines from the American Heart Association: a guideline from the American Heart Association Rheumatic Fever, Endocarditis, and Kawasaki Disease Committee, Council on Cardiovascular Disease in the Young, and the Council on Clinical Cardiology, Council on Cardiovascular Surgery and Anesthesia, and the Quality of Care and Outcomes Research Interdisciplinary Working Group. *Circulation* 2007, **116**, 1736–1754.

53 Snyder J, Bratton B. Antimicrobial prophylaxis for gastrointestinal procedures: current practices in North American academic pediatric programs. *J Pediatr Gastroenterol Nutr* 2002, **35**, 564–569.

54 Buderus S, Sonderkotter H, Fleischhack G, Lentze MJ. Diagnostic and therapeutic endoscopy in children and adolescents with cancer. *Pediatr Hematol Oncol* 2012, **29**, 450–460.

55 Bianco JA, Pepe MS, Higano C, Applebaum FR, McDonald GB, Singer JW. Prevalence of clinically relevant bacteremia after upper gastrointestinal endoscopy in bone marrow transplant recipients. *Am J Med* 1990, **89**, 134–136.

56 Allison MC, Sandoe JA, Tighe R, Simpson IA, Hall RJ, Elliott TS. Antibiotic prophylaxis in gastrointestinal endoscopy. *Gut* 2009, **58**, 869–880.

57 ASGE Standards of Practice Committee, Anderson MA, Fisher L, *et al*. Complications of ERCP. *Gastrointest Endosc* 2012, **75**, 467–473.

Part Three

Pediatric GI Pathologies and the Role of Endoscopy in Their Management

20

Esophagitis

Mário C. Vieira, Luciana B. Mendez Ribeiro, and Sabine Krüger Truppel

 KEY POINTS

- "Esophagitis" is really an histological term and the endoscopic description should probably better use nomenclature such as "erosive esophageal appearances." However, "esophagitis" is a term readily used by endoscopists to describe the macroscopic appearances of apparent esophageal inflammation.
- Esophagitis is multietiological and the causes are defined in this chapter.

- The endoscopist should be reminded to obtain multiple biopsies from different levels of the esophagus, and sending biopsies for microbiological and virological assessment, preferably in appropriate media, is an important step, where deemed appropriate.
- Macroscopic appearances are not a reliable indicator of microscopic inflammation or pathology.

Introduction

The term *esophagitis* has many clinical and pathological connotations and may describe different chemical, immunological, infectious, and ischemic disorders. Gastroesophageal reflux disease (GERD) and eosinophilic esophagitis, which are the major causes of esophagitis in children, as well as chemical injuries of the esophagus, are topics covered in other chapters of this book. In this chapter, less common causes, such as infectious disorders, epidermolysis bullosa, inflammatory bowel disease, chemotherapy and radiation-induced inflammation, which are also part of the injury panel of esophageal mucosa, will be reviewed [1,2].

Infectious esophagitis

Infectious esophagitis is a disease observed, in most cases, in immunocompromised patients. It may occur in patients infected by the human immunodeficiency virus (HIV), undergoing chemotherapy, receiving treatment with immunosuppressive drugs and those under prolonged therapy with antibiotics or corticosteroids [2].

The most common symptoms of esophageal infections are odynophagia, dysphagia, retrosternal chest pain, nausea, vomiting, and fever. Symptoms may lead to worsening of nutritional status and increased mortality of associated diseases. Infectious esophagitis, under special conditions, may present with

Practical Pediatric Gastrointestinal Endoscopy, Third Edition. Edited by George Gershman and Mike Thomson.
© 2021 John Wiley & Sons Ltd. Published 2021 by John Wiley & Sons Ltd.
Companion website: www.wiley.com/go/gershman3e

serious complications such as gastrointestinal bleeding, strictures, fistulae or perforation [2].

Upper gastrointestinal (GI) endoscopy is the gold standard for the diagnosis of esophageal lesions. It is the most sensitive and specific method, since it allows macroscopic evaluation of the mucosa and collection of samples for analysis through biopsies and cytology brushings. There is increased sensitivity if polymerase chain reaction (PCR), viral tissue culture, and immunohistochemistry tests are performed on the samples obtained through endoscopy [1,2].

Esophagitis associated with HIV

Infections of the digestive tract affect most HIV-infected patients. The most common pathogens involved are yeasts (*Candida* sp.), viruses (cytomegalovirus [CMV], herpes simplex virus [HSV], Epstein–Barr virus [EBV], human papillomavirus [HPV]), bacteria and protozoa (*Cryptosporidium* sp. and *Pneumocystis carinii*), which are usually associated with systemic disease. Infections may be isolated or co-existent [2]. Antiretroviral therapy has enabled viral load control and improvement of the immune function, with a significant reduction in the incidence of these opportunistic complications, decreasing morbidity and mortality from HIV infection [3].

Infectious esophagitis is the second most common gastrointestinal manifestation in HIV-infected patients [4]. The most common agent is *Candida albicans* co-existing often with other pathogens, particularly CMV.

The presence of symptoms of esophageal disfunction in these patients is an indication for endoscopic evaluation for the detection of lesions in the esophageal mucosa and biopsies and/or brushing for differential diagnosis [5].

Erosive or ulcerated esophagitis is, in general, assigned to CMV infection [4,5].

Esophagitis caused by *Candida*

Candida albicans is a normal commensal agent in the GI tract. Esophageal candidiasis is a common fungal infection in immunocompromised patients and is rare in immunocompetent patients. There are several *Candida* species that may be involved, but *C. albicans* is the main etiological agent of infectious esophagitis and can occur with or without concomitant oropharyngeal infection [6].

The most common symptoms of esophageal candidiasis are sialorrhea, odynophagia, and retrosternal chest pain, and most patients present with concomitant oropharyngeal candidiasis. Rare complications include bleeding, stricture, and perforation [7].

Upper GI endoscopy reveals whitish pseudomembranous plaques adhered to the esophageal wall, extending from the proximal to the distal part of the esophagus. Friability, edema, and erythema of varying degrees eventually associated with ulcerations may be observed (Figure 20.1) [8]. The endoscopic aspect can be classified in grades from I to IV (Table 20.1) [9].

Histopathological analysis with routine stains confirms the diagnosis through the identification of spores, hyphae, and pseudo-hyphae compatible with *Candida* sp. Culture is not useful unless susceptibility testing is required for suspected resistant agents [6,10].

The treatment for esophageal candidiasis is fluconazole for 14–21 days, orally or intravenously, in cases of significant dysphagia. Amphotericin B may be an alternative for cases refractory to fluconazole [6].

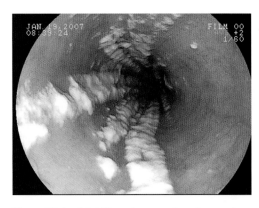

Figure 20.1 Friability, edema, and erythema of varying degrees eventually associated with ulceration.

Table 20.1 Endoscopic classification of esophageal candida

Grade	Description
I	A few small candida plaques up to 2 mm in size, with mucosal hyperemia but without edema or ulcerations
II	Multiple bigger white candida plaques with mucosal hyperemia and edema but without ulcerations
III	Confluent linear candida plaques with mucosal hyperemia and ulcerations
IV	As grade III but with constriction of the esophageal lumen

Source: Reproduced with permission from Kodsi et al. [9].

Esophagitis caused by CMV

Primary infection by CMV in immunocompetent patients is very frequent, occurring mainly in preschool children and young adults, and may be asymptomatic in most cases. In situ hybridization studies may show that CMV DNA may persist in a latent form in most organs. In the immunocompromised host, the latent virus may become reactivated and cause several diseases [11,12].

Cytomegalovirus esophagitis is rarely documented in immunocompetent patients [13,14]. It usually affects patients after organ or bone marrow transplantation, patients undergoing long-term dialysis, patients infected by HIV or those with acquired immunodeficiency syndrome (AIDS), patients with other debilitating diseases and those treated with immunosuppressive drugs [2,11,12]. The average time for the development of CMV esophagitis after solid organ transplantation is 5–7 months and after bone marrow transplantation is 2–3 months [11,12].

Nonspecific symptoms including nausea, vomiting, and fever are characteristic of the viral infection; however, odynophagia, dysphagia, chest pain, and bleeding may occur when there is esophageal involvement [2,12].

On upper GI endoscopy, diffuse erythema associated with small, shallow ulcers or multiple linear and deep ulcers with elevated margins may be observed, especially involving the middle and distal portions of the esophagus [12].

Biopsies should be performed in the central area of the lesion, as the cytopathic effects of the virus are not found in the squamous epithelium. Histological diagnosis is performed with the detection of large cells, mainly fibroblasts and endothelial cells, presenting, typically, bulky nuclei with viral inclusions and peripheral light halo ("owl's eye"). In addition to histological analysis, the specimens should be subjected to antigen detection and viral culture [15].

The first-line treatment is intravenous ganciclovir 10 mg/kg/day for 14–21 days.

Esophagitis caused by HSV

Primary infection by the herpes simplex virus is common in childhood, and there are positive antibody titers for HSV in 90% of adolescents. The most common presentation of the infection is gingivostomatitis, and some patients with severe involvement of the oropharyngeal wall may present with esophagitis. In immunocompetent children, herpes esophagitis is rare but should be considered in patients with odynophagia, even in those without skin or oropharyngeal lesions. Esophagitis is mainly caused by HSV type 1, by direct propagation of oral infection [16,17].

The typical clinical picture of herpetic esophagitis includes the triad of acute odynophagia, retrosternal pain, and fever. Hematemesis may occur in approximately 5% of patients. Esophageal perforation, systemic infection, food impaction, and tracheoesophageal fistula formation rarely occur. There are descriptions of herpetic esophagitis associated with eosinophilic esophagitis but the relationship between these two disorders has not yet been elucidated [18,19].

The endoscopic characteristics of herpes esophagitis are mucosal friability and small rounded vesicles or well-delimited shallow ulcers, typically affecting the middle and distal esophagus (Figures 20.2 and 20.3). Biopsies should be collected from the ulcer's edge as the agent is present in squamous epithelium [17,20].

Differential diagnosis of the lesions includes other infections (CMV, HIV, *Candida* sp. and bacteria); caustic ingestion; Behçet's disease, Crohn's disease and lesions due to pill ingestion [16].

Histology reveals signs of acute inflammation, ulceration and abnormalities of epithelial cells suggestive of viral infection, including ballooning degeneration and necrosis. The

nuclei present a "ground-glass" aspect, with multinucleated cells and nuclear molding. To increase the sensitivity of the histological findings, it is ideal to perform immunohistochemistry, in situ hybridization or tissue culture [20,21].

Treatment is based on maintaining hydration, nutrition and adequate analgesia, including acid suppression therapy. The use of intravenous aciclovir in immunocompetent patients is controversial but may be considered in patients with severe odynophagia [22].

Esophagitis caused by tuberculosis

The GI tract is the sixth site of extrapulmonary tuberculosis infection. Esophageal involvement is an extremely rare form of infection, accounting for only 0.2–1% of the GI manifestations of the disease. Primary esophageal tuberculosis is uncommon and rarely affects immunocompetent patients [23]. The most frequent symptoms are odynophagia, retrosternal pain, and weight loss followed by dysphagia and hematemesis [24].

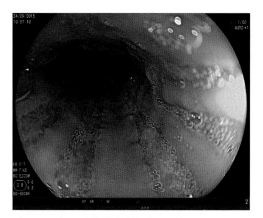

Figure 20.2 Endoscopic characteristics of herpes esophagitis including mucosal friability and small rounded vesicles or well-delimited shallow ulcers, typically affecting the middle and distal esophagus.

The typical lesion of esophageal tuberculosis is a solitary ulcer, with irregular margins, in the middle third of the esophagus. Complications such as bleeding, fistulae, and perforation are more frequent in tuberculosis

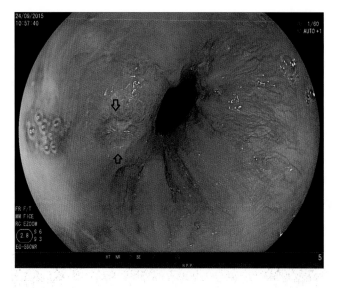

Figure 20.3 Similar characteristics are shown in this figure.

esophagitis than in other infectious esophagitis. Histology confirms the diagnosis when *Mycobacterium tuberculosis* or evidence of classic caseous granuloma is identified [25].

Other esophageal infections

Other viral infections rarely affect the esophagus in immunocompetent children. Among them, herpes zoster and EBV infections are reported as causes of ulcerative esophagitis in isolated cases [6]. The involvement of the esophagus by other fungal infections such as blastomycosis and histoplasmosis is reported sporadically in immunocompetent patients [2].

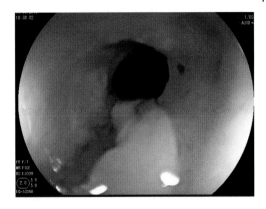

Figure 20.4 In epidermolysis bullosa, narrowing of the esophagus is more pronounced in the upper third, related to the intake of food that causes direct damage to the esophageal mucosa.

Epidermolysis bullosa

Epidermolysis bullosa (EB) is a hereditary rare disease, characterized by the development of blisters on the skin or mucous membranes with minimal trauma. The onset of the lesions usually occurs in early childhood [26,27].

The disease is classified into three major groups according to the form of genetic inheritance, specific clinical features and distribution of lesions, mucosal involvement and morbidity associated with the disease: EB simplex, junctional EB, and dystrophic EB [26,27].

The involvement of the GI tract is more frequent in patients with the recessive dystrophic form than other subtypes of EB. The intraluminal blisters, as they heal, can lead to single or multiple, short or long esophageal strictures, resulting in dysphagia, odynophagia, severe nutritional impairment, refractory anemia, hypoalbuminemia, malabsorption, and failure to thrive [26–28].

The onset of symptoms occurs up to the age of 10 in more than half of cases. Narrowing of the esophagus is more pronounced in the upper third, related to the intake of food that causes direct damage to the esophageal mucosa (Figure 20.4). The more distal strictures may be precipitated or exacerbated by gastroesophageal reflux. Radiological contrast studies provide additional information for planning the therapeutic strategy [26,28].

The goal of treatment is to facilitate swallowing and improve the nutritional status of the patient. Initial measures include dietary changes and nutritional supplementation associated with corticosteroid therapy, but only a few cases respond satisfactorily. When these measures are not sufficient to ensure adequate nutritional intake, esophageal dilation is necessary [26,28,29].

Endoscopic hydrostatic balloon dilation under direct visualization under fluoroscopic guidance is the preferred method. Balloon dilation produces radial force in the areas of stenosis and the localized lacerations are significantly smaller and therefore less likely to cause additional damage to the mucosa and esophageal perforation [26,29–31].

In situations where dilation of the esophagus is not available or in cases that do not respond satisfactorily to the procedure, a variety of surgical procedures may be used, but these procedures are complex and have high morbidity and mortality rates. Therefore, these procedures should be reserved for situations where the most conservative approach was ineffective [31].

Esophagitis in Crohn's disease

Crohn's disease can affect the entire GI tract. The esophagus is affected in approximately 3% of patients with ileocolonic disease, but isolated esophageal involvement is rare [32].

Esophageal symptoms range from odynophagia, heartburn, and chest pain to mild to severe dysphagia. In severe cases, bronchoesophageal or esophagogastric fistulae may develop [32].

Upper GI endoscopy reveals aphthous ulcerations and erosions usually located in the proximal esophagus, which helps in differentiating from peptic esophagitis (Figure 20.5). The typical histological finding is the presence of non-caseating granulomas, but this feature occurs in only 10% of patients [33].

Chemotherapy and radiotherapy-induced esophagitis

Esophageal disease is present in most patients undergoing chemotherapy and has been reported as the most troubling symptoms experienced by these patients [34,35]. Different chemotherapeutic agents (5-fluorouracil, methotrexate, vincristine, dactinomycin, bleomycin, daunorubicin, cytarabine) may induce esophageal damage, usually associated with severe oropharyngeal mucositis [36].

Thoracic irradiation-induced esophageal injury may also occur either by direct toxicity or by the radiosensitizing action of agents previously used for chemotherapy [37].

Patients receiving chemotherapy or radiation therapy are also at risk of presenting concomitant infectious (viral or fungal) esophagitis which must be considered in the differential diagnosis.

Symptoms of dysphagia and odynophagia that impair proper oral feeding should raise the suspicion of esophageal inflammation in these patients.

Endoscopy plays a role in the diagnosis, allowing sampling of the mucosa for identification of co-existing infections (e.g., cytological brushings, biopsy). However, a risk–benefit analysis for performing the procedure must consider patient factors (e.g., thrombocytopenia, neutropenia). Friability, edema, and erosions or ulcers are often found, with stricture formation as a further complication. The effectiveness of different treatment regimens for chemotherapy or radiation-induced esophagitis has not been properly evaluated. Acid suppression, topical anesthetics (e.g., viscous lidocaine),

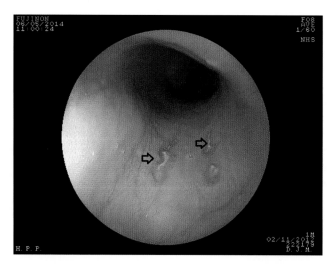

Figure 20.5 Crohn's esophageal involvement is usually with aphthoid ulceration and erosions can be seen throughout the esophagus, often located in the proximal esophagus, which helps in differentiating from peptic esophagitis.

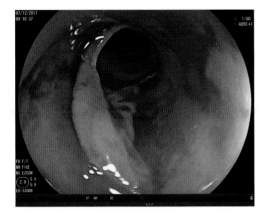

Figure 20.6 Radiation- or chemotherapy-induced esophagitis can be significant and can be treated with balloon dilation if strictures are identified.

steroids or narcotic analgesics have been routinely utilized to alleviate symptoms [38]. When identified, strictures are managed with endoscopic dilation (Figure 20.6).

Final considerations

Injury to the esophagus may result from a variety of causes including infection, medical treatment (chemotherapy and radiation therapy), or systemic illness. Endoscopy can be useful for diagnosing esophagitis, although a specific pattern is not identified in all cases and sampling of the mucosa may be useful in identifying the etiology of the injury.

Although other etiologies of esophageal injury occur less frequently than GERD in the pediatric population, pediatricians should be aware that esophageal symptoms may be the presenting feature of one of these conditions.

 • See companion website for videos relating to this chapter topic: www.wiley.com/go/gershman3e

REFERENCES

1 Noyer CM, Simon D. Oral and esophageal disorders. *Gastroenterol Clin North Am* 1997, **26**, 241–257.

2 Patel NC, Caicedo RA. Esophageal infections: an update. *Curr Opin Pediatr* 2015, **27**, 642–648.

3 Takahashi Y, Nagata N, Shimbo T, *et al.* Upper gastrointestinal symptoms predictive of candida esophagitis and erosive esophagitis in HIV and non-HIV patients. *Medicine* 2015, **94**, 2138.

4 Wang HW, Kuo CJ, Lin RW, *et al.* The clinical characteristics and manifestations of cytomegalovirus esophagitis. *Dis Esophagus* 2016, **29**, 392–399.

5 Werneck-Silva AL, Prado IB. Role of upper endoscopy in diagnosing opportunistic infections in human immunodeficiency virus-infected patients. *World J Gastroenterol* 2009, **15**, 1050–1056.

6 Zahmatkeshan M, Najib K, Geramizadeh B, Fallahzadeh E, Haghighat M, Hadi Imanieh M. Clinical characteristics of pediatric esophagitis in Southern Iran: a single-center experience. *Iran J Med Sci* 2013, **38**, 169–173.

7 Asayama N, Nagata N, Shimbo T, *et al.* Relationship between clinical factors and severy of esophageal candidiasis according to Kodsi's classification. *Dis Esophagus* 2014, **27**, 214–219.

8 Wilcox CM. Overview of infectious esophagitis. *Gastroenterol Hepatol* 2013, **9**, 517–519.

9 Kodsi BE, Wickremesinghe PC, Kozinn PJ, Iswara K, Goldberg PK. Candida esophagitis: a prospective study of 27 cases. *Gastroenterology* 1976, **71**, 715–719.

10 Kliemann DA, Pasqualotto AC, Falavigna AM, Giaretta T, Severo LC. Candida esophagitis: species distribution and risk factors for infection. *Rev Inst Med Trop Sao Paulo* 2008, **50**, 261–263.

11 Lemonovich TL, Watkins RR. Update on cytomegalovirus infections of the gastrointestinal system in solid organ transplant recipients. *Curr Infect Dis Rep* 2012, **14**, 33–40.

12 Wang HW, Cuo GJ, Lin WR, *et al.* The clinical characteristics and manifestations of cytomegalovirus esophagitis. *Dis Esophagus* 2016, **29**, 392–399.

13 Lim DS, Lee TH, Jin SY, Lee JS. Cytomegalovirus esophagitis in an immunocompetent patient: case report. *Turk J Gastroenterol* 2014, **25**, 571–574.

14 Hashimoto R, Chonan A. Esophagitis caused by cytomegalovirus infection in an immune-competent patient. *Clin Gastroenterol Hepatol* 2016, **14**, 143–144.

15 Maguire A, Sheahan K. Pathology of oesophagitis. *Histopathology* 2011, **60**, 864–979.

16 Al-Hussaini AA, Fagih MA. Herpes simplex ulcerative esophagitis in healthy children. *Saudi J Gastroenterol* 2011, **17**, 353–356.

17 Tzouvala M, Gaglia A, Papantoniou N, Triantafyllou K, Karamanolis G. Herpes simplex vírus eophagitis in an immunocompetent patient with Epstein–Barr virus infection. *Case Rep Gastroenterol* 2008, **2**, 451–455.

18 Castillero EC, Durán FG, Cabello N, Martínez JG. Herpes esophagitis in healthy adults and adolescents: report of 3 cases and review of the literature. *Medicine* 2010, **89**, 204–210.

19 Zimmermann D, Criblez DH, Dellon ES, *et al.* Acute herpes simplex viral esophagitis occurring in 5 immunocompetent individuals with eosinophilic esophagitis. *ACG Case Rep J* 2016, **3**, 165–168.

20 Wang H, Kuo CJ, Lin WR, *et al.* Clinical characteristics and manifestation of herpes esophagitis: one single-center experience in Taiwan. *Medicine* 2016, **95**, 3187.

21 Jibaly R, LaChance J, Abuhammour W. Herpes simplex esophagitis: report of 4 pediatric cases in immunocompetent patients. *J Pediatr Infect Dis* 2011, **6**, 205–209.

22 Lee B, Caddy G. A rare cause of dysphagia: herpes simplex esophagitis. *World J Gastroenterol* 2007, **13**, 2756–2757.

23 Vidal AP, Pannain VL, Bottino AM. Esophagitis in patients with acquired human immunodeficiency syndrome: a histological and immunohistochemistry study. *Arq Gastroenterol* 2007, **44**, 309–314.

24 Kumar S, Minz M, Sinha SK, *et al.* Esophageal tuberculosis with coexisting opportunistic infections in a renal allograft transplant recipient. *Transpl Infect Dis* 2017, **19**, 12640.

25 Jain SK, Jain S, Jain, M, Yaduvanshi A. Esophageal tuberculosis: is it so rare? Report of 12 cases and review of the literature. *Am J Gastroenterol* 2002, **97**, 287–291.

26 Castillo RO, Davies YK, Lin YC, Garcia M, Young H. Management of esophageal strictures in children with recessive dystrophic epidermolysis bullosa. *J Pediatr Gastroenterol Nutr* 2002, **34**, 535–541.

27 Fipe JD, Bruckner-Tuderman L, Eady RA, *et al.* Inherited epidermolysis bullosa: update recommendations on diagnosis and classification. *J Am Acad Dermatol* 2014, **70**, 1103–1126.

28 Ksia A, Mosbahi, S, Brahim MB. *et al.* Esophageal strictures in children with epidermolysis bullosa. *Arch Pediatr* 2012, **19**, 1325–1329.

29 Dall'Oglio L, Caldaro T, Foschia F, *et al.* Endoscopic management of esophageal stenosis in children: new and traditional treatments. *World J Gastrointest Endosc* 2016, **8**, 212–219.

30 Gollu G, Ergun E, Ates U, Can OS, Dindar H. Ballon dilatation in esophageal strictures in epidermolysis bullosa and the role of anesthesia. *Dis Esophagus* 2017, **30**, 1–6.

31 De Angelis P, Caldaro T, Torroni F, *et al.* Esophageal stenosis in epidermolysis bullosum: a challenge for the endoscopist. *J Pediatr Surg* 2011, **46**, 842–847.

32 Naranjo-Rodríguez A, Solórzano-Peck A, López-Rubio G, *et al.* Isolated oesophageal involvement of Crohn's disease. *Eur J Gastroenterol Hepatol* 2003, **15**, 1123–1126.

33 Grossi L, Ciccaglione AF, Marzio L. Esophagitis and it causes: who is "guilty" when acid is found "not guilty"? *World J Gastroenterol* 2017, **23**, 3011–3016.

34 Auguste LJ, Nava H. Postchemotherapy esophagitis: the endoscopic diagnosis and its impact on survival. *J Surg Oncol* 1986, **33**, 254–258.

35 Bellm LA, Epstein JB., Rose-Ped A, Martin P, Fuchs HJ. Patient reports of complications of bone marrow transplantation. *Support Care Cancer* 2000, **8**, 33–39.

36 Davila M, Bresalier RS. Gastrointestinal complications of oncologic therapy. *Nat Clin Pract Gastroenterol Hepatol* 2008, **5**, 682–696.

37 Werner-Wasik M, Yu X, Marks LB, Schultheiss TE. Normal-tissue toxicities of thoracic radiation therapy: esophagus, lung, and spinal cord as organs at risk. *Hematol Oncol Clin North Am* 2004, **18**, 131–160.

38 Berkey FJ. Managing the adverse effects of radiation therapy. *Am Fam Physician* 2010, **82**, 381–388, 394.

21

Eosinophilic esophagitis

Calies Menard-Katcher, Glenn T. Furuta, and Robert E. Kramer

 KEY POINTS

- The only currently available investigation which accurately diagnoses eosinophilic esophagitis (EE) and differentiates it from other esophageal pathologies is upper GI endoscopy with multiple biopsies.
- A pH study should usually accompany an upper GI endoscopy as reflux often co-exists with EE.

- At least two biopsies should be taken from the distal, middle, and proximal esophagus.
- EE strictures can be safely dilated with balloon dilation despite the apparent mucosal trauma elicited.
- About a quarter of EE cases have no macroscopically observable abnormality.

Introduction

Over the last decade, eosinophilic esophagitis (EoE) has emerged as one of the most common, if not the most common, causes of food impaction in children and adults. The diagnosis of EoE depends on the presence of symptoms and an abnormal esophageal biopsy that contains greater than 15 eosinophils per high-power field (HPF). Other causes for symptoms and esophageal eosinophilia need to be considered and ruled out prior to assigning the diagnosis of EoE. To date, no peripheral biomarker has been identified that could replace mucosal eosinophilia as a diagnostic benchmark. While there are several efforts to introduce less invasive methods of monitoring of mucosal inflammation once EoE is diagnosed, esophageal endoscopy continues to be essential to the diagnosis and management of EoE.

Endoscopy is not only helpful in its ability to obtain biopsies but also serves in several other ways. First, it helps to exclude other causes for presenting symptoms. Second, assessment of the esophageal mucosa by means of a validated endoscopic assessment score (EREFS) helps in determining the likelihood of identifying inflammation on biopsy and of response to treatment [1,2]. Endoscopy can also be a necessary method to retrieve foreign bodies and dislodge impacted food. Finally, it may be used to perform dilation in patients with EoE-related stricture(s) or long segment narrowing. This chapter will review each of these topics.

Mucosal biopsy procurement

Biopsies are obtained for three reasons in patients with EoE. At the initial presentation, they are obtained to verify or exclude the

---

Practical Pediatric Gastrointestinal Endoscopy, Third Edition. Edited by George Gershman and Mike Thomson.
© 2021 John Wiley & Sons Ltd. Published 2021 by John Wiley & Sons Ltd.
Companion website: www.wiley.com/go/gershman3e

presence of mucosal eosinophilia. Biopsies are procured from the proximal and distal esophagus and two studies in adults and children suggest that three biopsies from each site raises the probability of establishing the diagnosis to over 95% [3,4].

Biopsies have also been obtained to monitor disease activity. Several studies provide supporting evidence that reducing inflammation may reflect better outcomes [5] and, to date, using symptoms reported in the clinical setting as a primary assessment of treatment response does not appear to reliably correspond to presence or absence of mucosal eosinophilia. Since the reduction in mucosal eosinophilia may reflect better outcomes, surveillance endoscopic and histologic assessment has been deemed critical in therapeutic studies as well as clinical practice. Follow-up endoscopy for assessment of mucosal response to treatment is generally performed at approximately 8–12 weeks, though further studies will hopefully provide insight into the optimal timing of follow-up endoscopic assessment.

Finally, if patients with EoE develop unexpected symptoms while on treatment, endoscopy with biopsy assessment can help to assess for potential opportunistic infection, such as candida or herpes esophagitis.

Assessment of esophageal gross findings

To date, mucosal eosinophil enumeration has served as a biomarker for disease activity and therapeutic success. Since the esophageal biopsy represents less than 1% of the total surface area and counting eosinophils can be fraught with intraobserver variability, alternative methods have been sought. One of these focuses on the gross appearance of the esophageal mucosa and encompasses endoscopic features presently associated with EoE. The Eosinophilic Esophagitis Endoscopic Reference Score (EREFS) documents the presence or absence and severity of mucosal edema, rings,

exudate, furrows, and stricture [1] (Figures 21.1–21.4). While EREFS has not replaced the utility and specificity of histology assessment in either the clinical setting or in therapeutic trials, at least two studies have shown that its results can be used reliably to assess disease activity. Separate studies in adults and later in children and adolescents

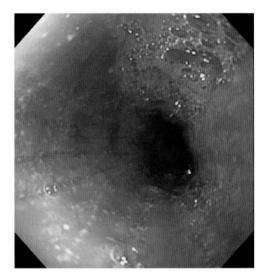

Figure 21.1 Exudate – whitish coating on the esophageal surface. Exudate represents eosinophilic purulent material.

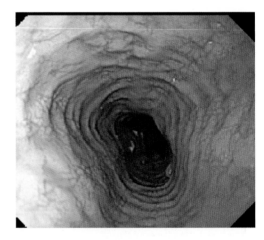

Figure 21.2 Circumferential rings along the length of the esophagus. This finding is representative of chronic remodeling.

determined that the EREFS classification system identified patients with EoE with an AUC of 0.93 [2,6].

A common language describing the endoscopic appearance allows clinicians and researchers to provide a more global assessment of changes seen in response to treatment. It also allows one to describe the possible progression of fibrostenotic complications that occur with chronic inflammation such as corrugated rings, stricture, and narrowing. This becomes important as we attempt to monitor patients over time in their response to treatment.

Therapeutic uses for endoscopy

Since patients with EoE can develop the complications of food impaction (Figure 21.5) and esophageal stricture, endoscopy is a necessary tool in both circumstances. Food impaction occurs in 33–55% of children and adults with EoE and often is the presenting feature [7]. Methods to remove food range from using single or multiple devices, including snare, net retriever, tripod grasper, rat tooth forceps, biopsy forceps, and suction. Due to the frequent need for multiple passes of the endoscope to fully remove an impaction, use of an overtube can be considered in children large enough to accommodate them, potentially to minimize the trauma of repeated esophageal intubation. Suction using a transparent suction cap secured to the end of the endoscope

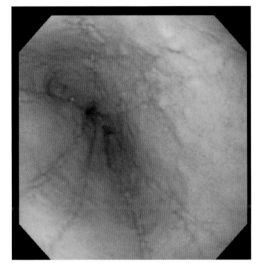

Figure 21.3 Mucosal edema and linear furrows. These finding are representative of mucosal edema with loss of vascular pattern.

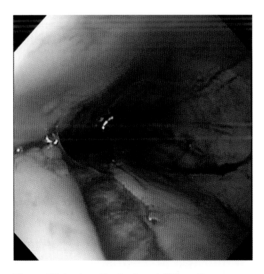

Figure 21.4 Longitudinal rent. This split can occur with the passage of the endoscope or dilator and represents fragility of the esophageal mucosa. It is also termed crepe paper esophagus or fragile esophageal mucosa.

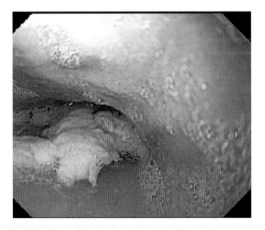

Figure 21.5 Food impaction present in the esophageal lumen. Mucosa is edematous.

has been shown to be effective and may reduce procedure time compared to other pull removal techniques [8]. Newer devices that combine a modified snare and a suction cap have been developed specifically to aid in the removal of impacted food. Often, difficult impactions require the use of multiple tools as they are rarely removed as a single piece. While gentle pressure to "push" the impaction into the stomach has been reported, extreme caution should be exercised as it often unknown if there may be a more distal stricture and longitudinal tearing of the mucosa due to crepe paper esophagus may occur.

Timing of this procedure is acute if there is drooling or other evidence of complete esophageal obstruction that puts the patient at risk for aspiration. For this reason, it should be done with endotracheal intubation. Even if the patient is able to manage their own secretions, removal of the impacted food bolus should be performed within 24 hours from the onset of symptoms to avoid tissue necrosis and decrease the risk of perforation during the procedure.

Focal strictures or long segment narrowings occur in a subset of children and many adults with EoE. Strictures may be isolated and focal but can also occur in a discontinuous or long segment fashion. The strictures or narrowing that occur in EoE can be detected by endoscopy but often require a high index of suspicion, complete esophageal insufflation and experience with EoE-related strictures. Studies in both children and adults demonstrate that narrowing can be missed in up to 55% of patients if endoscopy alone is used as a diagnostic tool, compared to barium esophagram and endoscopy together [9,10]. If a patient has solid food dysphagia, particularly when it persists after initiating EoE-directed treatment, performance of a barium esophagram, often with a coated pill, can be helpful in planning endoscopic interventions.

The method of performing dilation of the EoE-related narrowing can be different from that used for peptic or caustic strictures. More frequently, EoE-related strictures are long segment or diffuse, making them more amenable to bougie dilation with either Maloney or wire-guided Savary dilators. When focal strictures exist, balloon dilation is a reasonable approach and has the benefit of offering direct visualization during dilation as well as directing all the force radially. Bougie dilation directs some of the dilating force tangentially, which has lead to some concern that perforation risk is increased with this method, though there has not been clear evidence to support this contention. A balloon pull-through technique has also been described for adults in the management of EoE narrowing [11].

Complications include bleeding and esophageal perforation but several studies in adults and children have found these complications to be rare and no more frequent than in esophageal dilations for other underlying etiologies [12,13]. A systemic review of dilation in EoE and a metaanalysis comparing dilation method found that perforation from esophageal dilation in EoE is rare, and no evidence of a significant difference in perforation risk related to dilator type has been found [14]. Postoperative chest pain, however, is expected and can be preemptively treated with over-the-counter pain medications [12].

Dilation can improve dysphagia when used in the appropriate patient but it should not be viewed as an alternative to medication or dietary management of EoE – strategies that are directed at targeting the chronic inflammation. When inflammation is controlled, patients require fewer dilations to achieve a similar improvement in esophageal diameter [15]. When patients have fibrostenotic features and require dilation, more than half of patients – both adolescents and adults – will require repeated dilation in their management, often within a year of initial dilation [13,16].

Future alternative devices for mucosal assessment

While endoscopy will likely remain a critical and necessary part of EoE diagnosis, several approaches have been developed with the goal of either minimizing the invasive nature of repeat endoscopy used in monitoring response to treatment or providing an alternate global assessment of the esophagus in EoE.

Unsedated transnasal endoscopy is currently being used to sample the mucosa for histology [17]. This allows the patient to avoid anesthesia or sedation which may minimize cost and/or the time our patients need to take for procedures. Even less invasive are approaches that assess the esophageal mucosa without the need for sedation or biopsy, including the Esophageal String Test [18], Cytosponge™ [19], and confocal microscopy [20]. These approaches ideally will allow assessment of histological response to treatment without the use of endoscopy.

The EndoFlip® (Medtronic), a novel device used during endoscopy to identify the distensibility of the esophagus, may provide an outcome measure that more closely associates with patient outcomes. An adult study identified differences in patients with EoE compared to normal and it may be able to predict the likelihood of having a food impaction [21]. Differences in distensibility have also been seen in the pediatric EoE population and appear to be associated with clinical fibrostenotic features [22]. Future studies will be needed to show how these new tools will complement or be incorporated into current management approaches in EoE.

Acknowledgments

This work was supported by NIH 1K24DK100303 (Furuta) and Consortium for Gastrointestinal Eosinophilic Researchers (CEGIR). CEGIR (U54 AI117804) is part of the Rare Diseases Clinical Research Network (RDCRN), an initiative of the Office of Rare Diseases Research (ORDR), NCATS, and is funded through collaboration between NIAID, NIDDK, and NCATS and the support patient advocacy groups APFED, CURED and EFC (Furuta). NIH K23DK109263 (Menard-Katcher).

 • See companion website for videos relating to this chapter topic: www.wiley.com/go/gershman3e

REFERENCES

1 Hirano I, Moy N, Heckman MG, Thomas CS, Gonsalves N, Achem SR. Endoscopic assessment of the oesophageal features of eosinophilic oesophagitis: validation of a novel classification and grading system. *Gut* 2013, **62**, 489–495.

2 Dellon ES, Cotton CC, Gebhart JH, *et al.* Accuracy of the eosinophilic esophagitis endoscopic reference score in diagnosis and determining response to treatment. *Clin Gastroenterol Hepatol* 2016, **14**, 31–39.

3 Gonsalves N, Policarpio-Nicolas M, Zhang Q, Rao MS, Hirano I. Histopathologic variability and endoscopic correlates in adults with eosinophilic esophagitis. *Gastrointest Endosc* 2006, **64**, 313–319.

4 Shah A, Kagalwalla AF, Gonsalves N, Melin-Aldana H, Li BUK, Hirano I. Histopathologic variability in children with eosinophilic esophagitis. *Am J Gastroenterol* 2009, **104**, 716–721.

5 Kuchen T, Straumann A, Safroneeva E, *et al.* Swallowed topical corticosteroids reduce the risk for long-lasting bolus impactions in eosinophilic esophagitis. *Allergy* 2014, **69**, 1248–1254.

6 Wechsler JB, Bolton SM, Amsden K, Wershil BK, Hirano I, Kagalwalla AF. Eosinophilic esophagitis reference score accurately identifies disease activity and treatment effects in children. *Clin Gastroenterol Hepatol* 2018, **16**, 1056–1063.

7 Desai TK, Stecevic V, Chang CH, Goldstein NS, Badizadegan K, Furuta GT. Association of eosinophilic inflammation with esophageal food impaction in adults. *Gastrointest Endosc* 2005, **61**, 795–801.

8 Ooi M, Young EJ, Nguyen NQ. Effectiveness of a cap-assisted device in the endoscopic removal of food bolus obstruction from the esophagus. *Gastrointest Endosc* 2018, **87**, 1198–1203.

9 Gentile N, Katzka D, Ravi K, *et al.* Oesophageal narrowing is common and frequently under-appreciated at endoscopy in patients with oesophageal eosinophilia. *Aliment Pharmacol Ther* 2014, **40**, 1333–1340.

10 Menard-Katcher C, Swerdlow MP, Mehta P, Futura GT, Fenton LZ. Contribution of esophagram to the evaluation of complicated pediatric eosinophilic esophagitis. *J Pediatr Gastroenterol Nutr* 2015, **61**, 541–546.

11 Madanick RD, Shaheen NJ, Dellon ES. A novel balloon pull-through technique for esophageal dilation in eosinophilic esophagitis (with video). *Gastrointest Endosc* 2011, **73**, 138–142.

12 Schoepfer AM, Gonsalves N, Bussmann C, *et al.* Esophageal dilation in eosinophilic esophagitis: effectiveness, safety, and impact on the underlying inflammation. *Am J Gastroenterol* 2010, **105**, 1062–1070.

13 Menard-Katcher C, Furuta GT, Kramer RE. Dilation of pediatric eosinophilic esophagitis: adverse events and short-term outcomes. *J Pediatr Gastroenterol Nutr* 2017, **64**, 701–706.

14 Dougherty M, Runge TM, Eluri S, Dellon ES. Esophageal dilation with either bougie or balloon technique as a treatment for eosinophilic esophagitis: a systematic review and meta-analysis. *Gastrointest Endosc* 2017, **86**, 581–591.

15 Runge TM, Eluri S, Woosley JT, Shaheen NJ, Dellon ES. Control of inflammation decreases the need for subsequent esophageal dilation in patients with eosinophilic esophagitis. *Dis Esophagus* 2017, **30**, 1–7.

16 Runge TM, Eluri S, Cotton CC, *et al.* Outcomes of esophageal dilation in eosinophilic esophagitis: safety, efficacy, and persistence of the fibrostenotic phenotype. *Am J Gastroenterol* 2016, **111**, 206–213.

17 Friedlander JA, DeBoer EM, Soden JS, *et al.* Unsedated transnasal esophagoscopy for monitoring therapy in pediatric eosinophilic esophagitis. *Gastrointest Endosc* 2016, **83**, 299–306.

18 Furuta GT, Kagalwalla AF, Lee JJ, *et al.* The oesophageal string test: a novel, minimally invasive method measures mucosal inflammation in eosinophilic oesophagitis. *Gut* 2013, **62**, 1395–1405.

19 Katzka DA, Smyrk TC, Alexander JA, *et al.* Accuracy and safety of the cytosponge for assessing histologic activity in eosinophilic esophagitis: a two-center study. *Am J Gastroenterol* 2017, **112**, 1538–1544.

20 Tabatabaei N, Kang DK, Kim M, *et al.* Clinical translation of tethered confocal microscopy capsule for unsedated diagnosis of eosinophilic esophagitis. *Sci Rep* 2018, **8**, 2631.

21 Nicodème F, Hirano I, Chen J, *et al.* Esophageal distensibility as a measure of disease severity in patients with eosinophilic esophagitis. *Clin Gastroenterol Hepatol* 2013, **11**, 1101–1107.

22 Menard-Katcher C, Benitez AJ, Pan Z, *et al.* Influence of age and eosinophilic esophagitis on esophageal distensibility in a pediatric cohort. *Am J Gastroenterol* 2017, **112**, 1466–1473.

22

Gastritis and gastropathy

Shishu Sharma and Mike Thomson

 KEY POINTS

- "Gastritis" is a term used when histological confirmation of gastric inflammation is identified and is not an endoscopic term.

- There are many different causes of "gastropathy" which may or may not include inflammation and *H. pylori* is a diminishing cause in children.

Introduction

In the pediatric population the prevalence of *Helicobacter pylori*-related gastritis is in decline due to changes in overall global socioeconomic status, better diagnostic techniques, and effective treatment. Henc,e the other causes of gastritis and gastropathy have become more relevant and will be discussed in this chapter.

Gastritis and gastropathy are two terms which are inappropriately used interchangeably. The term *gastritis* should be used if there is an inflammation or gastric mucosal injury. *Gastropathy* should be used when there is gastric mucosal disorder without any inflammation or with negligible inflammation. The mucosal disorder can further be defined as epithelial cell injury which may be followed by regeneration [1]. Gastritis and gastropathy can be classified according to morphological features or based on etiology (Table 22.1).

Infective gastropathy

Helicobacter pylori has traditionally been the most common cause of gastritis in children [2] but with better socioeconomic conditions, early diagnosis and effective treatment, there has been a steady decline in its prevalence [3]. Hence there is increased reporting of non-*Helicobacter pylori* gastritis [4]. Besides *H. pylori*, *H. heilmanii* (previously called *Gastrospirillium hominis*), which is a spiral bacterium, can also cause chronic gastritis [5]. This bacterium is transmitted to humans via cats and dogs [6,7].

Gastric tuberculosis usually develops secondary to other primary lesions but sporadic primary gastric tuberculosis has been reported [8,9]. This can present as pyrexia of unknown origin [10], gastric outlet obstruction [11], benign peptic ulcer [12], stomach perforation [13], and gastric carcinoma [14]. The lesions are primarily present in the antrum

Practical Pediatric Gastrointestinal Endoscopy, Third Edition. Edited by George Gershman and Mike Thomson.
© 2021 John Wiley & Sons Ltd. Published 2021 by John Wiley & Sons Ltd.
Companion website: www.wiley.com/go/gershman3e

Table 22.1 Classification of gastropathy. Gastritis and gastropathy can be classified according to morphological features or based on etiology

Infective	Immune-mediated gastropathy
Helicobacter pylori	Autoimmune gastropathy
Non-*H. pylori* helicobacter species	Autoimmune endocrinopathies
Phlegmonous/suppurative	Graft-versus-host disease
Mycobacterial	
Viral	
Cytomegalovirus	
Epstein–Barr virus	
Human herpes virus 6	
Hepatitis C	
Measles	
Varicella	
Influenza	
Parasitic	
Giardia	
Ascariasis	
Cryptosporidium	
Toxoplasma	
Leishmaniasis	
Fungal	
Treponemal	
Granulomatous gastropathy	Vascular
Noninfectious	Henoch–Schönlein purpura
Crohn's disease	Portal hypertensive gastropathy
Sarcoidosis	Gastric antral vascular ectasia
Infectious	
Idiopathic	
Reactive and drug-induced gastropathy	Ischemic
NSAIDs	Trauma
Iron salts	Prolapse
Alendronate (bisphosphonates)	Burns
Sodium phosphate	Sepsis
Ethanol	Hypovolemia
Bile reflux	Cocaine
Corrosive	
Radiation	
Stress and exercise	
Allergic and eosinophilic	Others
Lymphocytic gastropathy	Collagenous
Celiac disease	Uremic gastropathy
	Hyperplastic gastropathy

NSAID, nonsteroidal antiinflammatory drug.

and prepyloric region. The endoscopic findings could be solitary or multiple ulcer or hypertrophic nodular lesions or pyloric stenosis.

Cytomegalovirus (CMV) gastritis is primarily but not exclusively seen in immunocompromised children [15]. It is also associated with childhood Menetrier's disease [16]. The endoscopic findings can include congested mucosa, swollen rugal folds with multiple erosions or ulcerations [17] and primarily it affects the gastric body and fundus. CMV DNA polymerase chain reaction (PCR) from biopsy samples is more sensitive than serology and also aids in disease localization [18,19]. Though spontaneous recovery usually occurs within 1–2 months, early detection and antiviral therapy can reduce morbidity and mortality in high-risk cases [20].

Other viruses that can cause gastritis are Epstein–Barr virus (EBV), herpes virus, hepatitis C, measles, varicella, and influenza, especially influenza A which can cause hemorrhagic diffuse gastritis.

The two most common gastritides caused by parasites are those ascribed to giardiasis and ascariasis. Giardiasis is associated with conditions causing hypochlorhydria such as biliary reflux, atrophic gastritis, partial gastrectomy or use of proton pump inhibitors (PPI). In such situations, correction of gastric pH, for example by discontinuation of PPI, can lead to decolonization of *Giardia* without any specific therapy [21].

Cryptosporidium, *Toxoplasma*, and *Leishmania* are other parasites causing gastritis, particularly in immunocompromised patients [22–24].

Fungal gastritis is seen in children with faltering growth, burns or those who are immunocompromised. The main pathogens are *Candida*, *Aspergillus*, *Histoplasma*, and mucormycosis.

Phlegmonous or suppurative gastritis is a rare rapidly progressive bacterial infection of the gastric submucosa leading to gangrene/necrosis or emphysema [25] which can occur predominantly in immunocompromised patients [26–28]. The main pathogens are alpha- and beta-hemolytic streptococci, although *Pneumococcus*, *E. coli*, *Staphylococcus aureus*, *Proteus*, and *Clostridium welchii* may also be implicated. The treatment includes aggressive use of antibiotics and very occasionally gastrectomy.

Reactive gastropathy

Reactive gastropathy or type C gastritis is the most common histological finding on gastric biopsies in North America [29]. There are no known specific endoscopic findings, but histologically it is characterized by foveolar hyperplasia, edema, smooth muscle hyperplasia and congestion of superficial capillaries in the lamina propria in absence of significant inflammation [30,31]. It occurs in response to long-term exposure to irritants such as bile, NSAIDs, corrosives, and other drugs.

It is important to highlight here the term *acute hemorrhagic erosive gastropathy* which develops shortly after exposure of gastric mucosa to various injurious irritants or may be due to significantly diminished gastric mucosal blood flow, leading to disruption of the gastric protective barrier, or occasionally viruses such as influenza A. Endoscopy shows multiple petechial hemorrhages and erosions [32], which are usually confined to the fundus and body in stress-related lesions (Curling's ulcers) or could be widespread, as with NSAIDs or ethanol [33].

Stress-induced gastritis (stress-related erosive syndrome) is associated with massive burn injury, head injury, sepsis, trauma and multiple system organ failure. A cohort of 1006 consecutive admissions enrolled in a pediatric intensive care unit reported upper GI bleeding in 10.2% admissions with 1.6% having significant upper GI bleed [34]. Although there is a clear guideline on stress-related prophylaxis for adults admitted to intensive care, unfortunately no such standardized guideline exists for the pediatric population [35].

Duodenogastric reflux (DGR) leading to biliary gastropathy could primarily occur due to motility issues or it could be secondary to surgery of the stomach, duodenum or gallbladder [36]. Therapeutic options are limited. Ursodeoxycholic acid is effective in reducing pain, nausea and vomiting [37]. Ursodeoxycholic acid is not proved to be effective in resolution of endoscopic or histological findings, but sucralfate does improve histological features [38]. Colestyramine can also be helpful by binding bile acids.

Accidental corrosive ingestion leading to gastropathy is a common problem in children worldwide [39]. In a review of 156 children with caustic ingestion, 11% had esophageal and gastric burns and 9% had gastric burns only [40]. Gastric injury is more likely to occur after ingestion of liquid rather than solid alkali [41]. The North American Society for Pediatric Gastroenterology Hepatology and Nutrition (NASPGHAN) has published guidelines for management of corrosive ingestion in the pediatric population [42].

Other causes of gastropathy are summarized in Table 22.1.

Conclusion

The etiology of pediatric gastropathy is different from that seen in adults and thus requires a tailored approach. Endoscopy and histopathology play a pivotal role in defining the etiology, localization, and extent of injury. As the prevalence of *H. pylori* declines, more emphasis is being placed on other causes of gastropathy. There is a need to develop an acceptable pediatric guideline for prophylaxis of stress-related gastropathy in an ICU setting and also in stress-inducing operations such as big orthopedic procedures – PPI prophylaxis is indicated in these situations.

 • See companion website for videos relating to this chapter topic: www.wiley.com/go/gershman3e

REFERENCES

1 Glickman JN, Antonioli DA. Gastritis. *Gastrointest Endosc Clin North Am* 2001, **11**, 717–740.

2 Drumm B, Sherman P, Cutz E, Karmali M. Association of Campylobacter pylori on the gastric mucosa with antral gastritis in children. *N Engl J Med* 1987, **316**, 1557–1561.

3 Genta RM, Lash RH. Helicobacter pylori-negative gastritis: seek, yet ye shall not always find. *Am J Surg Pathol* 2010, **34**, e25–e34.

4 Elitsur Y, Lawrence Z. Non-Helicobacter pylori related duodenal ulcer disease in children. *Helicobacter* 2001, **6**, 239–243.

5 Oliva MM, Lazenby AJ, Perman JA. Gastritis associated with Gastrospirillum hominis in children. Comparison with Helicobacter pylori and review of the literature. *Mod Pathol* 1993, **6**, 513–515.

6 Thomson MA, Storey P, Greer R, Cleghorn GJ. Canine-human transmission of

Gastrospirillum hominis. *Lancet* 1994, **344**, 1097–1098.

7 Lavelle JP, Landas S, Mitros FA, Conklin JL. Acute gastritis associated with spiral organisms from cats. *Dig Dis Sci* 1994, **39**, 744–750.

8 Subei I, Attar B, Schmitt G, Levendoglu H. Primary gastric tuberculosis: a case report and literature review. *Am J Gastroenterol* 1987, **82**, 769–772.

9 Brody JM, Miller DK, Zeman RK, *et al.* Gastric tuberculosis: a manifestation of acquired immunodeficiency syndrome. *Radiology* 1986, **159**, 347–348.

10 Salpeter SR, Shapiro RM, Gasman JD. Gastric tuberculosis presenting as fever of unknown origin. *West J Med* 1991, **155**, 412–413.

11 Gupta B, Mathew S, Bhalla S. Pyloric obstruction due to gastric tuberculosis – an endoscopic diagnosis. *Postgrad Med J* 1990, **66**, 63–65.

12 Rathnaraj S, Singh SK, Verghese M. Gastric tuberculosis presenting with hematemesis. *Indian J Gastroenterol* 1997, **16**, 110–111.

13 Sharma BC, Prasad H, Bhasin DK, Singh K. Gastroduodenal tuberculosis presenting with massive hematemesis in a pregnant woman. *J Clin Gastroenterol* 2000, **30**, 336.

14 Khan FY, AlAni A, Al-Rikabi A, Mizrakhshi A, Osman ME. Primary gastric fundus tuberculosis in immunocompetent patient: a case report and literature review. *Braz J Infect Dis* 2008, **12**, 453–455.

15 Hinnant KL, Rotterdam HZ, Bell ET, Tapper ML. Cytomegalovirus infection of the alimentary tract: a clinicopathological correlation. *Am J Gastroenterol* 1986, **81**, 944–950.

16 Hoffer V, Finkelstein Y, Balter J, Feinmesser M, Garty BZ. Ganciclovir treatment in Menetrier's disease. *Acta Paediatr* 2003, **92**, 983–985.

17 Emory TS, Gostout CJ, Carpenter HA. *Atlas of Gastrointestinal Endoscopy & Endoscopic Biopsies*. American Registry of Pathology, Washington, DC, 2000.

18 Andrade J de S, Bambirra EA, Lima GF, Moreira EF, de Oliveira CA. Gastric cytomegalic inclusion bodies diagnosed by histologic examination of endoscopic biopsies in patients with gastric ulcer. *Am J Clin Pathol* 1983, **79**, 493–496.

19 Bonnet F, Neau D, Viallard JF, *et al.* Clinical and laboratory findings of cytomegalovirus infection in 115 hospitalized non-immunocompromised adults. *Ann Med Intern* 2001, **152**, 227–235.

20 Goodrich JM, Mori M, Gleaves CA, *et al.* Early treatment with ganciclovir to prevent cytomegalovirus disease after allogeneic bone marrow transplantation. *N Engl J Med* 1991, **325**, 1601–1607.

21 Reynaert H, Fernandes E, Bourgain C, Smekens L, Devis G. Proton-pump inhibition and gastric giardiasis: a causal or casual association? *J Gastroenterol* 1995, **30**, 775–778.

22 Lumadue JA, Manabe YC, Moore RD, Belitsos PC, Sears CL, Clark DP. A clinicopathologic analysis of AIDS-related cryptosporidiosis. *AIDS* 1998, **12**, 2459–2466.

23 Kofman E, Khorsandi A, Sarlin J, Adhami K. Gastric toxoplasmosis: case report and review of the literature. *Am J Gastroenterol* 1996, **91**, 2436–2438.

24 Laguna F, García-Samaniego J, Soriano V, *et al.* Gastrointestinal leishmaniasis in human immunodeficiency virus-infected patients: report of five cases and review. *Clin Infect Dis* 1994, **19**, 48–53.

25 Kussin SZ, Henry C, Navarro C, Stenson W, Clain DJ. Gas within the wall of the stomach report of a case and review of the literature. *Dig Dis Sci* 1982, **27**, 949–954.

26 Panieri E, Krige J. Phlegmonous gastritis. *Dig Surg* 1997, **14**, 210.

27 Mittleman RE, Suarez RV. Phlegmonous gastritis associated with the acquired immunodeficiency syndrome/pre-acquired immunodeficiency syndrome. *Arch Pathol Lab Med* 1985, **109**, 765–767.

28 Miller AI, Smith B, Rogers AI. Phlegmonous gastritis. *Gastroenterology* 1975, **68**, 231–238.

29 Carpenter HA, Talley NJ. Gastroscopy is incomplete without biopsy: clinical relevance of distinguishing gastropathy from gastritis. *Gastroenterology* 1995, **108**, 917–924.

30 Appelman HD. Gastritis: terminology, etiology, and clinicopathological correlations: another biased view. *Hum Pathol* 1994, **25**, 1006–1019.

31 Dixon MF, O'Connor HJ, Axon AT, King RF, Johnston D. Reflux gastritis: distinct histopathological entity? *J Clin Pathol* 1986, **39**, 524–530.

32 Sloan JM. Acute haemorrhagic gastritis and acute infective gastritis, gastritis caused by physical agents and corrosive, uremic gastritis. In: Whitehead R (ed.). *Gatrointestinal and Oesophageal Pathology*. Churchill Livingstone, Edinburgh, 1989, p. 385.

33 Sugawa C, Lucas CE, Rosenberg BF, Riddle JM, Walt AJ. Differential topography of acute erosive gastritis due to trauma or sepsis, ethanol and aspirin. *Gastrointest Endosc* 1973, **19**, 127–130.

34 Chaibou M, Tucci M, Dugas MA, Farrell CA, Proulx F, Lacroix J. Clinically significant upper gastrointestinal bleeding acquired in a pediatric intensive care unit: a prospective study. *Pediatrics* 1998, **102**, 933–938.

35 Spirt MJ, Stanley S. Update on stress ulcer prophylaxis in critically ill patients. *Crit Care Nurse* 2006, **26**, 18–20.

36 Bonavina L, Incarbone R, Segalin A, Chella B, Peracchia A. Duodeno-gastro-esophageal reflux after gastric surgery: surgical therapy and outcome in 42 consecutive patients. *Hepatogastroenterology* 1999, **46**, 92–96.

37 Stefaniwsky AB, Tint GS, Speck J, Shefer S, Salen G. Ursodeoxycholic acid treatament of bile reflux gastritis. *Gastroenerology* 1985, **89**,1000–1004.

38 Buch KL, Weinstein WM, Hill TA, *et al.* Sucralfate therapy in patients with symptoms of alklaine reflux gastritis. A randomized, double-blind study. *Am J Med* 1985, **79**, 49–54.

39 Buntain WL, Cain WC. Caustic injuries to the esophagus: a pediatric overview. *South Med J* 1981, **74**, 590–593.

40 Previtera C, Giusti F, Guglielmi M. Predictive value of visible lesions (cheeks, lips, oropharynx) in suspected caustic ingestion: may endoscopy reasonably be omitted in completely negative pediatric patients? *Pediatr Emerg Care* 1990, **6**, 176–178.

41 Weigert A. Caustic ingestion in children. *Contin Educ Anaesth Crit Care Pain* 2005, **5**, 5–8.

42 Kramer RE, Lerner DG, Lin T, *et al.* Management of ingested foreign bodies in children: a clinical report of the NASPGHAN Endoscopy Committee. *J Pediatr Gastroenterol Nutr* 2015, **60**, 562–574.

23

Celiac disease

Alina Popp, Vasile Daniel Balaba, and Markku Mäki

 KEY POINTS

- Macroscopic evidence of likely celiac disease includes a mosaic appearance of the duodenal mucosa, so-called "scalloping" of the duodenal folds, and a serrated appearance of the folds.
- At least four biopsies from the duodenum distal to the second part and two biopsies from the first part of the duodenum should be obtained and ideally orientated on card in the endoscopy room.

- Endoscopic confirmation of the diagnosis of manifest celiac disease may now not be needed if the tTG IgA is greater than 10× the upper limit of normal, the antiendomysial IgA is positive, and the patient is symptomatic. Additional HLA DQ2 and/or DQ8 positivity may not be required.

Introduction

Celiac disease (CD) is an immune-mediated, systemic disease triggered and driven by an environmental insult, for example by gluten ingestion in genetically susceptible individuals. As the autoimmune process primarily involves the small intestine, leading to the pathognomonic gluten-triggered and gluten-dependent villous atrophy and crypt hyperplasia, examination and sampling of the duodenal mucosa by means of endoscopy is an important part of the diagnosis.

From the old days of Margot Shiner's jejunal biopsy tube and Watson and Crosby capsules [1], when we were blindly sampling the intestinal mucosa, we now have the opportunity to do in vivo a presumptive visual diagnosis by analyzing the villous surface with novel endoscopic techniques such as water immersion, chromoendoscopy, magnification or confocal laser endomicroscopy, followed by histopathological evaluation of sampled biopsy specimens. Although in adult CD histological assessment of enterobiopsy samples is currently the gold standard for diagnosis, in pediatric CD there has been a possibility to perform a nonbiopsy diagnosis, when following certain rules: the patient should have symptoms that could be attributable to CD, serum transglutaminase 2 antibody (TG2-ab) titers >10 times upper limit of normality, be endomysial antibody positive and carry human leukocyte antigen (HLA) DQ2 or DQ8 molecules [2].

Here we discuss the strengths and weaknesses of small intestinal endoscopic diagnosis and pitfalls in sampling and reading of biopsy specimens.

Practical Pediatric Gastrointestinal Endoscopy, Third Edition. Edited by George Gershman and Mike Thomson.
© 2021 John Wiley & Sons Ltd. Published 2021 by John Wiley & Sons Ltd.
Companion website: www.wiley.com/go/gershman3e

Visual diagnosis, biopsy sampling, handling, and histopathology

Despite the nonbiopsy strategy adopted in recent years for symptomatic patients, endoscopy remains essential for most children suspected for CD – for patients with no or vague symptoms, with signs of malabsorption without symptoms, with extraintestinal manifestations, in risk groups and healthy family members. However, compared to adults, where endoscopy can also be considered a case finding tool, its role in pediatric CD has been merely for mucosal sampling to get biopsy specimens for diagnosis. The same endoscopic features of CD that have been described in adult patients have been reported in children also – mucosal mosaic pattern, scalloping, visible vascular pattern or reduction of duodenal folds; these endoscopic markers however have low sensitivity in children with CD [3,4].

Over the years, endoscopic visualization of the duodenal mucosal pattern has improved, so that today one can see the villi up close, with the aid of advanced endoscopic techniques, as is the case with water immersion images as shown in Figures 23.1a and 23.1b, corresponding to histopathological views of normal mucosal morphology (Figure 23.1c) and subtotal villous atrophy. Also demonstrated is the pathognomonic feature of a manifest lesion in CD (Figure 23.1e). Endoscopists may nowadays set a real-time diagnosis of clear villous atrophy, confirming, correcting or even replacing the pathologist's work. However, endoscopy cannot assess for crypt hyperplasia thus missing early developing disease with villi still normal looking and tall (Figure 23.1a and 23.1d). This was true also for properly oriented biopsies evaluated under liquid surface using high-power dissecting microscope showing the mucosal morphology continuum from normal to "flat" (Figure 23.1a–d). Crypt hyperplasia may already be occurring when the mucosa is visually evaluated as "normal" (Figure 23.1a and 23.1b). At a later stage when crypt hyperplasia is more prominent, the villi merge and convolute to low villous ridges (Figure 23.1c) and further to the gluten-induced so-called "flat" lesion, the endstage of the mucosal pathology continuum (Figure 23.1d). When biopsies showing low villous ridges are cut wrongly (tangentially), artificially tall villi are seen on histology slides, evaluated to represent normal mucosa of grade Marsh 0 or I when actually being Marsh 3b or 3c [5] (Figure 23.1e). Studies correlating visual endoscopic appearance to proper morphometric evaluations are lacking.

Gluten-induced duodenal mucosal lesions can be patchy, depending on the time and amount of gluten ingestion. This is where novel endoscopic techniques such as chromoendoscopy come in, allowing for targeted biopsies in the diseased mucosa. In routine clinics the diagnosis is based on the most severe lesions of the sampled biopsies.

Visualization of villi using modern endoscopic techniques is not widely available, and also because of missing comparative studies, traditional histological assessment of biopsies is needed. CD guidelines support a multiple biopsy protocol, two specimens from the bulb and four from the distal part of the duodenum, but these recommendations are poorly followed in routine practice [6–9], mostly because of prolonged procedural time [8,10]. Therefore a multibite biopsy technique has been suggested, but a study in adults proved that the single-biopsy technique is preferred, yielding a higher proportion of well-oriented duodenal biopsy specimens [11]. As mentioned, the orientation and correct vertical cutting of biopsy specimens are of paramount importance as neither morphometric results nor Marsh class can be given if crypts are cut in cross-section only.

Biopsy orientation on acetate cellulose filters in the endoscopy room has been recommended [12] but again, it is not enough to blindly press the biopsy on a filter strip resulting in messy fixed biopsies; proper orientation is needed (Figure 23.2). Recuttings are often demanded to find a representative number of intact villus-crypt units to allow evaluation, so

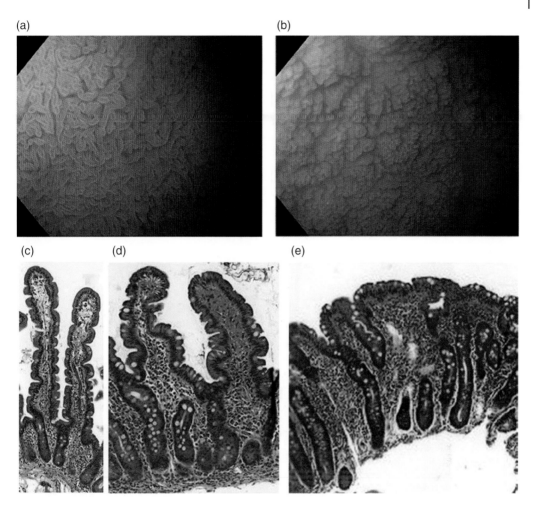

Figure 23.1 (a) Endoscopy with water immersion showing normal villus pattern of the duodenal mucosa, in a healthy patient (Marsh grade 0). (b) Endoscopy with water immersion showing blunted villi, in a CD patient with subtotal villous atrophy (Marsh grade 3b or 3c). (c) Histology appearance of (a), tall villi and low crypts with a villus height (VH):crypt depth (CrD) ratio of 3.15. (d) Histology appearance of a similar visual mucosal appearance of intact villi as in (a); villi appear tall but there is a clear crypt hyperplasia, VH:CrD of 1.57, i.e., diseased mucosa representing Marsh grade 3a. (e) Histology appearance of a pathognomonic celiac disease crypt hyperplastic lesion, VH:CrD 0.2, corresponding to Marsh grade 3c.

biopsies should be processed separately, not placed in the same paraffin block.

Duodenal bulb biopsies have been traditionally avoided because of concerns regarding their difficult interpretation due to histological confounders such as peptic injury, gastric metaplasia, Brunner's glands or lymphoid follicles [13]. Current guidelines recommend taking biopsies from the proximal mucosa and the bulb, resulting in a diagnosis called ultra-short

CD [14]. However, a pediatric CD study has shown that bulb specimens are frequently of poor quality, tiny or having many Brunner artefacts, rendering them unreadable. Further morphological injury, even with crypt hyperplasia, is common in the duodenal bulb in nonceliacs, leading to false-positive diagnoses [15]; for these situations, evaluation for bulb TG2-targeted IgA subepithelial deposits is a powerful tool to confirm CD [15]. If bulb

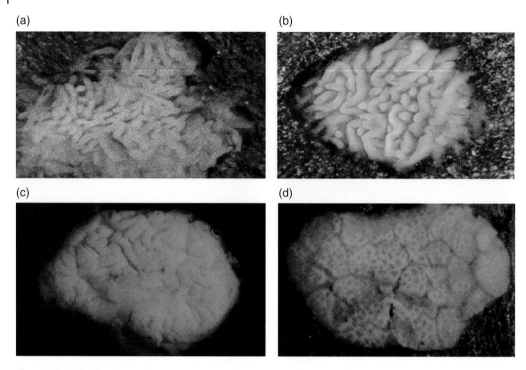

Figure 23.2 (a) Duodenal biopsy specimen with bottom opened and oriented on a filter paper with villi upwards. The biopsy is inspected under a dissection microscope under liquid surface, still in its fixative. Villi are slender and tall, mostly leaf-like but also finger-like. A presumptive diagnosis of normal mucosa can be made. (b) Villi are still finger-like and quite tall also tall villus ridges; both villi and ridges are thickened. Presumptive diagnosis of early-stage disease. Histopathology also showed crypt hyperplasia. (c) The disease is progressing, villi have merged and convoluted to low villus ridges, indicating clear disease. Wrong tangential cutting of low villus ridges results in histological appearance of artificial tall villi. (d) Full-blown celiac disease, gluten-induced manifest mucosa, so-called "flat" lesions with crypt openings seen at the surface.

biopsies are taken, they should not be put in the same fixative vial with the distal duodenal biopsies.

Future of endoscopy in pediatric CD

The insufficient number, poor quality and bad orientation of biopsies, disease patchiness, caution regarding bulb samples, low sensitivity of endoscopic markers, and, most importantly, bad interobserver agreement between pathologists [16] have all cast a shadow on the use of endoscopy in the routine diagnosis of CD, despite efforts in overcoming each of them. The trend towards a nonendoscopic nonbiopsy diagnosis of CD is catching on, so that the future of endoscopy in CD might be limited for selected cases. One future need in children will be clinical drug trials using gluten-induced mucosal injury as the primary outcome [17]. Modern endoscopy techniques with visual evaluation of the duodenal mucosa, including correlation with histopathology, determining the extent of the lesion, and evaluating the percentage of the lesioned mucosa, warrant further studies.

 • See companion website for videos relating to this chapter topic: www.wiley.com/go/gershman3e

REFERENCES

1 Paveley WF. From Aretaeus to Crosby: a history of coeliac disease. *BMJ* 1988, **297**, 1646–1649.

2 Husby S, Koletzko S, Korponay-Szabó IR. ESPGHAN Working Group on Coeliac Disease Diagnosis; ESPGHAN Gastroenterology Committee; European Society for Pediatric Gastroenterology, Hepatology, and Nutrition. European Society for Pediatric Gastroenterology, Hepatology, and Nutrition guidelines for the diagnosis of coeliac disease. *J Pediatr Gastroenterol Nutr* 2012, **54**, 572–573.

3 Ravelli MA, Tobanelli P, Minelli L, Villanacci V, Cestari R. Endoscopic features of celiac disease in children. *Gastrointest Endosc* 2001, **54**, 736–742.

4 Ozçay F, Demir H, Saltik IN. Low sensitivity of endoscopic markers in children with celiac disease. *Gastrointest Endosc* 2002, **56**, 321.

5 Taavela J, Koskinen O, Huhtala H, *et al.* Validation of morphometric analyses of small-intestinal biopsy readouts in celiac disease. *PloS One* 2013, **8**, e76163.

6 Wallach T, Genta RM, Lebwohl B, Green PH, Reilly NR. Adherence to celiac disease and eosinophilic esophagitis biopsy guidelines is poor in children. *J Pediatr Gastroenterol Nutr* 2017, **65**, 64–68.

7 Ofei S, Boyle B, Ediger T, Hill I. Adherence to endoscopy biopsy guidelines for celiac disease: a pediatric institutional analysis. *J Pediatr Gastroenterol Nutr* 2015, **61**, 440–444.

8 Rostami-Nejad M, Villanacci V, Hogg-Kollars S, *et al.* Endoscopic and histological pitfalls in the diagnosis of celiac disease: a multicentre study assessing the current practice. *Rev Esp Enferm Dig* 2013, **105**, 326–333.

9 Lebwohl B, Genta RM, Kapel RC, *et al.* Procedure volume influences adherence to celiac disease guidelines. *Eur J Gastroenterol Hepatol* 2013, **25**, 1273–1278.

10 Lebwohl B, Kapel RC, Neugut AI, Green PH, Genta RM. Adherence to biopsy guidelines increases celiac disease diagnosis. *Gastrointest Endosc* 2011, **74**, 103–109.

11 Latorre M, Lagana SM, Freedberg DE, *et al.* Endoscopic biopsy technique in the diagnosis of celiac disease: one bite or two? *Gastrointest Endosc* 2015, **81**, 1228–1233.

12 Ravelli A, Villanacci V. Tricks of the trade: how to avoid histological pitfalls in celiac disease. *Pathol Res Pract* 2012, **208**, 197–202.

13 Gonzalez S, Gupta A, Cheng J, *et al.* Prospective study of the role of duodenal bulb biopsies in the diagnosis of celiac disease. *Gastrointest Endosc* 2010, **72**, 758–765.

14 Mooney PD, Kurien M, Evans KE, *et al.* Clinical and immunologic features of ultra-short celiac disease. *Gastroenterology* 2016, **150**, 1125–1134.

15 Taavela J, Popp A, Korponay-Szabó IR, *et al.* A prospective study on the usefulness of duodenal bulb biopsies in celiac disease diagnosis in children: urging ution. *Am J Gastroenterol* 2016, **111**, 124–133.

16 Werkstetter K, Korponay-Szabó IR, Popp A, *et al.* Accuracy in diagnosis of celiac disease without biopsies in clinical practice. *Gastroenterology* 2017, **153**, 924–993.

17 Mäki M. Celiac disease treatment: gluten-free diet and beyond. *J Pediatr Gastroenterol Nutr* 2014, **59**, S15–S17.

24

Role of endoscopy in inflammatory bowel disease including scoring systems

Salvatore Oliva, Mike Thomson, David Wilson, and Dan Turner

 KEY POINTS

- Upper GI endoscopy (EGD) can help to discern the distribution of inflammatory bowel disease (IBD) and also in some cases differentiate the type of IBD and should occur in all patients at initial evaluation.
- Inflammation of the stomach is seen in ulcerative colitis as well as in Crohn's disease.
- Terminal ileal (TI) intubation is important in differentiating the type of IBD and the TI may in some cases be the only area affected.
- Panenteric assessment may occasionally be necessary with wireless video capsule endoscopy and tissue acquisition by enteroscopy.
- A recent change in approach in Crohn's disease management is now more focused on mucosal

- healing – hence endoscopic frequency and reliance upon it may increase in established disease, although mucosal healing may lag behind clinical response.
- The Pediatric Ulcerative Colitis Activity Index (PUCAI) seems to be adequate for making decisions on management changes in UC rather than repetitive endoscopy.
- Validated scoring systems in adults can be utilized and help to diminish interobserver variability in disease description, but these are yet to be fully validated in pediatric IBD.
- Multiple biopsies from the TI and at least four sites from the colon should occur during ileocolonoscopy.

Introduction

There is a widely held view that endoscopy has revolutionized the approach to patients with inflammatory bowel diseases (IBD) as a pivotal tool in different steps of patient management. In the last few decades, gastrointestinal (GI) endoscopy has undergone significant developments in pediatrics in terms of technology and availability of pediatric-size equipment, enabling comprehensive investigation of the GI tract in children.

Reporting of endoscopic disease activity should always include accurate descriptors of any abnormalities in each segment. However, due to variability between different operators, the scoring of endoscopic disease activity is becoming an important endpoint in clinical trials as well as in clinical practice. A wider application of the scoring system and the development of newer scores will help in management of pediatric IBD patients.

Diagnosis

Endoscopy remains the fundamental diagnostic tool for IBD in both adults and children. Ileocolonoscopy (IC) should include complete colonoscopy, and ileal intubation should

Practical Pediatric Gastrointestinal Endoscopy, Third Edition. Edited by George Gershman and Mike Thomson.
© 2021 John Wiley & Sons Ltd. Published 2021 by John Wiley & Sons Ltd.
Companion website: www.wiley.com/go/gershman3e

always be advocated [1]. Sigmoidoscopy and partial colonoscopy are insufficient to explore disease extent and reach a definite diagnosis. Endoscopy of the ileocolon should be deferred in cases of toxic megacolon, while in cases of acute severe colitis, sigmoidoscopy or partial/full ileocolonoscopy might be considered in expert hands.

The Porto Criteria and ESPGHAN Paediatric Endoscopy Guidelines indicate on a strong evidence base that EGD should be performed in all children at the initial evaluation of disease irrespective of the presence or absence of upper gastrointestinal symptoms [2]. Endoscopic procedures in children should be performed according to recent ESPGHAN/ESGE recommendations [1]. As stated in the ECCO guidelines for histopathology in IBD, multiple biopsies from at least four sites along the colon (cecum, trasverse colon, sigmoid colon, rectum) and terminal ileum should be obtained and placed immediately in separate vials, accompanied by clinical information [3]. Multiple biopsies imply a minimum of two representative samples from each segment, including macroscopically normal segments. The Porto criteria also advocate multiple biopsies from esophagus, stomach, and duodenum in the EGD for all children with IBD irrespective of upper symptoms [2].

Establishing a definite and accurate diagnosis in a patient suspected of having IBD is mandatory. Therefore, a complete work-up should be advocated. In patients transferred to a pediatric IBD unit without previously fulfilling Porto Criteria properly, a future strategy to complete the diagnostic work-up should be planned, especially when a full ileocolonoscopy has not been performed. If successful treatment has been adequately initiated after the first endoscopy, complete fulfillment of the Porto Criteria could be postponed. Endoscopic findings can change over short periods of time. When a colonoscopy has shown only nonspecific findings, due to interruption or dissociation between endoscopy and histology, a new endoscopy should be completed, in order to better characterize the disease.

Monitoring

The usefulness of endoscopic reassessment should be individualized according to the disease type, severity, risk of relapse and risk of progression and in general, when a significant change in medical management is contemplated. Indeed, in pediatric IBD, the overall rate of management change after endoscopy can be up to 42% of cases [4]. Unfortunately, the appropriateness of periodic endoscopic reassessment after index ileocolonoscopy has never been formally studied and the value of it is much debated, especially in pediatric ulcerative colitis (UC). Indeed, treatment changes based on endoscopy are more frequent in children with Crohn's disease (CD) than UC [5]. Clinical judgment and Pediatric Ulcerative Colitis Activity Index (PUCAI) have shown to be adequate for the evaluation of disease activity in pediatric patients. A PUCAI <10 has been closely associated with mucosal healing and not inferior to endoscopic evaluation in predicting clinically important outcomes [6,7]. Endoscopic appearance lags behind clinical improvement and may thereby underestimate response to treatment [8].

It does not seem justified to routinely recommend endoscopic assessment in pediatric UC solely for assessing disease activity, response to treatment or at relapse. Even though endoscopy is still considered the standard for evaluating disease activity in IBD, and used to confirm mucosal healing, it is invasive and costly [9]. However, endoscopic evaluation is mandatory in any case before major treatment changes (escalating and deescalating treatment strategies), for diagnosing complications (e.g., stenosis, dysplasia) and to exclude other diagnoses, such as ischemia and rarely infection, such as CMV [10].

In *Clostridium difficile* infection, evaluation by colonic endoscopy may be misleading in active colitis as typical pseudomembranes are commonly absent [11,12]. Moreover, full ileocolonoscopy is not recommended in severe colitis as the risk for serious complications, such as perforation, is higher even though it may be attempted safely in expert hands [13].

In colectomized patients, initial clinical suspicion of pouchitis should be confirmed by endoscopic evaluation of the pouch with mucosal biopsies. A clinical pattern of "irritable pouch syndrome" is characterized by increased stool frequency and cramping with normal pouch endoscopy and histology [14].

The benefit of postoperative endoscopy in CD has not been prospectively evaluated in children. A recent Australian study demonstrated that adults who underwent colonoscopy six months after surgery to decide on treatment adjustment had a considerably lower relapse at 18 months after surgery [15]. Extrapolation from these data in adults suggests that a similar protocol may also be necessary in pediatric patients to monitor for postoperative recurrence and treatment aimed at relapse prevention [16].

Reporting of endoscopic disease activity should always include accurate descriptors of any abnormalities in each segment [17]; however, due to the variability between different operators, the scoring of endoscopic disease activity is becoming an important endpoint in clinical trials [18–20]. Although validated endoscopic indexes are used in adults with IBD to assess mucosal healing, pediatric endoscopic endpoints to assess efficacy of medications in clinical trials are not clear. Validated scoring systems will be essential as investigators become more familiar with enrolling children into studies with endoscopic endpoints, such as mucosal healing. The distribution and severity of inflammation noted during endoscopy of children early in the course of IBD may be patchy, with a pattern that is less commonly seen in adults with IBD. For this reason, scoring systems used in adults may not easily be extrapolated to children.

However, despite their limitations, the use of endoscopic scoring systems can aid in reporting endoscopic findings and allow for easy comparisons between a patient's current and previous endoscopy result. If it is feasible, the use of scores in clinical practice is recommended. However, documentation of endoscopic disease activity remains generally subjective in children. For this reason, if the endoscopic scoring systems are not used, it is important to report the following findings in each segment of the bowel, extent and location of inflammation; if bowel involvement is continuous or involves skip areas; presence of erythema; loss of vascular pattern; bleeding (contact or spontaneous); presence of erosions or ulceration (superficial or deep); and the presence of strictures or fistulae. In addition, on follow-up endoscopy, it is important to note the degree of change of endoscopic activity since the previous evaluation.

A wider application of the scoring system and the development of newer scores will help with the comparison between drug efficacies and optimize a treat-to-target treatment algorithm in patient management of pediatric IBD.

Scoring systems

Ulcerative colitis

There are currently no validated scoring systems of endoscopic activity for pediatric patients with UC. Several endoscopic scoring systems and indices have been developed over recent years and many are used as clinical trial outcome measures. Few have been rigorously validated in adults and there is no reference standard for scoring endoscopic activity in UC. Some indices form part of composite scores that integrate clinical information (e.g., the Mayo endoscopic subscore and the Ulcerative Colitis Disease Activity Index). Definitions of endoscopic disease activity (remission, mild, moderate, and severe disease) and the ability of specific indices to reliably detect meaningful endoscopic changes have not been either rigorously validated or available. In addition, clinical endoscopic and histological assessments do not always correlate. Furthermore, most scoring systems use the appearance of the rectosigmoid mucosa rather than the entire colon and do not take segmental differences throughout the colon into consideration, including endoscopic rectal sparing.

Despite the relative simplicity of scoring and category definitions, intraobserver and inter-observer differences among experts remain a significant weakness in current scoring systems. Several scores include mucosal friability, which is subject to intraobserver and interobserver variation in definition and interpretation.

Mayo score

The Mayo score is a composite that includes clinical and endoscopic elements in the assessment of disease activity. The four variables are stool frequency, rectal bleeding, physician's global assessment, and changes in the rectosigmoid mucosa at flexible endoscopy. The endoscopic subsection has a four-point grading scale for categories ranging from normal to severe disease (0 – normal/inactive disease; 1 – mild disease: erythema, reduced vascular pattern, mild friability; 2 – moderate disease: marked erythema, absent vascular pattern, friability, mucosal erosions; 3 – severe disease: spontaneous bleeding, ulceration). Although the score itself was not validated prior to its introduction in 1987, it is widely accepted and utilized in several landmark trials [21].

This score includes variable degrees of friability in the score of 1 and 2, which results in high interobserver discrepancy and inconsistent results. The strengths of the Mayo endoscopic subscore lie in the frequency and ease of its use in clinical trials. Its weakness lies in its lack of validation, the fact that it does not distinguish between deep and superficial ulceration and that the score only reflects the most severely affected segment of the bowel visualized without giving any indication of the extent or distribution of mucosal inflammation and setting no minimal insertion length [22].

Reasonable concordance ($\kappa = 0.58$; 0.26–0.89) between the PUCAI and endoscopic Mayo subscores was demonstrated in a post hoc analysis of the pediatric trial of infliximab in ulcerative colitis [7].

Ulcerative Colitis Endoscopic Index of Severity (UCEIS)

This index has been developed prospectively and recently validated [23,24]. From 10 initial descriptors, the UCEIS was constructed using regression modeling around three descriptors: vascular patterning, bleeding, and erosions/ulcers. Severity, in terms of UCEIS scores, was compared to a visual analogue scale of overall endoscopic severity. Mucosal friability is not included as an element of this score following results of prior analyses showing significant inter- and intraobserver variation of this item. Subsequent validation studies have shown good inter- and intraobserver reliability. The UCEIS correlated well with both full and partial Mayo scores as well as a global rating of endoscopic severity based on a visual analogue scale. Indeed, the UCEIS is currently the most cited tool for assessing endoscopic severity of UC in adults. Nevertheless, further studies are required to establish thresholds and the clinical relevance of different UCEIS scores and explore more deeply its sensitivity to change [25]. Interestingly, prior knowledge of clinical data had only a modest effect on UCEIS scores apart from the description of bleeding at endoscopy.

Ulcerative Colitis Colonoscopic Index of Severity (UCCIS)

This index has been developed prospectively and encompasses assessments of four mucosal variables: vascular pattern; granularity; bleeding/friability; and ulceration in five colonic segments along the entire colon [24,26]. Interobserver variability was greater in the cecum/ascending colon than in distal segments whereas bleeding and friability showed only moderate correlation in the descending and sigmoid colon segments. The index correlated well with clinical and laboratory parameters of disease activity. This index has not been validated in multicenter international studies that include nonambulatory patients and cut-off values for meaningful change, remission, mild, moderate and severe disease activity have yet to be defined.

Crohn's disease

Crohn's Disease Endoscopic Index of Severity (CDEIS)

The CDEIS was first developed by the Groupe d'Étude Thérapeutique des Affections Inflammatories Digestives (GETAID) [27]. This index scores the presence of superficial or deep ulcers present in each examined segment (rectum, sigmoid and left colon, transverse colon, right colon, and ileum). The affected and ulcerated areas are assessed using two visual-analogue scales (VAS).

The CDEIS is often considered the gold standard for classifying endoscopic disease activity in CD. It is highly reproducible and sensitive to changes in endoscopic mucosal appearance and healing [28]. The CDEIS is the most commonly used endoscopic tool to assess disease activity in clinical trials although there is no agreement or formal validation regarding cut-off values for defining endoscopic response to treatment, endoscopic remission or mucosal healing and no data available on long-term clinical outcomes, especially in children. The main limitation of the CDEIS is that it is a complex tool that requires training and experience to utilize, reserving its use mostly for clinical trials [29].

Simple Endoscopic Score for CD (SES-CD)

The SES-CD score was developed to simplify the CDEIS without losing precision and reproducibility [30]. It was shown to have a close correlation with CDEIS (Spearman's rank order correlation coefficient 0.938, p <0.0001). The most relevant updates were (i) changes in the definition of ulcers (aphthous, large and very large ulcers); (ii) establishment of a functional definition of narrowing instead of ulcerated or not ulcerated stenosis; (iii) change from VAS to four-modality Likert scales to assess the affected and ulcerated surfaces. There are two major limitations of this score: (i) the absence of formally validated cut-off values for inactive, mild, moderate, or severe endoscopic activity; and (ii) the lack of interobserver agreement.

Rutgeerts score

The Rutgeerts score is used for assessing endoscopic activity in the neoterminal ileum after ileocecal resection. Although it has not been fully prospectively validated, the severity of Rutgeerts score on endoscopy in an asymptomatic patient within 12 months of ileocolonic resection has been shown to predict the risk of clinical recurrence (low risk with grade 0 or 1; high risk with grade 3 or 4) [16].

 • See companion website for videos relating to this chapter topic: www.wiley.com/go/gershman3e

REFERENCES

1 Thomson M, Tringali A, Landi R, *et al.* Pediatric gastrointestinal endoscopy: European Society of Pediatric Gastroenterology Hepatology and Nutrition (ESPGHAN) and European Society of Gastrointestinal Endoscopy (ESGE) guidelines. *J Pediatr Gastroenterol Nutr* 2017, **64**, 133–153.

2 Levine A, Koletzko S, Turner D, *et al.* ESPGHAN Revised Porto Criteria for the diagnosis of inflammatory bowel disease in children and adolescents. *J Pediatr Gastroenterol Nutr* 2014, **58**, 795–806.

3 Magro F, Langner C, Driessen A, *et al.* European consensus on the histopathology of inflammatory bowel disease. *J Crohns Colitis* 2013, **7**, 827–851.

4 Thakkar K, Lucia CJ, Ferry GD, *et al.* Repeat endoscopy affects patient management in pediatric inflammatory bowel disease. *Am J Gastroenterol* 2009, **104**, 722–727.

5 Ho GT, Mowat C, Goddard CJ, *et al.* Predicting the outcome of severe ulcerative colitis: development of a novel risk score to aid early selection of patients for second-line medical therapy or surgery. *Aliment Pharmacol Ther* 2004, **19**, 1079–1087.

6 Schechter A, Griffiths C, Gana JC, *et al.* Early endoscopic, laboratory and clinical predictors of poor disease course in paediatric ulcerative colitis. *Gut* 2015, **64**, 580–588.

7 Turner D, Griffiths AM, Veerman G, *et al.* Endoscopic and clinical variables that predict sustained remission in children with ulcerative colitis treated with infliximab. *Clin Gastroenterol Hepatol* 2013, **11**, 1460–1465.

8 Beattie RM, Nicholls SW, Domizio P, Williams CB, Walker-Smith JA. Endoscopic assessment of the colonic response to corticosteroids in children with ulcerative colitis. *J Pediatr Gastroenterol Nutr* 1996, **22**, 373–379.

9 Fefferman DS, Farrell RJ. Endoscopy in inflammatory bowel disease: indications, surveillance, and use in clinical practice. *Clin Gastroenterol Hepatol* 2005, **3**, 11–24.

10 Turner D, Levine A, Escher JC, *et al.* Management of pediatric ulcerative colitis: joint ECCO and ESPGHAN evidence-based consensus guidelines. *J Pediatr Gastroenterol Nutr* 2012, **55**, 340–361.

11 Issa M, Vijayapal A, Graham MB, *et al.* Impact of clostridium difficile on inflammatory bowel disease. *Clin Gastroenterol Hepatol* 2007, **5**, 345–351.

12 Rahier JF, Magro F, Abreu C, *et al.* Second European evidence-based consensus on the prevention, diagnosis and management of opportunistic infections in inflammatory bowel disease. *J Crohns Colitis* 2014, **8**, 443–468.

13 Turner D, Travis SP, Griffiths AM, *et al.* Consensus for managing acute severe ulcerative colitis in children: a systematic review and joint statement from ECCO, ESPGHAN, and the Porto IBD Working Group of ESPGHAN. *Am J Gastroenterol* 2011, **106**, 574–588.

14 Shen B, Achkar JP, Lashner BA, *et al.* Irritable pouch syndrome: a new category of diagnosis for symptomatic patients with ileal pouch-anal anastomosis. *Am J Gastroenterol* 2002, **97**, 972–977.

15 De Cruz P, Kamm MA, Hamilton AL, *et al.* Crohn's disease management after intestinal resection: a randomised trial. *Lancet* 2015, **385**,1406–1417.

16 Rutgeerts P, Geboes K, Vantrappen G, Kerremans R Coenegrachts JL, Coremans G. Natural history of recurrent Crohn's disease at the ileocolonic anastomosis after curative surgery. *Gut* 1984, **25**, 665–672.

17 Annese V, Daperno M, Rutter MD, *et al.* European evidence-based consensus for endoscopy in inflammatory bowel disease. *J Crohns Colitis* 2013, **7**, 982–1018.

18 Dulai PS, Levesque BG, Feagan BG, D'Haens G, Sandborn WJ. Assessment of mucosal healing in inflammatory bowel disease: review. *Gastrointest Endosc* 2015, **82**, 246–255.

19 Samaan MA, Mosli MH, Sandborn WJ, *et al.* A systematic review of the measurement of endoscopic healing in ulcerative colitis clinical trials: recommendations and implications for future research. *Inflamm Bowel Dis* 2014, **20**, 1465–1471.

20 Khanna, R., Khanna R, Bouguen G, *et al.* A systematic review of measurement of endoscopic disease activity and mucosal healing in Crohn's disease: recommendations for clinical trial design. *Inflamm Bowel Dis* 2014, **20**, 1850–1861.

21 Schroeder KW, Tremaine WJ, Ilstrup DM. Coated oral 5-aminosalicylic acid therapy for mildly to moderately active ulcerative colitis. A randomized study. *N Engl J Med* 1987, **317**, 1625–1629.

22 Mazzuoli S, Guglielmi FW, Antonelli E, Salemme M, Bassotti G, Villanacci V. Definition and evaluation of mucosal healing in clinical practice. *Dig Liver Dis* 2013, **45**, 969–977.

23 Travis SP, Schnell D, Krzeski P, *et al.* Developing an instrument to assess the endoscopic severity of ulcerative colitis: the Ulcerative Colitis Endoscopic Index of Severity (UCEIS). *Gut* 2012, **61**, 535–542.

24 Samuel S, Bruining DH, Loftus EV Jr, *et al.* Validation of the ulcerative colitis colonoscopic index of severity and its correlation with disease activity measures. *Clin Gastroenterol Hepatol* 2013, **11**, 49–54.

25 Vuitton L, Peyrin-Biroulet L, Colombel JF, *et al.* Defining endoscopic response and remission in ulcerative colitis clinical trials: an international consensus. *Aliment Pharmacol Ther* 2017, **45**, 801–813.

26 Thia KT, Loftus EV Jr, Pardi DS, *et al.* Measurement of disease activity in ulcerative colitis: interobserver agreement and predictors of severity. *Inflamm Bowel Dis* 2011, **17**, 1257–1264.

27 Mary JY, Modigliani R. Development and validation of an endoscopic index of the severity for Crohn's disease: a prospective multicentre study. Groupe d'Etudes Therapeutiques des Affections Inflammatoires du Tube Digestif (GETAID). *Gut* 1989, **30**, 983–989.

28 Rutgeerts P, Diamond RH, Bala M, *et al.* Scheduled maintenance treatment with infliximab is superior to episodic treatment for the healing of mucosal ulceration associated with Crohn's disease. *Gastrointest Endosc* 2006, **63**, 433–442.

29 Sanborn WJ, Feagan BG, Hanauer SB, *et al.* A review of activity indices and efficacy endpoints for clinical trials of medical therapy in adults with Crohn's disease. *Gastroenterology* 2002, **122**, 512–530.

30 Daperno M, d'Haens G, van Assche G, *et al.* Development and validation of a new, simplified endoscopic activity score for Crohn's disease: the SES-CD. *Gastrointest Endosc* 2004, **60**, 505–512.

Part Four

Therapeutic Pediatric Endoscopy

25

Endoscopic management of esophageal strictures

Michael Manfredi, Frederick Gottrand, Luigi Dall'Oglio, Mike Thomson,
George Gershman, Antonio Quiros, and Thierry Lamireau

 KEY POINTS

- Different esophageal strictures origin and their different management
- How to dilate and how to avoid stricture relapse
- How to avoid complications and their management.

Stricture presentation

Congenital esophageal strictures (CES) are caused by a malformation of the esophageal wall leading to narrowing of the esophageal lumen [1,2]. Four types are described: membranous; web or diaphragm (MD); fibromuscular stenosis (FMS); and tracheobronchial remnants (TBR). Congenital stenosis may also be revealed by progressive dysphagia with semisolid foods or even liquids and episodes of food impaction. Symptoms like regurgitation and aspiration are frequent, leading to cough, respiratory distress or choking during feeds. Feeding refusal or apnea can occur in small babies. Contrast esophagogram reveals abrupt stenosis of varying length, mostly located in the distal esophagus. Endoscopy confirms the stenosis, which can be tight, preventing the passage of the endoscope. Thoracic CT can also be helpful.

Acquired strictures are mostly secondary to surgical repair of an esophageal atresia, occur-

ring in up to 80% of cases in some series [3,4]. Factors implicated in the pathophysiology of anastomotic strictures include the creation of a long gap esophageal atresia leading to high-tension esophageal anastomosis, ischemia, two suture layer anastomosis, use of silk suture material, anastomotic leak, and gastroesophageal reflux. Children with long gap esophageal atresia are especially at risk of stricture of the anastomosis and sometimes of the colonic segment used for esophagoplasty. Stricture is usually diagnosed on systematic contrast esophagogram performed in the follow-up of these children. It is also suspected in case of feeding difficulties occurring sometimes early after surgical repair, with regurgitations and feeding refusal in small babies. It can be associated with aspiration, leading to cough, respiratory distress or choking during feeds. When feeding is impossible, nutrition via a gastrostomy is mandatory. Feeding difficulties are more often revealed at the time of transition to a more solid diet, with regurgitation, dysphagia

---

Practical Pediatric Gastrointestinal Endoscopy, Third Edition. Edited by George Gershman and Mike Thomson.
© 2021 John Wiley & Sons Ltd. Published 2021 by John Wiley & Sons Ltd.
Companion website: www.wiley.com/go/gershman3e

with semisolid foods, and impaction of solid foods like meat in older children. Contrast esophagogram confirms the stricture at the location of the anastomosis.

Caustic ingestion can be responsible for severe burning lesions Children with grade 2 or 3 caustic lesions of the esophagus often develop multiple or long strictures [5]. Ingestion of a button battery can lead to severe ulceration of the esophagus, sometimes leading to stenosis. These strictures are usually diagnosed on systematic contrast esophagogram performed during the follow-up of these children. This is dealt with in more detail in Chapter 26.

Peptic stenosis has become rare since proton pump inhibitors are now largely used in the treatment of gastroesophageal reflux, but it can occur in some children like those with cerebral palsy [6]. Eosinophilic esophagitis can be responsible for esophageal stenosis requiring dilation. Stenosis can also complicate esophageal involvement associated with skin diseases, such as dystrophic epidermolysis bullosa or Stevens–Johnson syndrome.

Classification

For purposes of characterization and treatment planning, esophageal strictures may be differentiated into two structural types: simple and complex. Strictures that are short (<2 cm), focal, not angulated, and permitting the passage of an endoscope can be labeled as simple strictures. This type of stricture is amenable to through-the-scope (TTS) balloon dilation. Simple strictures tend to be due to peptic esophagitis, Schatzki's ring and esophageal web. Complex strictures are those that are angulated, long (>2 cm), irregular and have a very narrow lumen (Figure 25.1). Complex strictures are more commonly seen in children with caustic ingestions, anastomotic strictures, post radiofrequency ablation and chest radiation therapy.

ESPGHAN–ESGE guidelines on diagnostic and therapeutic endoscopy in pediatrics suggest the following definitions of refractory and recurrent esophageal strictures: "inability to successfully remediate the anatomic problem to obtain age-appropriate feeding possibilities after a maximum of 5 dilation sessions with maximal 4-week intervals" for refractory strictures and "inability to maintain a satisfactory luminal diameter for 4 weeks once the age-appropriate feeding diameter has been achieved" for recurrent strictures [7–9].

Diagnosis

The evaluation and classification of esophageal stenosis requires a multimodal approach. Contrast radiological studies provide information about the stricture's shape, location, length, diameter of the residual lumen as well

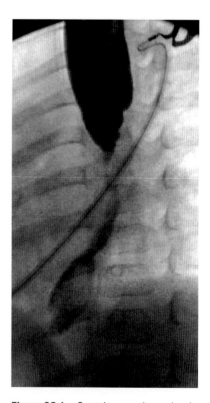

Figure 25.1 Complex esophageal stricture secondary to caustic ingestion.

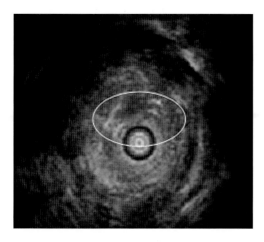

Figure 25.2 Congenital esophageal stenosis with tracheal remnants.

as associated anomalies, while endoscopy clarifies the etiology of the stricture: CES versus peptic, eosinophilic or corrosive esophagitis, and allows instant endoscopic treatment. However, even high-resolution computed tomography is not sensitive enough for diagnosis of TBR in the esophageal wall, or to differentiate TBR from FMS prior to endoscopic or surgical intervention.

With the advent of endoscopic ultrasonography (EUS), definitive diagnosis of FMS and TBR became feasible (Figure 25.2) [10–13]. The resolution of the high-frequency EUS (15–30 MHz) miniprobe allows discrimination of cartilaginous tissue, fluid-filled lesions, thickened muscular layer or external "compressing" vascular structures which is very helpful in guiding therapy. In addition, transendoscopic EUS is useful in assessing severity and degree of submucosal scarring in children with eosinophilic esophagitis (EE). It is also useful in selection of patients with EE and significant scarring who may carry an increased risk of perforation after dilation (see Chapter 21).

Differential diagnosis

Symptoms like dysphagia, regurgitation, feeding difficulties, and even food impaction may be caused by numerous diseases of the esophagus even in the absence of stenosis.

Gastroesophageal reflux is frequently responsible for feeding difficulties. Complications such as peptic esophagitis have become rare and peptic stenosis exceptional since the widespread use of proton pump inhibitors. However, they may be encountered in children with repaired esophageal atresia and cerebral palsy.

Eosinophilic esophagitis must be sought in atopic children presenting with persistent manifestations of gastroesophageal reflux, feeding difficulties or food impaction [14]. Endoscopy may show white deposits and a linear pseudotracheal appearance. Diagnosis will be confirmed by the presence of numerous eosinophils in the mucosae.

Infectious esophagitis can occur in cases of primary or secondary immunodeficiency syndrome. Dysphagia and feeding difficulties are usually associated with painful deglutition. Endoscopy shows an inflammatory mucosa and biopsies reveal the microorganism.

Achalasia is a rare condition which can be difficult to differentiate from stenosis of the distal esophagus. It can be isolated or associated with Sjögren's syndrome, triple A syndrome (achalasia, alacrimia, and ACTH insensitivity), familial dysautonomia, and Ondine's syndrome. Children present with progressive dysphagia with solid food or liquids, regurgitation, vomiting, and weight loss. Respiratory symptoms are frequent in small children, with nocturnal cough, chronic bronchopathy, and aspiration pneumonia responsible for delayed diagnosis [15]. Contrast esophagogram reveals a dilated esophagus, with a narrowed termination. Esophageal manometry demonstrates dyskinesia or akinesia of the corpus esophagus and increased pressure of the lesser esophageal sphincter associated with a fault in relaxation (see Chapter 27).

Dysmotility of the esophagus is constant in children with repaired esophageal atresia, and can be responsible for dysphagia and food impaction in the absence of anastomotic stenosis. Other motor dysfunctions of the esophagus can occur in rare conditions, such as diabetic neuropathy, scleroderma, and infection with *Trypanosoma cruzei*. Tumors of the esophagus, such as leiomyoma, are exceptional in children.

Treatment

Bougie dilation

There are two types of bougie dilators: guidewire and nonguidewire types. The guidewire ones are tapered cylindrical flexible tubes made of polyvinyl chloride with a central channel to accommodate a guidewire. These dilators have variable length of tapered portion and also radiopaque markers for fluoroscopic guidance (e.g., Savary-Gilliard® dilators, Cook Medical, Eder-Puestow, or American Dilators and SafeGuide®). The nonguidewire tungsten dilators weighted for gravity assistance are inserted when patients are in an upright position. The two commonly used nonguidewire bougie dilators are Hurst and Maloney dilators. The Hurst dilators have a rounded blunt tip, while the Maloney dilators have a tapered tip. Both dilators were designed for self-dilation at home. Another type of mechanical dilator is the Tucker dilator designed for patients with gastrostomy. Tucker dilators can remain inside the patient for periodic serial dilations [9,16–21].

The basic technique of mechanical dilation involves the passage of a bougie across the stricture. This results in both longitudinal shearing force as well as radial force on the stricture area. The goal of mechanical dilation is to pass serial bougie dilators of incremental size across the stricture site. Although fluoroscopy can be helpful for confirming the position and progression of the bougie dilator, it is not mandatory. It is generally recommended to use fluoroscopy in complex strictures. Mechanical dilation requires training the

appreciate the feel of resistance while advancing the bougie across the stricture site. The goal is to feel and then overcome the resistance from the stricture with the minimal force. Once this goal is achieved, it is generally recommended to pass no more than three consecutive dilators in increments of 1 mm in a single session for a total of 3 mm. This approach, known as the "rule of 3," is well established for mechanical dilation.

Balloon dilation

Balloon dilators deliver equal radial force across the entire length of the stricture. They are designed to pass through the endoscope with or without a guidewire. Through-the-scope dilation allows the endoscopist to directly visualize the stricture during and immediately after dilation. However, through-the-scope balloon dilation requires endoscopes with a working channel of ≥2.8 mm. This can be problematic for infants under 10 kg. In this case, a 0.035 mm or smaller guidewire can be passed into the stomach either through the biopsy channel, using the "exchange" technique leaving the wire in place as the scope is removed, or under fluoroscopic guidance. The balloon is then passed over the wire.

The first step of balloon dilation is estimation of the stricture size. The golden rule of the procedure is application of the balloons by 1 mm increments up to 3 mm above the diameter of the stricture. It is also interpreted as three times the diameter of the stricture, such that a 3 mm stricture should not be dilated more than 9 mm, etc. The middle portion of the balloon is centered across the stricture with either endoscopic and/or fluoroscopic guidance. Introducing into the balloon dilator water-soluble contrast and the use of fluoroscopy allow one to observe the disappearance of the waist of the stricture which is a sign of successful dilation (Figure 25.3). In the setting of a complex stricture, fluoroscopy is useful in advancing the wire and balloon safely across the stricture. An immediate esophagogram

(a) (b)

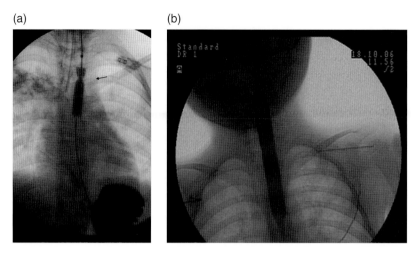

Figure 25.3 (a) Fluoroscopic appearance of a balloon waist. The arrow shows the balloon being pinched by the esophageal stricture. (b) Disappearance of the stricture waist.

under fluoroscopy post dilation can be useful for detecting and managing an early esophageal leak [9,16–21].

Adjunct therapies

Intralesional steroid injection

Despite more than half a century of endoscopic steroid injection as adjunct therapy to balloon dilation of esophageal strictures, the available data and recommendations remain controversial. Potential benefits have been linked to several biological properties of steroids: interference with collagen synthesis, fibrosis, and chronic scarring processes [22,23].

The preferred steroid for intralesional injection is triamcinolone acetate or acetonide (10–40 mg/mL solution). Betamethasone and dexamethasone preparations have also been used.

The technique of intralesional injection is not standardized, especially in pediatrics. Currently, ESGE–ESPGHAN guidelines for pediatric gastrointestinal endoscopy do not support routine use of intralesional steroid injection for refractory esophageal stenosis in children [9].

Mitomycin C

Mitomycin C, an antifibrotic, has been proposed as an adjunct treatment to manage esophageal strictures [24–29]. Mitomycin C has mainly been used topically but there are also reports of injection of mitomycin C [27]. There are numerous methods of topical application of mitomycin C: soaking pledgets or cotton swab placement on the stricture area, dripping via an injection needle onto the affected area, and using a spray catheter. The dose of mitomycin C used in these studies is also variable, ranging from 0.004 mg/mL to 1 mg/mL. We use 0.5–1.0 mg/mL on 1–3 separate occasions and shield the normal tissue from the soaked cotton swab using a plastic sheath over the tip of the endoscope whilst holding the swab in place with biopsy forceps [24,25].

The effect of monotherapy with mitomycin C in comparison with dilation has been assessed in 30 children with caustic strictures [23]. Although this study was not blinded and does not appear to be randomized, there was a statistically significant improvement in dysphagia score ($p = 0.005$), and increased median interval between dilations in mitomycin C group [26].

In another retrospective study, the efficacy of topical application of mitomycin C as adjunct therapy to endoscopic dilation in preventing recurrence of anastomotic strictures after surgical repair was analyzed in 21 children with esophageal atresia (EA). Eleven children received mitomycin C concurrently with endoscopic dilations [29]. The authors documented no benefit of adding mitomycin C treatment in the resolution of the stricture compared with repeated esophageal dilations alone in historical controls. There is a hypothetical risk of secondary malignancy with mitomycin C, therefore long-term follow-up with esophageal biopsies at the site of mitomycin C application should be recommended.

Incisional therapy

Endoscopic electrocautery incisional therapy (EIT) has been reported as an alternative treatment for refractory strictures in a small number of adult series. There are variations in the EIT technique reported in the literature. The technique involves the use of a needle knife to make incisions into a stricture at its densest points. Typically, multiple radial incisions are made around the stricture site (Figure 25.4). An electrosurgical generator applies a cut current to make the incision. One approach is to make several incisions in the stricture site followed up with balloon dilation. The balloon allows for preferential tearing along the incision site.

A large pediatric experience looking at EIT in the treatment of refractory anastomotic strictures reported a 61% success rate. In this study of 36 refractory strictures, the median number of dilations prior to EIT was eight. This group had a median of two dilations in the two years post EIT. In this same study, EIT was performed on 22 nonrefractory strictures with 100% success. The median number of dilations prior to EIT was three and the median number of dilations in the two years after EIT was one. In this study the severe adverse event rate was 2.3% with three perforations [30].

Electrocautery incisional therapy shows promise as a treatment option for pediatric refractory strictures and may be considered prior to surgical resection even in severe cases. The complication rate, albeit low, is significant and EIT should only be considered in experienced hands with surgical consultation. Further prospective longitudinal studies are needed to validate this treatment.

Esophageal stenting

Endoscopic dilations are the mainstay of the conservative approach for esophageal strictures of any etiology. However, some patients may experience recurrent or refractory esophageal stricture despite multiple dilation sessions and therefore further treatments are needed [9,31–38].

Even though primarily used as a palliative procedure to relieve dysphagia associated with malignant esophageal strictures, temporary stent placement has increasingly been used as a conservative treatment for refractory and recurrent benign esophageal strictures in adults – and recently in children (Figure 25.5). To date, no evidence-based indications exist about the timing of stent placement, but most experts agree that stent placement should be considered when other treatment options have failed [9].

The rationale for esophageal stenting for recalcitrant strictures is that continuous radially oriented pressure over a long period allows the esophagus to maintain luminal patency while simultaneously stretching the stricture. Remodeling of scar tissue may occur while the

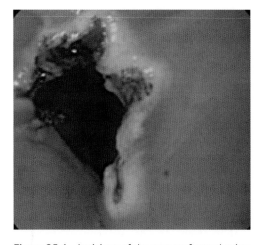

Figure 25.4 Incisions of the scar performed using a needle knife and a cutting electric current.

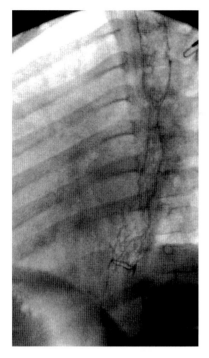

Figure 25.5 Two-year-old boy with complex esophageal stricture due to caustic ingestion was treated with a fully covered GORE® VIABIL® biliary endoprosthesis and regained the ability to eat blended food.

stent is in place, which can result in persistent luminal patency and reduced risk of recurrent stricture formation.

Multiple types of stents are commercially available from various manufacturers. These devices differ in material (metal, plastic or biodegradable polymer), luminal diameter, and flexibility and have the same conceptual design: exert centrifugal force on the esophageal wall while allowing the passage of food into the stent lumen.

Unfortunately, appropriately sized esophageal stents designed for small pediatric patients are lacking, therefore airway or biliary stents use has been reported in children [31]. Currently, three main categories of esophageal stents are commercially available: self-expandable metal stents (SEMSs), self-expandable plastic stents (SEPSs), and biodegradable stents (BDSs).

Self-expandable metal stents

Self-expandable metal stents consist of woven, knitted, or laser-cut metal mesh cylinders that exert self-expansive forces until their maximum fixed diameter is reached. All SEMSs are made of nitinol, a nickel and titanium alloy that has unique properties of shape memory and superelasticity. To prevent tissue ingrowth through the stent mesh, SEMSs can be fully or partially covered by a plastic membrane or silicone. In fully covered SEMs (FCSEMSs), the entire length of the stent is covered while in partially covered SEMs (PCSEMSs), the proximal and distal ends of the stent are devoid of covering. Partial or fully covered SEMSs are currently recommended for palliation of malignant dysphagia; only fully covered stent designs can safely be removed after a prolonged time of stenting [38].

Self-expandable metal stents can be placed under endoscopic and/or fluoroscopic guidance. After endoscopic and/or fluoroscopic assessment of length and degree of stricture, a guidewire is passed endoscopically, the SEMS delivery system is advanced over the wire and then deployed across the stricture under continuous fluoroscopic monitoring. To guide accurate stent placement, the proximal and distal ends of the stenotic tract should be marked appropriately with radiopaque markers (metal or plastic radiopaque bands placed on the patient's skin, hemoclips deployed endoscopically, or submucosal injection of a radiopaque agent). To decrease the risk of migration, stent length should be 4 cm longer than the stricture.

The ESGE suggests that FCSEMSs should be preferred over PCSEMSs for the treatment of refractory benign esophageal stricture in adults, because of their lack of embedment and ease of removability. Indeed, hyperplastic tissue reaction of the esophageal mucosa to the bare metal mesh may preclude safe stent removal.

Self-expandable plastic stents

Self-expandable plastic stents are constituted by a woven polyester skeleton completely covered with a silicone membrane. Radiopaque markers are positioned at the middle and ends of the stent to assist fluoroscopy-guided delivery. To reduce the risk of migration, SEPSs are designed to have a wider proximal flange.

Compared to SEMSs, complete silicone coating prevents granulation tissue growing through SEPSs, allowing for easier removal even after they have been in place for several months [9,38].

Biodegradable stents

Biodegradable stents are made of biomaterial composed of synthetic polymers (generally polydioxanone) that are free of toxic effects (including carcinogenicity, immunogenicity, teratogenicity), are completely degraded or absorbed by the body and hence do not have to be removed.

The polydioxanone BDS lasts for about three weeks and begins to degrade in 11–12 weeks. As for SEPS, BDSs are radiolucent but have radiopaque markers at both ends and in the middle and need to be assembled and loaded onto the delivery system prior to insertion. Placement technique is similar to that previously described for SEMSs and SEPSs.

The theoretical advantage over SEMS and SEPS is that BDSs do not require removal.

Dynamic Stent

The Dynamic Stent® (DS) consists of a silicone tube of varying sizes coaxially built over a nasogastric tube. The main difference with previously described stents is that instead of passing within the lumen of the stent, foods pass between the stent and the esophageal wall. This new concept in stent design derives from the thirty years' experience of the inventors. Since 1988, the Digestive Surgery and Endoscopy Unit of Bambino Gesù Children's Hospital in Rome has produced the DS manually, using silicone tubes of increasing size coaxially overlapped on each other to fashion the stent until the desired size is reached (7, 9 or 12.7 mm outer diameter) (Figure 25.6). To ensure correct

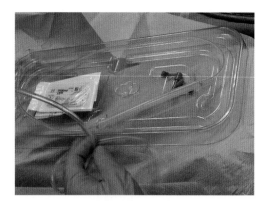

Figure 25.6 The Dynamic Stent®.

positioning of the stent over the stricture, the device is mounted on a nasogastric tube (Figure 25.7). The DS is currently undergoing the European CE medical device approval process; a commercial version will be available in the market in the next few years [36].

The placement technique is comparable to that of previous stents. The stent, customized according to stricture size, is inserted through the mouth and advanced over a guidewire under endoscopic and fluoroscopic guidance through the stricture (skin markers and radiopaque markers at both ends of the stent are used as reference point). The nasogastric tube of the stent is passed with a backward movement through the nasopharynx and nose, and then fixed externally. The DS should remain in place for at least eight weeks, but according to patient tolerability, longer durations (up to six months) are advocated to achieve better results. Indeed, passing the food between the esophageal wall and the stent, there is no risk of tissue reaction and stent embedment [9,31–38].

Outcome

The ESGE clinical guideline for esophageal stenting in adults suggests consideration of temporary stent placement for refractory benign esophageal strictures. Although only SEPSs have received formal approval for this indication in adults, the guideline does not

(a)

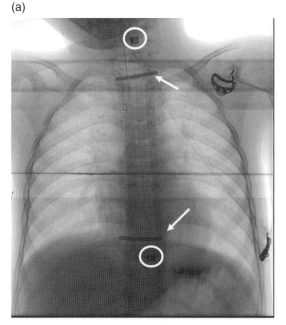

(b)

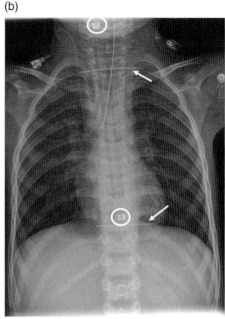

Figure 25.7 (a) The Dynamic Stent® in correct position. The two radiopaque bars (*arrows*) are at the level of the proximal and distal ends of the stricture. The two Dynamic Stent radiopaque ends are in the circles. (b) Partial Dynamic Stent proximal dislocation in the same patient. The two radiopaque bars (*arrows*) are at the level of the proximal and distal ends of the stricture. The two Dynamic Stent radiopaque ends are in the circles. In this position, respiratory distress can be caused by stent laryngeal compression.

recommend a specific type of expandable stent (SEMS, SEPS, BDS) because none has been shown to be superior to any other. However, the ESGE suggests that FCSEMSs be preferred over PCSEMSs because of their lack of embedment and ease of removability. Moreover, although no studies have compared different strategies in terms of stenting duration, the ESGE guideline suggests that stents should remain in place for at least 6–8 weeks and no more than 12 weeks, to maximize success and minimize the risk of hyperplastic tissue reaction and stent embedment.

Overall, pediatric data on stricture resolution are scarce and heterogeneous, reported success rates ranging from 26% to 86%. In a study by Manfredi et al., 24 children with esophageal atresia underwent a total of 41 stent placement (SEPSs 14, FCSEMSs 27), with a success rate of 39% and 26% at ≥30 and ≥90 days after stent removal, respectively. The

mean duration of stent placement was 9.7 days (range 2–30 days). In this study, the authors reported that esophageal stenting is a safe and effective approach in closing esophageal perforations, especially post dilation [30]. In a series of predominantly small children (median age 1 year old), Best et al. reported that esophageal stenting using an airway FCSEMS was successful in all seven patients (five esophageal atresia, one battery ingestion and one major congenital cardiac anomaly) [37]. Lange et al. published their experience with FCSEMS (biliary, bronchial and colonic stents) use in 11 children with esophageal strictures of different etiologies. Median duration of stent placement was 29 days (range 17–91 days). Six children (55%) were successfully treated without any further intervention, two needed one single dilation after stent removal, while two did not improve and required surgery [38]. Recent ESPGHAN-ESGE guidelines for pediatric gastrointestinal endoscopy suggest temporary stent placement (or application of topical mitomycin C) for refractory esophageal stenosis in children [9].

In relation to the Dynamic Stent, the group at the Bambino Gesù Children's Hospital reported an overall success rate of 89% in a series of 79 children, mostly with caustic strictures.

High-dose systemic steroid therapy (dexamethasone 2 mg/kg/day for three days) was administered in all children after stent placement [36].

 • See companion website for videos relating to this chapter topic: www.wiley.com/go/gershman3e

REFERENCES

1 Michaud L, Coutenier F, Podevin G, *et al.* Characteristics and management of congenital esophageal stenosis: findings from a multicenter study. *Orphanet J Rare Dis* 2013, **8**, 186.

2 Nihoul-Fékété C, De Backer A, Lortat-Jacob S, Pellerin D. Congenital esophageal stenosis: a review of 20 cases. *Pediatr Surg Int* 1987, **2**, 86–92.

3 Pinheiro PF, Simões e Silva AC, Pereira RM. Current knowledge on esophageal atresia. *World J Gastroenterol* 2012, **18**, 3662–3672.

4 Baird R, Laberge JM, Lévesque D. Anastomotic stricture after esophageal atresia repair: a critical review of recent literature. *Eur J Pediatr Surg* 2013, **23**, 204–213.

5 de Jong AL, Macdonald R, Ein S, Forte V, Turner A. Corrosive esophagitis in children: a 30-year review. *Int J Pediatr Otorhinolaryngol* 2001, **57**, 203–211.

6 Pearson EG, Downey EC, Barnhart DC, *et al.* Reflux esophageal stricture – a review of 30 years' experience in children. *J Pediatr Surg* 2010, **45**, 2356–2360.

7 Lew RJ, Kochman ML. A review of endoscopic methods of esophageal dilation. *J Clin Gastroenterol* 2002, **35**, 117–126.

8 Shah JN. Benign refractory esophageal strictures: widening the endoscopist's role. *Gastrointest Endosc* 2006, **63**, 164–167.

9 Thomson M, Tringali A, Dumonceau JM, *et al.* Paediatric gastrointestinal endoscopy: European Society for Paediatric Gastroenterology Hepatology and Nutrition and European Society of Gastrointestinal Endoscopy Guidelines. *J Pediatr Gastroenterol Nutr* 2017, **64**, 133–153.

10 Quiros JA, Urayama S. EUS in the diagnosis and management of esophageal pathology in children. *Gastrointest Endosc* 2004, **59**, 144.

11 Quiros JA, Hirose S, Patino M, Lee H. Esophageal tracheobronchial remnant, endoscopic ultrasound diagnosis, and surgical management. *J Pediatr Gastroenterol Nutr* 2013, **56**, e14.

12 Dall'Oglio L, Caldaro T, Foschia F, *et al.* Endoscopic management of esophageal stenosis in children: new and traditional treatments. *World J Gastrointest Endosc* 2016, **8**, 212–219.

13 Usui N, Kamata S, Kawahara H, *et al.* Usefulness of endoscopic ultrasonography in the diagnosis of congenital esophageal stenosis. *J Pediatr Surg* 2002, **37**, 1744–1746.

14 Liacouras CA, Furuta GT, Hirano I, *et al.* Eosinophilic esophagitis: updated consensus recommendations for children and adults. *J Allergy Clin Immunol* 2011, **128**, 3–20.

15 Hallal C, Kieling CO, Nunes DL, *et al.* Diagnosis, misdiagnosis, and associated diseases of achalasia in children and adolescents: a twelve-year single center experience. *Pediatr Surg Int* 2012, **28**, 1211–1217.

16 Siddiqui UD, Banerjee S, Barth B, *et al.* Tools for endoscopic stricture dilation. *Gastrointest Endosc* 2013, **78**, 391–404.

17 Manfredi MA. Endoscopic management of anastomotic esophageal strictures secondary

to esophageal atresia. *Gastrointest Endosc Clin North Am* 2016, **26**, 201–219.

18 Siersema PD, de Wijkerslooth LR. Dilation of refractory benign esophageal strictures. *Gastrointest Endosc* 2009, **70**, 1000–1012.

19 Manfredi MA. Endoscopic management of anastomotic esophageal strictures secondary to esophageal atresia. *Gastrointest Endosc Clin North Am* 2016, **26**, 201–219.

20 Tambucci R, Angelino G, De Angelis P, *et al*. Anastomotic strictures after esophageal atresia repair: incidence, investigations, and management, including treatment of refractory and recurrent strictures. *Front Pediatr* 2017, **5**, 120.

21 Michaud L, Gottrand F. Anastomotic strictures: conservative treatment. *J Pediatr Gastroenterol Nutr* 2011, **52**, S18–S19.

22 Berenson GA, Wyllie R, Caulfield M, Steffen R. Intralesional steroids in the treatment of refractory esophageal strictures. *J Pediatr Gastroenterol Nutr* 1994, **18**, 250–252.

23 Kochhar R, Ray JD, Sriram PV, Singh K. Intralesional steroids augment the effects of endoscopic dilation in corrosive esophageal strictures. *Gastrointest Endosc* 1999, **49**, 509–513.

24 Afsal N, Lloyd-Thomas A, Albert D, Thomson M. A child with oesophageal strictures. *Lancet* 2002, **359**, 1032.

25 Rosseneau S, Yerushalmi B, Ibaguen-Secchia E, *et al*. Topical application of Mitomycin C in esophageal strictures. *J Pediatr Gastroenterol Nutr* 2007, **44**(3), 336–341.

26 Uhlen S, Fayoux P, Vachin F, *et al*. Mitomycin C: an alternative conservative treatment for refractory esophageal stricture in children? *Endoscopy* 2006, **38**, 404–407.

27 Spier BJ, Sawma VA, Gopal DV, Reichelderfer M. Intralesional mitomycin C: successful treatment for benign recalcitrant esophageal stricture. *Gastrointest Endosc* 2009, **69**, 152–153.

28 Berger M, Ure B, Lacher M. Mitomycin C in the therapy of recurrent esophageal

strictures: hype or hope? *Eur J Pediatr Surg* 2012, **22**, 109–116.

29 Chapuy L, Pomerleau M, Faure C. Topical mitomycin-C application in recurrent esophageal strictures after surgical repair of esophageal atresia. *J Pediatr Gastroenterol Nutr* 2014, **59**, 608–611.

30 Manfredi MA, Clark SJ, Medford S, *et al*. Endoscopic electrocautery incisional therapy as a treatment for refractory benign pediatric esophageal strictures. *J Pediatr Gastroenterol Nutr* 2018, **67**, 464–468.

31 Kramer RE, Quiros JA. Esophageal stents for severe strictures in young children: experience, benefits, and risk. *Curr Gastroenterol Rep* 2010, **12**, 203–210.

32 Spaander MC, Baron TH, Siersema PD, *et al*. Esophageal stenting for benign and malignant disease: European Society of Gastrointestinal Endoscopy (ESGE) Clinical Guideline. *Endoscopy* 2016, **48**, 939–948.

33 Varadarajulu S, Banerjee S, Barth B, *et al*. Enteral stents. *Gastrointest Endosc* 2011, **74**, 455–464.

34 Tokar JL, Banerjee S, Barth BA, *et al*. Drug-eluting/biodegradable stents. *Gastrointest Endosc* 2011, **74**, 954–958.

35 De Peppo F, Zaccara A, Dall'Oglio L, *et al*. Stenting for caustic strictures: esophageal replacement replaced. *J Pediatr Surg* 1998, **33**, 54–57.

36 Foschia F, De Angelis P, Torroni F, *et al*. Custom dynamic stent for esophageal strictures in children. *J Pediatr Surg* 2011, **46**, 848–853.

37 Best C, Sudel B, Foker JE, Krosch TC, Dietz C, Khan KM. Esophageal stenting in children: indications, application, effectiveness, and complications. *Gastrointest Endosc* 2009, **70**, 1248–1253.

38 Lange B, Kubiak R, Wessel LM, Kähler G. Use of fully covered self-expandable metal stents for benign esophageal disorders in children. *J Laparoendosc Adv Surg Tech A* 2015, **25**, 335–341.

26

Endoscopic management of caustic ingestion

Erasmo Miele and Samy Cadranel

 KEY POINTS

- Mucosal injury begins within minutes of caustic ingestion.
- Alkali ingestion has a greater risk of transmural damage.
- Endoscopy should ideally occur within 6–12 hours of the ingestion and if performed more than 48 hours following ingestion, it increases the risk of perforation.
- Various treatments have been proposed to prevent esophageal strictures, including ipecac, oral dilutions, neutralizing agents, antacids, antibiotics, and systemic corticosteroids, but

the optimal management strategy remains controversial.
- If a stricture develops then balloon or bougie dilation should occur.
- If repeated dilation (more than two times) is needed then postdilation topical application of the antifibrotic mitomycin C is indicated.
- Caustic ingestion increases the risk of carcinoma formation (both adenocarcinoma and squamous cell carcinoma) with an incidence of 2–8% and some suggest endoscopic surveillance after the age of 20 years.

Introduction

Ingestion of caustic agents can induce severe esophageal and gastric lesions, including necrosis, sometimes leading to life-threatening acute complications [1]. In contrast with deliberate ingestion in adults and adolescents, in children younger than 6 years (with peak incidence at 2 years) the small amount of corrosive substances, usually ingested accidentally, causes mild and superficial lesions [2]. Preventive measures implemented in industrialized countries have significantly reduced caustic injuries whereas this objective has yet to be realized in many developing countries [3].

Epidemiology

Caustic ingestion in children remains a worldwide problem, with an incidence ranging from 5 to 518 per 100 000 children per year [3], with more than 40 000 cases reported yearly in England and Wales [4]. In 2014, the annual report of the American Association of Poison Control Centers documented more than 1 million substance exposures in children younger than 5 years, representing 50% of all exposures, with a male/female predominance of 1.3:1. However, only one out of the 25 fatalities was due to a caustic agent, sodium hypochlorite [5].

Practical Pediatric Gastrointestinal Endoscopy, Third Edition. Edited by George Gershman and Mike Thomson.
© 2021 John Wiley & Sons Ltd. Published 2021 by John Wiley & Sons Ltd.
Companion website: www.wiley.com/go/gershman3e

Pathophysiology

The severity of lesions depends on the type, quantity, concentration, and time of contact of the caustic substance with the mucosa [6]. Strong alkali (pH >11) causes tissue injury by liquefactive necrosis, a process that involves saponification of fats and solubilization of proteins. Cell death occurs from emulsification and disruption of cellular membranes. This leads to deeper penetration into tissues with a greater likelihood of transmural injury. Alkali absorption leads to thrombosis of blood vessels impeding blood flow to the already damaged tissue [7]. The higher surface tension of alkalis permits a longer contact time with esophageal tissues. In addition, the stomach and duodenum could be affected [8].

The mode of tissue injury with acids is coagulation necrosis. The coagulum prevents the corrosive agent from spreading transmurally, hence reducing the incidence of full-thickness injury. Its lower surface tension and the formation of protective esophageal eschar allow acids to bypass the esophagus rapidly without much damage while affecting the stomach more severely [9]. Mucosal injury begins within minutes of caustic ingestion, characterized by necrosis and hemorrhagic congestion secondary to the formation of thrombosis in the small vessels. These events continue in the next several days until approximately 4–7 days, leading to mucosal sloughing, bacterial invasion, granulation tissue, and collagen deposition. The healing process typically begins three weeks after ingestion. By the third week, scar retraction occurs and may continue for a few more months until stricture formation occurs.

Clinical presentation

Corrosive ingestion may be deduced from oral burns, including lip or tongue erythema and edema, leukoplakia, or ulceration [10]. Most common symptoms are dysphagia, drooling, feeding refusal, retrosternal pain, abdominal pain, and vomiting. Minor symptoms do not rule out the presence of relevant injury, but increased number of symptoms correlates with a likelihood of significant injury [7]. Rarely, children develop airway symptoms, such as shortness of breath or hypoxia and, in severe cases, hemodynamic instability and/or circulatory collapse, although none of these symptoms is completely predictive of esophageal injury [11]. Beware of symptoms of sepsis, indicative of esophageal perforation which requires emergent surgical debridement and/ or esophagectomy [10].

Assessment and management

Suspicion of caustic ingestion needs prompt evaluation in the closest emergency department and requires a detailed history, verification of the nature of the ingested product, ideally with the container brought by whoever brings the child. If the ingestion is doubtful, without oral lesions, and the patient is asymptomatic, observation by the physician can be sufficient, providing adequate follow-up is ensured [12]. Symptomatic children should be kept nil by mouth on intravenous maintenance fluid until further investigations are performed; broad-spectrum antibiotics are indicated if there are signs of perforation, and may be given empirically for patients with suspected bacteremia or aspiration pneumonia or pneumonitis [13]. Chest and abdominal radiographs and standard blood tests should be obtained to detect metabolic acidosis, leukocytosis, hemolysis or signs of coagulopathy [14]. Every child suspected of caustic ingestion and with symptoms/signs (e.g., oral lesions, vomiting, drooling, dysphagia, hematemesis, dyspnea, abdominal pain, etc.) needs an early upper GI endoscopy (UGE) to identify all digestive tract lesions [12].

Endoscopy

Endoscopy should be performed within the first 24 hours, preferably 6–12 hours after ingestion in order to observe any severe complications while stabilizing the child. A too early endoscopy may not show the extent of the burns whereas an endoscopy done after 48 hours increases the risk of perforation. UGE is performed in the operating room, under general anesthesia and a protected airway, with minimal air insufflations [10] and great caution taken to avoid advancing blindly. If an adequate view cannot be achieved or severe circumferential injury is detected, endoscopy should be terminated [3]. Careful examination of the esophagus, stomach, and duodenum determines the degree and extent of tissue damage (Table 26.1, Figures 26.1–26.4) and the necessity for nasogastric feeding tube placement to facilitate enteral feeding and patency of esophageal lumen in children with severe esophageal damage and high risk of stricture [10,12,14].

Table 26.1 Endoscopic classification of caustic injuries

Grade	Features
Grade 0	Normal
Grade I	Superficial mucosal edema and erythema
Grade II	Mucosal and submucosal ulcerations
Grade IIa	Superficial ulcerations, erosions, exudates
Grade IIb	Deep discrete or circumferential ulcerations
Grade III	Transmural ulcerations with necrosis
Grade IIIa	Focal necrosis
Grade IIIb	Extensive necrosis
Grade IV	Perforations

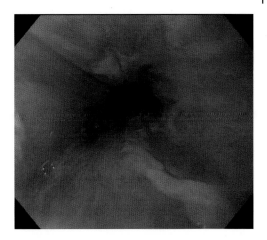

Figure 26.1 Grade I corrosive esophagitis with diffuse erythema and minimal mucosal sloughing.

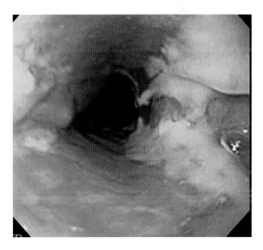

Figure 26.2 Grade IIa corrosive esophagitis: extensive mucosal sloughing.

Treatment

Most children affected by mild injuries (grade 0–IIa) need observation in hospital until full oral feeds are tolerated. Patients with more severe injuries (grade IIb and III) require accurate evaluation of probable development of strictures during initial hospitalization of 2–4 weeks. A liquid diet, orally or via nasogastric tube, may initially be necessary in as many as a quarter of patients [15] and efforts should be undertaken to prevent vomiting. Nothing

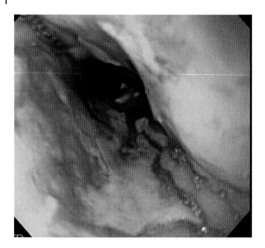

Figure 26.3 Grade IIb of corrosive esophagitis: multiple ulcerations.

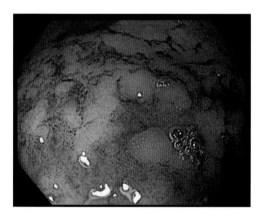

Figure 26.4 Corrosive gastritis.

should be given by mouth if perforation is suspected [12].

Various treatments have been proposed to prevent esophageal strictures, including ipecac, oral dilutions, neutralizing agents, antacids, antibiotics, and systemic corticosteroids, but the optimal management strategy remains controversial [16,17].

Induction of emesis with syrup of ipecac or liquids used to dilute or neutralize the caustic agent are strongly contraindicated because vomiting further exposes the esophagus to the caustic agent [10]. Broad-spectrum antibiotics are frequently prescribed in the acute phase, based on animal studies of increased

granulation with bacterial invasion of disrupted mucosa [18], although clinical evidence does not support its routine use [19]. To prevent stricture formation, corticosteroids have been used to reduce fibroblast proliferation in children, adults, and rabbits with grade II or III lesions [10,19–21]. Although corticosteroids did not show any benefit in metaanalysis, recent guidelines recommend the use of high doses of intravenous dexamethasone ($1\,g/1.73\,m^2$ per day) administration for a short period (three days) in IIb esophagitis early after corrosive ingestion [12,22]. There is no evidence of benefit from the use of corticosteroids in other grades of esophagitis (I, IIa, III) [12]. Use of PPIs is a widespread practice although there is no evidence suggesting that it effectively protects the esophageal mucosa and reduces the formation of stricture [3].

Long-term complications

The risk of esophageal stricture (Figure 26.5), the major complication following caustic ingestion, is as high as 77% in grade IIb lesions and may reach 100% in patients with grade III [1]. Stricture formation can occur as early

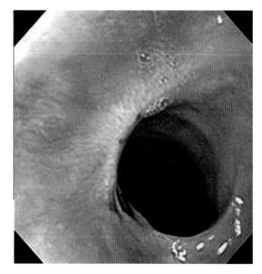

Figure 26.5 Esophageal stricture after lye ingestion.

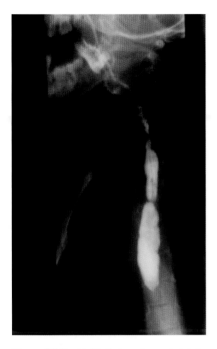

Figure 26.6 Multiple esophageal strictures two months after caustic ingestion.

as three weeks after ingestion, usually established in 80% of the patients who will develop stricture by eight weeks (Figure 26.6) [7].

Once strictures develop, repeated dilations are needed. Several methods can be used, including mercury-filled bougies, antegrade Maloney or retrograde Tucker dilators and dilators passed over a guidewire or pulled through a string left in situ between dilations [1]. Balloon dilation under endoscopic control has been successfully used in children [23].

After the dilation session, topical application (four minutes of 0.4 mg of mitomycin in 1 mL of vehicle) of mitomycin, an antibiotic with antineoplastic and antiproliferative properties that also inhibits RNA and protein synthesis, seems a promising strategy in reducing the number of dilations needed and stabilizing the scarring of the esophagus at an acceptable diameter [24].

Unfortunately, in some children, surgery is needed. Extensive necrosis noted on endoscopy and patients with evidence of perforation are indications for immediate surgical intervention. Esophagectomy, esophagogastrectomy or gastrectomy may be indicated if wide necrosis is confirmed or in case of long and tight strictures. Esophageal reconstruction may be achieved by small bowel or colon interposition and gastric transposition [1].

Caustic ingestion increases the risk of carcinoma formation (both adenocarcinoma and squamous cell carcinoma) with an incidence of 2–8% [25]. However, periodic surveillance for the development of dysplasia following caustic ingestion is controversial. It has been suggested that after the initial ingestion, periodic endoscopy should be considered in patients 20 years of age or older [26].

 • See companion website for videos relating to this chapter topic: www.wiley.com/go/gershman3e

REFERENCES

1 Elshabrawi M, A-Kader HH. Caustic ingestion in children. *Expert Rev Gastroenterol Hepatol* 2011, **5**, 637–645.

2 Hockenberry MJ, Wilson D. *Wong's Nursing Care of Infants and Children Multimedia Enhanced Version*, 9th edn. Elsevier, Mosby, 2013.

3 Arnold M, Numanoglu A. Caustic ingestion in children – a review. *Semin Pediatr Surg* 2017, **26**, 95–104.

4 Stiff G, Alwafi A, Rees B, Lari J. Corrosive injuries of the oesophagus and stomach: experience in management at a regional paediatric centre. *Ann R Coll Surg Engl* 1996, **78**, 119–123.

5 Mowry JB, Spyker DA, Brooks DE, McMillan N, Schauben J. 2014 Annual Report of the American Association of Poison Control Centers' National Poison Data System

(NPDS): 32nd annual report. *Clin Toxicol* 2015, **53**, 962–1147.

6 Osman M, Russell J, Shukla D, Moghadamfalahi M, Granger DN. Responses of the murine esophageal microcirculation to acute exposure to alkali, acid, or hypochlorite. *J Pediatr Surg* 2008, **43**, 1672–1678.

7 Kay M, Wyllie R. Caustic ingestions in children. *Curr Opin Pediatr* 2009, **2**, 651–654.

8 Karagiozoglou-Lampoudi T, Agakidis CH, Chryssostomidou S, Arvanitidis K, Tsepis K. Conservative management of caustic substance ingestion in a pediatric department setting, short-term and long-term outcome. *Dis Esophagus* 2011, **24**, 86–91.

9 Park KS. Evaluation and management of caustic injuries from ingestion of acid or alkaline substances. *Clin Endosc* 2014, **47**, 301–307.

10 Kurowski JA, Kay M. Caustic ingestions and foreign bodies ingestions in pediatric patients. *Pediatr Clin North Am* 2017, **64**, 507–524.

11 Dogan Y, Erkan T, Cokugras FC, Kutlu T. Caustic gastroesophageal lesions in childhood: an analysis of 473 cases. *Clin Pediatr* 2006, **45**, 435–438.

12 Thomson M, Tringali A, Dumonceau JM, *et al*. Paediatric gastrointestinal endoscopy: European Society for Paediatric Gastroenterology Hepatology and Nutrition and European Society of Gastrointestinal Endoscopy Guidelines. *J Pediatr Gastroenterol Nutr* 2017, **64**, 133–153.

13 Contini S, Scarpignato C. Caustic injury of the upper gastrointestinal tract: a comprehensive review. *World J Gastroenterol* 2013, **19**, 3918–3930.

14 Zargar SA, Kochhar R, Mehta S, Mehta SK. The role of fiberoptic endoscopy in the management of corrosive ingestion and modified endoscopic classification of burns. *Gastrointest Endosc* 1991, **37**, 165–169.

15 Sánchez-Ramírez CA, Larrosa-Haro A, Vásquez Garibay EM, Larios-Arceo F. Caustic ingestion and oesophageal damage in children: clinical spectrum and feeding practices. *J Paediatr Child Health* 2011, **47**, 378–380.

16 Uygun I. Caustic oesophagitis in children: prevalence, the corrosive agents involved, and management from primary care through to surgery. *Curr Opin Otolaryngol Head Neck Surg* 2015, **23**, 423–432.

17 Krey H. On the treatment of corrosive lesions in the oesophagus; an experimental study. *Acta Otolaryngol Suppl* 1952, **102**, 1–49.

18 Shub MD. Therapy of caustic ingestion: new treatment considerations. *Curr Opin Pediatr* 2015, **27**, 609–613.

19 Bautista A, Varela R, Villanueva A, Estevez E, Tojo R, Cadranel S. Effects of prednisolone and dexamethasone in children with alkali burns of the oesophagus. *Eur J Pediatr Surg* 1996, **6**, 198–203.

20 Bautista A, Tojo R, Varela R, Estevez E, Villanueva A, Cadranel S. Effects of prednisolone and dexamethasone on alkali burns of the esophagus in rabbit. *J Pediatr Gastroenterol Nutr* 1996, **22**, 275–283.

21 Usta M, Erkan T, Cokugras FC, *et al*. High doses of methylprednisolone in the management of caustic esophageal burns. *Pediatrics* 2014, **133**, E1518–E1524.

22 Fulton JA, Hoffman RS. Steroids in second degree caustic burns of the esophagus: a systematic pooled analysis of fifty years of human data: 1956-2006. *Clin Toxicol* 2007, **45**, 402–408.

23 Sato Y, Frey EE, Smith WL, Pringle KC, Soper RT, Franken EA Jr. Balloon dilatation of esophageal stenosis in children. *Am J Roentgenol* 1988, **150**, 639–642.

24 Afzal NA, Albert D, Thomas AL, Thomson M. A child with oesophageal strictures. *Lancet* 2002, **359**, 1032.

25 Ti TK. Esophageal carcinoma associated with corrosive injury: prevention and treatment by esophageal resection. *Br J Surg* 1983, **70**, 223–225.

26 Isolauri J, Markkula H. Lye ingestion and carcinoma of the esophagus. *Acta Chir Scand* 1989, **155**, 269–271.

27

Pneumatic balloon dilation and peroral endoscopic myotomy for achalasia

Valerio Balassone, Mike Thomson, and George Gershman

 KEY POINTS

- After the diagnosis is made, a number of therapeutic options are available. The aim is to decrease lower esophageal sphincter (LES) pressure, improve bolus clearance and, if present, reduce symptoms related to spasms (e.g., chest pain, dysphagia, and odynophagia).
- Pharmacological treatments such as calcium channel blockers or botulin toxin injection are rarely used in the pediatric population because of the short-term effectiveness and the risk of side effects.

- Pneumatic dilation (PD) is still the first procedure to be employed and after three failed PDs then laparoscopic Heller's myotomy (LHM) should be undertaken.
- Peroral endoscopic myotomy (POEM) is a recently established procedure in the adult population and experience with children is accumulating.
- Because of LES disruption, GERD may occur after any achalasia intervention.

Introduction

Achalasia is a life-long debilitating condition characterized by incomplete lower esophageal sphincter (LES) relaxation, increased LES tone and aperistalsis of the esophagus, which leads to slow or absent bolus transit into the stomach. Diagnosis of achalasia in children is generally made between 7 and 15 years of age. The incidence ranges between 0.1 and 0.18/100 000 children per year [1]. The etiology of achalasia is unknown. It is thought to be an autoimmune-mediated disease with a presumed correlation with viral infection and genetical susceptibility [2]. Achalasia may be part of the triple A syndrome (achalasia, alacrimia, and ACTH insensitivity) and an association with Down's syndrome is possible [3]. Main reported symptoms are vomiting/regurgitation (80%), dysphagia (75%) and weight loss or growth retardation (64%). Chest pain is also frequent. Severity of symptoms may be evaluated according to Eckardt's score. Unlike adults, children tend to experience more respiratory symptoms like chronic or night cough as well as extraesophageal complications (recurrent aspiration, tracheal compression by megaesophagus). Refusal of food and failure to thrive have been reported in infants with early achalasia [4].

Once the diagnosis has been established, therapeutic options are represented by medications, endoscopy, and surgery.

Practical Pediatric Gastrointestinal Endoscopy, Third Edition. Edited by George Gershman and Mike Thomson.
© 2021 John Wiley & Sons Ltd. Published 2021 by John Wiley & Sons Ltd.
Companion website: www.wiley.com/go/gershman3e

Diagnosis and management of achalasia

Clinical history, upper endoscopy, and esophagram are useful in suspected achalasia and to exclude an outlet obstruction, eosinophilic esophagitis or benign esophageal stricture. The gold standard for diagnosis is high-resolution manometry (HRM) which allows classification of the disorder according to the Chicago Classification (CC) into three subtypes of achalasia plus another separate group of esophageal spastic disorders [5].

A few CC parameters are necessary to classify achalasia subtypes: integrated relaxation pressure (IRP) is the most important. It is a complex metric depending on the adequacy of LES relaxation, crural contraction, and pattern and timing of distal esophageal contraction. An IRP >15 mmHg is present in each subtype of achalasia. In type I achalasia (Figure 27.1a), there is negligible pressurization in the esophageal body, evidentced by the absence of any area circumscribed by the 30 mmHg isobaric contour (black line). In type II (Figure 27.1b), panesophageal pressurization occurs, evident by the banding pattern of the 30 mmHg isobaric contour spanning from the upper esophageal sphincter (UES) to the esophagogastric junction (EGJ). Type III achalasia (Figure 27.1c) is characterized by spastic contractions with or without periods of compartmentalized pressurization.

Spastic esophageal disorders (SEDs) include spastic achalasia (type III), diffuse esophageal spasm (DES), and nutcracker/jackhammer esophagus (JH). Although treatment of type I and II achalasia is mainly focused on LES obliteration, management of SEDs may require adjunct treatments on esophageal body spasm.

Van Lennep *et al.* have recently proposed an updated management algorithm of achalasia in children (Figure 27.2) [6].

Therapeutic options

After diagnosis is made, a number of therapeutic options are available. The aim is to decrease LES pressure, improve bolus clearance and, if present, reduce symptoms related to spasms (i.e., chest pain). Pharmacological treatments such as calcium channel blocker or botulin toxin injection are rarely used in the pediatric population because of the short-term effectiveness and the risk of side effects [7,8]. Pneumatic dilation (PD) and surgical myotomy, namely laparoscopic Heller myotomy (LHM), are frequently employed. Peroral endoscopic myotomy (POEM) is a recently established procedure in the adult population but experience with children is limited. Because of LES disruption, GERD may occur after any achalasia intervention.

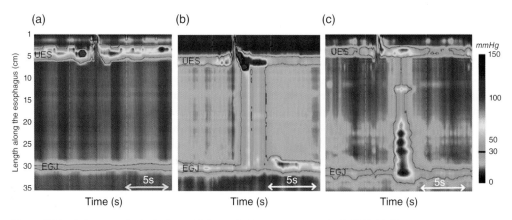

Figure 27.1 Subtypes of achalasia on high-resolution manometry: (a) I, (b) II, (c) III.

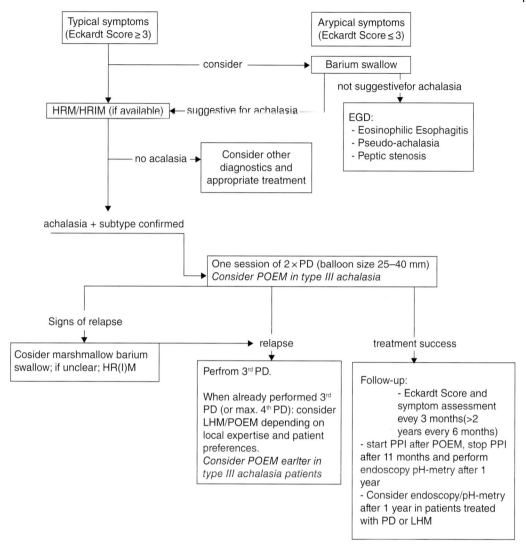

Figure 27.2 Diagnosis and treatment algorithm based on expert opinion and current knowledge from the literature. EGD, sophagogastroduodenoscopy; HRIM, high-resolution impedance manometry; HRM, high-resolution manometry; LHM, laparoscopic Heller myotomy; PD, pneumatic dilation; POEM, peroral endoscopic myotomy; PPI, proton pump inhibitors. *Source:* Van Lennep *et al.* [6].

Pneumatic balloon dilation

Use of PD in children is relatively uncommon. A practicing pediatric gastroenterologist usually lacks experience in PD in achalasia. Therefore, children with achalasia should be referred to high-volume centers of excellence. Pneumatic dilation works by stretching and rupturing fibers of the circular muscle of the LES. The degree of muscle rupture is related to pressure, diameter of the dilator and time of dilation. In general, high pressure associated with use of large balloons and prolonged duration of dilation increases the risk of perforation. Progressive ischemic necrosis of the esophageal mucosa could explain so-called delayed perforation and false-negative results of immediate postprocedure chest and abdominal films and an esophagogram with water-soluble contrast.

Two techniques of PD have been described: traditional, or so-called fluoroscopic-guided technique, and endoscope-guided PD without fluoroscopy, which is not validated in children.

The child should be well prepared before dilation to decrease the risk of aspiration with residual food in the dilated and poorly empty-ing esophagus. Liquid diet for 24 hours and overnight fasting are recommended.

Pneumatic dilation is quite painful so PD requires deep sedation or general anesthesia without muscle relaxant.

The initial steps are similar for fluoroscopic- and endoscope-guided PD.

1) Complete aspiration of residual liquid and solid food from the dilated esophagus.
2) Advancement of the endoscope into the middle of the gastric body.
3) Insertion of a guidewire into the antrum through the biopsy channel.
4) An "exchange" procedure: a guidewire is pushed slowly forward while the endoscope is pulled back synchronously until com-pletely removed from the mouth.

A few additional steps are involved in the fluoroscopic-guided technique. The Rigiflex® 30 mm diameter dilator (Boston Scientific, Boston, MA) (Figure 27.3) is primed by inject-ing a small amount of diluted water-soluble contrast into the balloon, dispersing it manu-ally and aspirating completely. Then the well-lubricated dilator is inserted into the mouth and slowly advanced into the esophagus over the guidewire under fluoroscopic guidance until two radiopaque markers in the middle of the balloon traverse the diaphragm.

Then, the dilator is pulled back slowly until the markers appear 1 cm above the diaphragm. The position of the balloon is secured by hold-ing the dilator firmly up against the bite block, preventing displacement of the balloon into the stomach.

During inflation, a high-pressure zone in the LES creates an hourglass-shaped fluoroscopic image of the balloon dilator. This so-called "waist" disappears once the pressure within the balloon reaches 7–12 psi.

Current data support the graded dilator approach. Initial dilation using a 30 mm bal-loon is recommended for most patients followed by symptomatic and objective assess-ment in 4–6 weeks. If patients continue to be symptomatic, the next size dilator may be employed. The safety and efficacy of the 35 mm dilator in children 8 years and older have been proved [9].

There is no consensus on the duration of inflation. However, longer sessions increase the risk of mucosal ischemia and subsequent perforation.

The endoscope-guided technique eliminates exposure to radiation. The technique requires a few additional steps.

1) Marking the midsection of the Rigiflex bal-loon dilator with a thick colored marker.
2) Passing the balloon over the guidewire into the stomach.
3) Reinsertion of the endoscope to control the position of the balloon in the esophagus.
4) Pulling the balloon back into the esophagus until the color mark reaches the gastroe-sophageal junction.

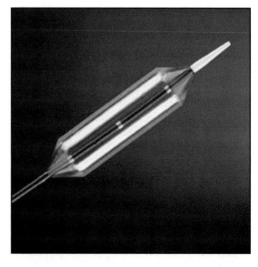

Figure 27.3 Rigiflex dilator.

5) Inflation of the balloon up to 12 psi and maintaining the balloon inflated until the appearance of the ischemic ring at the low esophageal sphincter.

Please note that this technique is not validated in children.

Careful observation for at least six hours and postprocedure chest X-ray and esophagogram with water-soluble contrast are mandatory to exclude esophageal perforation. Persistent chest pain for more than one hour and fever should be considered as red flags of complications and indication for treatment even without a proven pneumomediastinum or radiographic signs of perforation.

Immediate symptomatic improvement after the first dilation occurs in the majority of adults and children.

Multiple dilations are often required to achieve sustained relief of symptoms. Reported efficacy of multiple PDs ranges between 60% and 90% in the pediatric population. Type 2 achalasia (Chicago 3.0 Classification) is associated with better results of PD [10].

According to some adult studies, young age at presentation, classic achalasia, high LES pressure three months after PD, and incomplete obliteration of the balloon's waist during PD are the most important predicting factors of the need for repeated treatment during follow-up.

However different outcome measures have been employed to assess effectiveness, including Eckardt's score <3, need for repeat dilation or response evaluated by clinicians in various studies [11–13]. According to some studies, pneumatic dilation is an effective and safe initial treatment for achalasia and may spare children with achalasia an operation [14]. On the other hand, severe fibrosis generated by repeated PDs is associated with failure of surgical and endoscopic myotomy and increased morbidity [15]. Balloon dilation requires short length of stay and is generally cost-effective.

The major complication of PD is esophageal perforation. Over the last 15 years, the reported rate of this complication in children and adults has been under 2%. Conservative management of perforation with broad-spectrum antibiotics, proton pump inhibitors, withholding of oral feeds, and parenteral nutrition is very effective and carries less risk of morbidity associated with surgery [16].

Laparoscopic Heller myotomy should be considered after three failed PD attempts.

Peroral endoscopic myotomy

Peroral endoscopic myotomy (POEM) was introduced in Japan by Inoue in 2008 for non-sigmoid achalasia. Subsequently, the indication was extended to spastic esophageal disorders and sigmoid esophagus [17]. After a mucosal incision, a submucosal tunnel is created to reach the GEJ and to protect the mucosal flap from thermal damage (Figure 27.4–27.8).

A myotomy is performed for the total length of the submucosal tunnel. The mucosal incision is closed using standards clips. The tunnel can be created in the anterior (2 o' clock) or posterior (5 o' clock) wall of the esophagus according to the operator's preference. This possibility to choose between two alternative tunnel orientations is particularly useful in the management

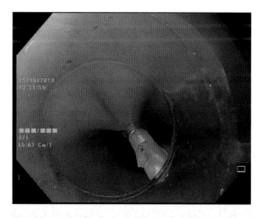

Figure 27.4 Submucosal injection of methylene blue prior to mucosotomy.

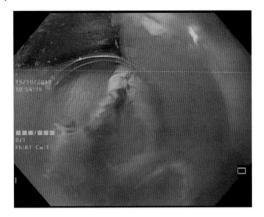

Figure 27.5 Lineal mucosal incision.

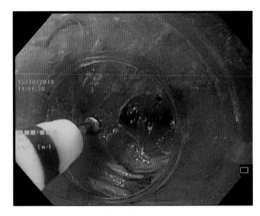

Figure 27.7 Creation of a tunnel using an electrical knife and pressure from the cup on the endoscope.

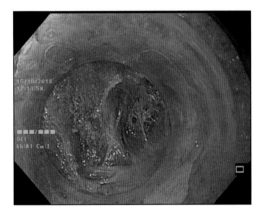

Figure 27.6 Initial stage of tunnel development.

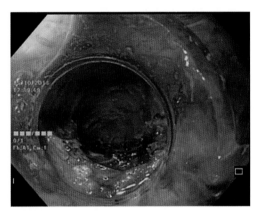

Figure 27.8 Completion of the tunnel with exposed circular muscle.

of recurrent symptoms after POEM or LHM as it avoids the fibrosis caused by previous myotomy [18]. Because no antireflux flap valve is created, GERD after POEM and PD is reported to be higher than LHM. Therefore, diligent follow-up with pH impedance monitoring and surveillance endoscopy of patients undergoing POEM or PD is required. On the other hand, management of recurrent symptoms is generally easier after POEM comparing to LHM because no flap valve can impair clearance of the esophagus with ineffective peristalsis. For this reason, many pediatric surgeons perform a Heller procedure without flap valve as first choice in children with achalasia and a second antireflux procedure only in selected patients with GERD unresponsive to proton pump inhibitor.

Midterm effectiveness results in adult are extremely satisfactory; Eckardt's score is less than 3 points in 98% of patients and postoperative stay is generally around 3–4 days. However, data in pediatric population are limited and less than 100 children have undergone POEM worldwide [19–22]. The safety profile in expert hands is extremely satisfactory; the most common complication is mucosal perforation that is reported in up to 3% of POEMs and is generally evident by the day after endoscopy or esophagram.

Management of mucosal perforation after POEM is generally conservative (prolonged fasting, antibiotics, endoscopic treatment).

Capnoperitoneum/capnomediastinum requiring decompression, pleural effusion, and submucosal bleeding have also been reported as major adverse events. No mortality or emergency surgery after POEM has been reported [14].

 • See companion website for videos relating to this chapter topic: www.wiley.com/go/gershman3e

REFERENCES

1 Smits M, van Lennep M, Vrijlandt R, *et al.* Pediatric achalasia in the Netherlands: incidence, clinical course, and quality of life. *J Pediatr* 2016, **169**, 110–115e3.

2 Eckardt AJ, Eckardt VF. Current clinical approach to achalasia. *World J Gastroenterol* 2009, **15**, 3969–3975.

3 Viegelmann G, Low Y, Sriram B, Chu HP. Achalasia and Down syndrome: a unique association not to be missed. *Singapore Med J* 2014, **55**, e107–e108.

4 Myers NA, Jolley SG, Taylor R. Achalasia of the cardia in children: a worldwide survey. *J Pediatr Surg* 1994, **29**, 1375–1379.

5 Roman S, Gyawali CP, Xiao Y, Pandolfino JE, Kahrilas PJ. The Chicago classification of motility disorders: an update. *Gastrointest Endosc Clin North Am* 2014, **24**, 545–561.

6 van Lennep M, van Wijk MP, Omari TI, Benninga MA, Singendonk MM. Clinical management of pediatric achalasia. *Expert Rev Gastroenterol Hepatol* 2018, **12**, 391–404.

7 Hurwitz M, Bahar RJ, Ament ME, *et al.* Evaluation of the use of botulinum toxin in children with achalasia. *J Pediatr Gastroenterol Nutr* 2000, **30**, 509–514.

8 Maksimak M, Perlmutter DH, Winter HS. The use of nifedipine for the treatment of achalasia in children. *J Pediatr Gastroenterol Nutr* 1986, **5**, 883–886.

9 Babu R, Grier D, Cusick E, Spicer RD. Pneumatic dilatation for childhood achalasia. *Pediatr Surg Int* 2001, **17**, 505–507.

10 Vaezi MF, Pandolfino JE, Vela MF. ACG Clinical Guideline: diagnosis and management of achalasia. *Am J Gastroenterol* 2013, **108**, 1238–1249.

11 Perisic VN, Scepanovic D, Radlovic N. Nonoperative treatment of achalasia. *J Pediatr Gastroenterol Nutr* 1996, **22**, 45–47.

12 Khan AA, Shah SW, Alam A, Butt AK, Shafqat F. Efficacy of rigiflex balloon dilatation in 12 children with achalasia: a 6-month prospective study showing weight gain and symptomatic improvement. *Dis Esophagus* 2002, **15**, 167–170.

13 Pastor AC, Mills J, Marcon MA, Himidan S, Kim PC. A single center 26-year experience with treatment of esophageal achalasia: is there an optimal method? *J Pediatr Surg* 2009, **44**, 1349–1354.

14 Zaheed Hussain S, Thomas R, Tolia V. A review of achalasia in 33 children. *Dig Dis Sci* 2002, **47**, 2538–2543.

15 Haito-Chavez Y, Inoue H, Beard KW, *et al.* Comprehensive analysis of adverse events associated with per oral endoscopic myotomy in 1826 patients: an international multicenter study. *Am J Gastroenterol* 2017, **112**, 1267–1276.

16 Gershman G, Ament ME, Vargas J. Frequency and medical management of esophageal perforation after pneumatic dilatation in achalasia. *J Pediatr Gastrolenterol Nutr* 1997, **25**, 548–553.

17 Bechara R, Ikeda H, Inoue H. Peroral endoscopic myotomy: an evolving treatment for achalasia. *Nat Rev Gastroenterol Hepatol* 2015, **12**, 410–426.

18 Ngamruengphong S, Inoue H, Ujiki MB, *et al.* Efficacy and safety of peroral endoscopic myotomy for treatment of achalasia after failed heller myotomy. *Clin Gastroenterol Hepatol* 2017, **15**, 1531–1537e3.

19 Chen WF, Li QL, Zhou PH, *et al.* Long-term outcomes of peroral endoscopic myotomy for achalasia in pediatric patients: a prospective, single-center study. *Gastrointest Endosc* 2015, **81**, 91–100.

20 Caldaro T, Familiari P, Romeo EF, *et al.* Treatment of esophageal achalasia in children: today and tomorrow. *J Pediatr Surg* 2015, **50**, 726–730.

21 Kethman WC, Thorson CM, Sinclair TJ, Berquist WE, Chao SD, Wall JK. Initial experience with peroral endoscopic myotomy for treatment of achalasia in children. *J Pediatr Surg* 2018, **53**, 1532–1536.

22 Li QL, Zhou PH. Perspective on peroral endoscopic myotomy for achalasia: Zhongshan experience. *Gut Liver* 2015, **9**, 152–158.

28

Endoscopic approaches to the treatment of gastroesophageal reflux disease

Mike Thomson and Chris Fraser

 KEY POINTS

- Evolution of this approach has occurred over the last 10 years and the present generation (transoral incisionless fundoplication) is safe and effective in adults and, in a small series, in children.
- With CO_2 insufflation, no adverse events have occurred. Air insufflation should not be used.
- One-year objective efficacy with pH studies and quality of life with standardized validated

- scoring systems have shown medium-term success in children.
- In the UK in day case procedures, this approach compares favorably with laparoscopic, and even more so with open, fundoplication.
- The technique at present is limited by the size of the patient to approximately 25 kg bodyweight.
- Clearly, this technique requires further evaluation but initial studies are encouraging.

Introduction

Gastroesophageal reflux disease (GERD) is symptomatic reflux associated with sequelae. These include failing to thrive, refractory wheezing, coughing aspiration, acute life-threatening events, apnea, chronic otitis media, sinusitis, hematemesis, anemia, esophageal strictures, and Barrett's esophagus. A follow-up of 126 children with GERD in infancy showed 55% were symptom free by 10 months and 81% by 18 months of age. However, those with frequent symptoms (>90 days) in the first two years of life are more likely to have symptoms by 9 years of age.

Gastroesophageal reflux treatment aims to achieve symptom relief while preventing complications. Patients who fail to achieve control with medical therapy may have persistent, severe esophagitis or become long-term dependent on antireflux treatments. In such cases, an antireflux procedure may be indicated. The principle of surgery in GERD is to form some kind of reconstruction of the antireflux barrier, although exactly how efficacy is achieved is not fully understood. Open Nissen's fundoplication has been the treatment of choice to date, but is invasive and associated with morbidity and mortality. In recent years, laparoscopic fundoplication has become popular and, in general, has replaced the open Nissen's procedure, although superior efficacy and safety have yet to be demonstrated. With the laparoscopic procedure, cosmesis is clearly superior, and in adult studies complications appear less common, with good success rates. It could be argued, therefore, that there remains little or no place for open antireflux procedures in pediatrics.

Practical Pediatric Gastrointestinal Endoscopy, Third Edition. Edited by George Gershman and Mike Thomson.
© 2021 John Wiley & Sons Ltd. Published 2021 by John Wiley & Sons Ltd.
Companion website: www.wiley.com/go/gershman3e

Three endoscopic techniques have been devised and used for treatment of pediatric GERD. These are described below.

Endoscopic suturing devices

Endoluminal gastroplication makes use of an EndoCinch® sewing machine attached to the endoscope (gastroscope) placing three pairs of stitches below the gastroesophageal junction to create three internal plications of the stomach. Plications may be applied either circumferentially or longitudinally dependent on operator preference. The authors have a preference for placing two plications circumferentially 1.5 cm below the gastroesophageal junction and one 0.5 cm below the gastroesophageal junction, which we believe may be anatomically superior to other formations (Figures 28.1–28.4).

Endoluminal gastroplication is now routinely carried out as a day-case procedure in adults. Preliminary studies have shown it to be quick, noninvasive, effective, and safe. Results are comparable to the laparoscopic fundoplication in adults, which has been studied as a preferable alternative choice to an open Nissen's fundoplication.

Recently, the authors have reported use of EndoCinch in the treatment of 17 children (eight males, median age 12.9 years, range 6.1–17.7, median weight 45 kg, range 16.5–75) with GERD refractory to or dependent on (>12 months) proton pump inhibitors. All patients showed posttreatment improvement in symptom severity, frequency, and validated reflux-related quality of life scores (p <0.0001) (Figure 28.5). At 36 months median follow-u,p 11 out of 17 patients were asymptomatic and no longer taking any antireflux medications.

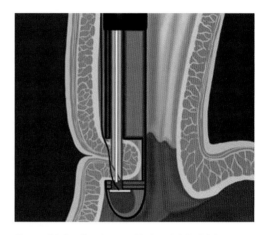

Figure 28.2 Suction applied and full-thickness tissue capture followed by needle and pusher wire placement of stitch.

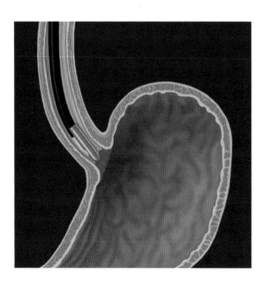

Figure 28.1 EndoCinch front-mounted on the endoscope.

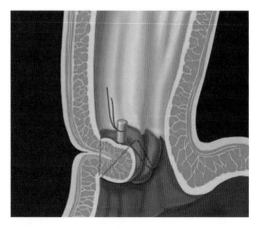

Figure 28.3 Endoscopic gastroplication. This figure shows the pattern of a zig-zag stich when applied with an EndoCinch sewing machine.

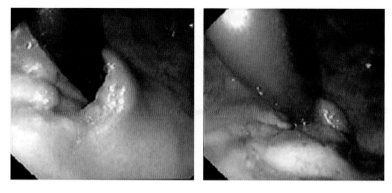

Figure 28.4 View (J manoeuver) of a lax GE junction in a child with major reflux after application of stitch with the EndoCinch.

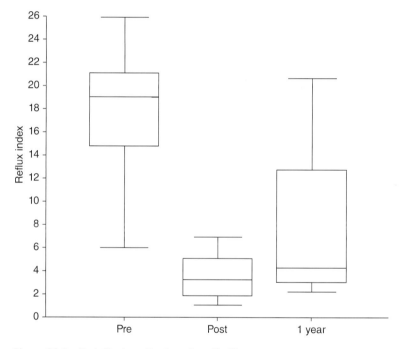

Figure 28.5 EndoCinch pediatric series pH efficacy at one year.

At 12 months follow-up, all pH parameters improved and had returned to normal in eight of nine patients who underwent pH studies (reflux index fell from 16.6% [0.9–67%] to 2.5% [0.7–15.7%], p <0.0001) (see Figure 28.5).

The duration of action is open to ongoing assessment and debate, and has not been particularly impressive in adult studies. The reasons for superior efficacy and duration in children may be conjectured and due to some or all of the following: three pairs versus two pairs of sutures; greater time and care taken by the operator allowed by general anesthetic with the added advantage of absence of movement or retching during the procedure; and lastly the relatively deeper suture depth in the thinner pediatric esophagus compared to the larger adult one. Data are now available indicating medium-term success in terms of reflux-related quality-of-life scoring at three years post EndoCinch and in terms of avoidance of PPI in the majority of patients. This is a small study but worthy of mention (Figure 28.6).

Despite the loss of sutures on observational follow-up studies, some efficacy has been maintained, and the human and porcine endoultrasound studies of Liu *et al.*, along with cadaveric analysis of the porcine model post EndoCinch, may throw some light on this observation. They suggest that the tissue remodeling in response to the foreign body, which is the suture, resulting in significant hypertrophy of the circular muscle layer of the esophagus may be the reason.

Nevertheless, EndoCinch has not maintained its initial enthusiastic uptake, and has been recently superseded by the next generation of full-thickness gastroplication transoral endoscopic techniques.

The next technique to appear was the Full-Thickness Plicator® (Ndo-Surgical). This is placed under direct vision with a neonatal size endoscope passed through a specially designed endoscopic delivery system with an outer diameter of more than 20 mm. The retroflexion of both allows observation firstly of the opening of the jaws of the device, followed by the insertion of the corkscrew into the fundal tissue, allowing capture of the fundus and withdrawal into the jaws which are then closed. A pretied full-thickness plication is then applied by the mechanism of shutting the jaws and a serosa-to-serosa plication is made (Figures 28.7–28.9). A multicenter adult study has shown acceptable efficacy and a reduction of PPI requirement in a small adult cohort, but further study is necessary before this can be applied to children – the device is size and age constrained due to its large outer diameter.

EsophyX®

This device is an alternative to the plicator technology along a similar theme, although not identical.

The novel Transoral Incisionless Fundoplication (TIF)® procedure using EsophyX (Texas Laparoscopic Consultants) mimics antireflux surgery in constructing an anterior partial fundoplication with tailored delivery of multiple fasteners during a single-device insertion (Figures 28.10 and 28.11). The TIF procedure was designed to restore the

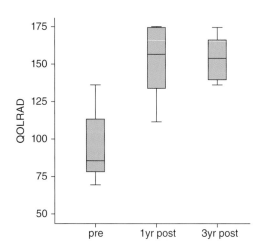

Figure 28.6 Significant improvement in the total QOLRAD score one and three years after gastroplication with the EndoCinch.

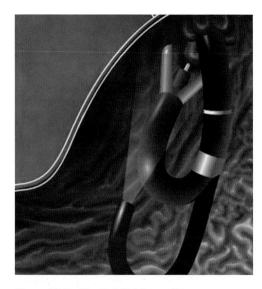

Figure 28.7 The Full-Thickness Plicator.

antireflux competency of the gastroesophageal junction by reducing small hiatal hernias, increasing LES resting pressure, narrowing the cardia, and recreation of the acute angle of His.

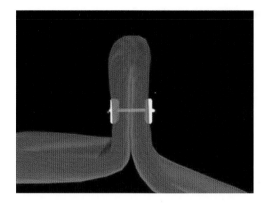

Figure 28.8 Application of the Full-Thickness Plicator.

Clinical results with TIF at one, two, and three years support its efficacy in eliminating heartburn and regurgitation, reducing the daily use of PPIs, normalizing esophageal acid exposure, and reducing proximal extent of refluxate. Based on one-year results, in September 2007 the FDA cleared EsophyX for the treatment of GERD and small (<2 cm) hiatal hernia.

The TIF procedure has been demonstrated to be safe in adults. Post-TIF adverse events are mild and transient and include musculoskeletal and epigastric pain, nausea, and dysphagia up to one week secondary to sore throat. Only three esophageal perforations have been reported to date for 3000 cases performed worldwide. None of the subjects experienced chronic dysphagia, gas bloating, or diarrhea at long-term follow-up.

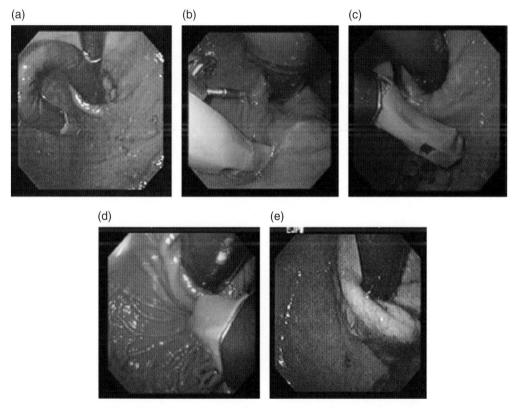

Figure 28.9 Retroverted views of stages of application of the Full-Thickness Plicator. (a) Plicator and gastroscope retroflexed to the GEJ. (b) Arms opened, tissue retractor advanced to serosa. (c) Gastric wall retracted. (d) Resulting full-thickness plication. (e) Arms closed, single pretied implant deployed.

(a)   (b)

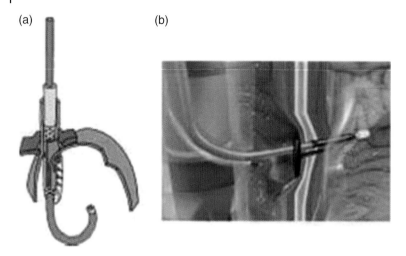

Figure 28.10 Distal end of the EsophyX device (a) and SerosaFuse fastener (b). The valve is constructed by drawing tissue into the device with the aid of a helical retractor. The tissue mold is then closed over the retracted tissue and the fasteners are deployed. The fastener is delivered by a pusher that slides over a stylet. Source: Reproduced with permission from Jobe BA, O'Rourke RW, McMahon BP, *et al.* Transoral endoscopic fundoplication in the treatment of gastroesophageal reflux disease: the anatomic and physiologic basis for reconstruction of the esophagogastric junction using a novel device. *Ann Surg* 2008, **248**, 69–76.

A feasibility study was started in December 2008 after obtaining appropriate training in the use of the EsophyX device in its second iteration – the so-called TIF2 procedure. The feasibility study was conducted with 12 children (eight male) with a median age of 12.25 years (range 8–18) years and weight of 38.2 kg (range 26–91). The median duration of GERD symptoms was 45 months (range 24–70) and all subjects were on GERD medication for more than six months. The median pre-TIF2 reflux index off treatment was 11.4% (range 6–48%). Hiatus hernia was present in 17% (2/12). Median operative time was 42 minutes (range 25–94). Adverse events were experienced by three subjects and consisted of mild or moderate pharyngeal irritation and epigastric pain. Two of the three subjects also had retrosternal chest pain and were subsequently found to have pneumomediastinum on CT chest but no leak on barium swallow. One of these two patients had pyrexia accompanying chest pain and was treated for possible mediastinitis and discharged home after five days of intravenous antibiotics. Subsequently, CO_2 insufflation was employed and more rapid absorption resulted in no further periprocedure mediastinal gas leak.

At six-month follow-up, all subjects (n = 10) discontinued PPIs, 80% were asymptomatic and 70% had normalized or clinically significantly reduced reflux index (10% time pH <4). The results of this feasibility study showed that the TIF procedure was feasible, safe (with CO_2 insufflation) and clinically effective in treating GERD in children. Ongoing studies are occurring. Furthermore, the speed of the procedure, the days of hospitalization, the relative cost-efficacy, and cost–benefit are identified in Figures 28.12–28.14.

Delivery of radiofrequency energy (Stretta® system)

The Stretta system has two parts – a catheter and a control module. The Stretta catheter is a flexible, hand-held, single patient-use device that delivers radiofrequency energy generated by the control module (Figure 28.15). It is

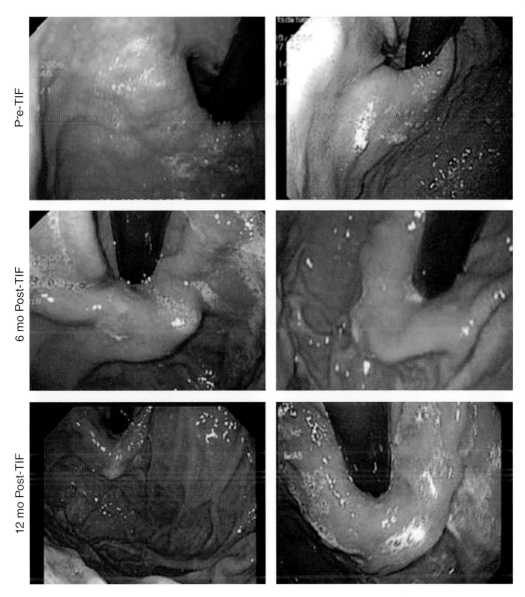

Figure 28.11 Endoscopic images of gastroesophageal valves from two subjects before and at six and 12 months following TIF. Source: Reproduced from Cadiere GB, Buset M, Muls V, *et al.* Antireflux transoral incisionless fundoplication using EsophyX: 12-month results of a prospective multicenter study. *World J Surg* 2008, **32**, 1676–1688, with kind permission from Springer Science+Business Media B.V.

inserted into the patient's mouth and advanced to the gastroesophageal junction. A balloon is inflated and needle electrodes are deployed into the tissue. Radiofrequency energy is delivered through the electrodes to create thermal lesions in the muscle of the lower esophageal sphincter and gastric cardia. As these lesions heal, the tissue contracts, resulting in a reduction of reflux episodes with improvement in symptoms. The Stretta control module delivers this radiofrequency while, at the same time, providing feedback to the physician regarding

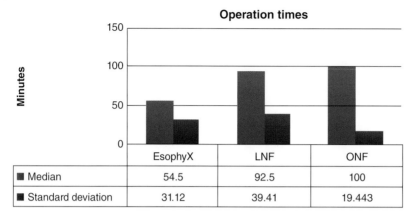

Figure 28.12 Operation times comparing endoscopic, laparoscopic. and open fundoplication.

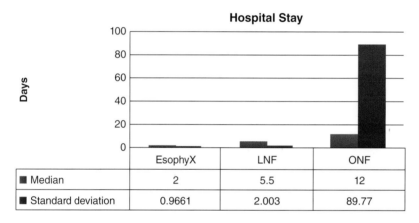

Figure 29.13 Hospital stay (days) comparing endoscopic, laparoscopic, and open fundoplication.

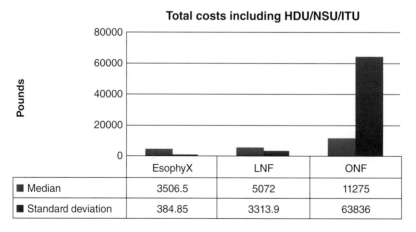

Figure 28.14 Total cost comparing endoscopic, laparoscopic, and open fundoplication (British pounds).

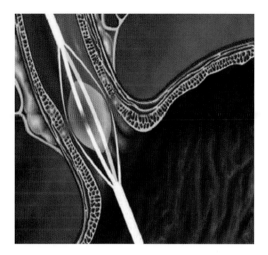

Figure 28.15 The Stretta system. Use of a balloon to deliver radiofrequency energy via needle electrodes to the mucosa.

treatment temperatures, tissue impedance values, elapsed time, catheter position measurement, and irrigation rate.

This treatment has been used in adults since 1999. Complications are rare but among those reported are ulcerative esophagitis with gastroparesis, esophageal perforation, and a case of aspiration following the procedure. Short-term (one year) success was reported in an open-label trial. In a prospective study (nonrandomized controlled trial) of 75 patients (age 49 +/− 14 years, 44% male, 56% female) undergoing laparoscopic fundoplication and 65 patient (age 46 +/− 12 years, 42%, 58% female) using the Stretta procedure, at six months 58% of Stretta patients were off PPIs and an additional 31% had reduced their dose significantly. In comparison, 97% of laparoscopic fundoplication patients were off PPIs. With long-term follow-up of the patients receiving the Stretta treatment, beyond two years, 56% had discontinued use of all antisecretory drugs.

This treatment has been reported in an uncontrolled study of eight children with a variable follow-up period of 5–15 months. It was reported that six of eight children improved, and the cohort included three neurologically impaired children who also had

concomitant PEG placement. One of this group had a postprocedure aspiration which was successfully treated. Of the two failures, one remained dependent on PPI and the other had a successful Nissen's fundoplication.

Pediatric gastroenterologists may be guarded in using this form of treatment as clearly, using thermal energy treatment in a 70 year old is different from using it in a child who may have unknown consequences in the long term. With the more recent and probably safer iterations of this technique, there are a number of studies occurring in pediatrics and these may provide positive results in due course.

Gastroesophageal biopolymer injection

In the Enteryx® (Boston Scientific) procedure, a liquid polymer is injected into the lower esophageal sphincter with a needle catheter via an endoscope. After the injection, the polymer solidifies into a sponge-like permanent implant. This improves the gastroesophageal junction, by supporting and improving its elasticity and therefore reducing the degree of gastroesophageal reflux (Figure 28.16).

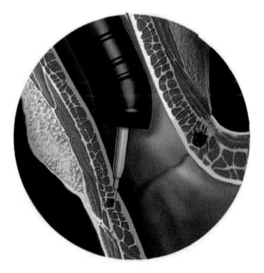

Figure 28.16 Injection of liquid polymer into the esophageal mucosa. The Enteryx procedure.

In an international open-label clinical trial on 144 patients, Cohen showed a greater than 50% reduction in PPI in 84% at the end of one year and 72% by two years, with elimination in 67% patients. In a prospective, randomized trial, endoluminal gastroplasty (EndoCinch) was compared with Enteryx in 51 consecutive patients dependent on PPI therapy. At six months, PPI therapy could be stopped or dosage was reduced by more than 50% in 20 of 26 (77%) EndoCinch-treated patients and in 20 of 23 patients treated by Enteryx (87%, p = 0.365). Approximately 25% of the patients in both groups required retreatment in an attempt to achieve symptom control. To date, an estimated 3800 patients have been treated with the Enteryx device, which was approved in 2003 by the FDA. To date, there are no published records of its use in pediatrics.

However, the FDA and Boston Scientific notified healthcare professionals and patients about serious adverse events, including death, occurring in patients treated with the Enteryx device. Based upon reports filed with the FDA, patients suffered leakage, swelling, and ulcers in the esophagus. One elderly patient died after some of the polymer had been injected into the woman's aorta, which ruptured, causing her to bleed to death.

On September 23, 2005, Boston Scientific ordered a recall of all Enteryx Procedure Kits and Enteryx Injector Single Packs from commercial distribution. The company's recall notice stated that some doctors accidentally punctured the wall of the esophagus while injecting the substance, causing adverse events. Additionally, Boston Scientific suspended sales of its Enteryx device after more than two dozen reports of problems. The notice was posted on the company's website during the week of September 19, 2005.

Conclusion

The most promising results seem to accrue in the mid-term with the suturing devices which attain full-thickness plications, increase the intraabdominal portion of the esophagus (most likely by plication tags inserting through the diaphragmatic crura as well as the full thickness of the esophageal wall, i.e., actual change in anatomy), and raised intrasphincteric length and resting pressure. Endoultrasound may provide a more controlled and sophisticated approach to this technology in the future.

 • See companion website for videos relating to this chapter topic: www.wiley.com/go/gershman3e

 FURTHER READING

Cadière GB, Rajan A, Germay O, Himpens J. Endoluminal fundoplication by a transoral device for the treatment of GERD: a feasibility study. *Surg Endosc* 2008, **22**, 333–342.

Cadière GB, Van Sante N, Graves JE, Gawlicka AK, Rajan A. Two-year results of a feasibility study on antireflux transoral incisionless fundoplication (TIF) using EsophyX. *Surg Endosc* 2009, **23**, 957–964.

Cohen LB, Johnson DA, Ganz RA, *et al.* Enteryx implantation for GERD: expanded multicenter trial results and interim postapproval follow-up to 24 months. *Gastrointest Endosc* 2005, **61**, 650–658.

Festen C. Paraesophageal hernia: a major complication of Nissen's fundoplication. *J Pediatr Surg* 1981, **16**, 496–499.

Filipi CJ, Lehman GA, Rothstein RI, *et al.* Transoral, flexible endoscopic suturing for treatment of GERD: a multicenter trial. *Gastrointest Endosc* 2001, **53**, 416–422.

Gotley DC, Smithers BM, Rhodes M, Menzies B, Branicki FJ, Nathanson L. Laparoscopic Nissen fundoplication – 200 consecutive cases. *Gut* 1996, **38**, 487–491.

Hyams JS, Ricci A Jr, Leichtner AM. Clinical and laboratory correlates of esophagitis in young children. *J Pediatr Gastroenterol Nutr* 1988, **7**, 52–56.

Islam S, Geiger JD, Coran AG, Teitelbaum DH. Use of radiofrequency ablation of the lower esophageal sphincter to treat recurrent gastroesophageal reflux disease. *J Pediatr Surg* 2004, **39**, 282–286.

Jobe BA, O'Rourke RW, McMahon BP, *et al.* Transoral endoscopic fundoplication in the treatment of gastroesophageal reflux disease: the anatomic and physiologic basis for reconstruction of the esophagogastric junction using a novel device. *Ann Surg* 2008, **248**, 69–76.

Liu DC, Somme S, Mavrelis PG, *et al.* Stretta as the initial antireflux procedure in children. *J Pediatr Surg* 2005, **40**, 148–151.

Liu JJ, Glickman JN, Carr-Locke DL, Brooks DC, Saltzman JR. Gastroesophageal junction smooth muscle remodeling after endoluminal gastroplication. *Am J Gastroenterol* 2004, **99**, 1895–1901.

Mahmood Z, McMahon BP, Arfin Q, *et al.* Endocinch therapy for gastro-oesophageal reflux disease: a one-year prospective follow-up. *Gut* 2003, **52**, 34–39.

Mahmood Z, Byrne PJ, McMahon BP, *et al.* Comparison of transesophageal endoscopic plication (TEP) with laparoscopic Nissen fundoplication (LNF) in the treatment of uncomplicated reflux disease. *Am J Gastroenterol* 2006, **101**, 431–436.

Martin AJ, Pratt N, Kennedy JD, *et al.* Natural history and familial relationships of infant spilling to 9 years of age. *Pediatrics* 2002, **109**, 1061–1067.

Mattioli G, Repetto P, Carlini C, *et al.* Laparoscopic vs open approach for the treatment of gastroesophageal reflux in children. *Surg Endosc* 2002, **16**, 750–752.

Park P, Kjellin T, Kadirkamanathan S, Appleyard M. Results of endoscopic gastroplasty for gastrooesophageal reflux disease. *Gastrointest Endosc* 2001, **53**, AB115.

Pleskow D, Rothstein R, Lo S, *et al.* Endoscopic full-thickness plication for the treatment of GERD: a multicenter trial. *Gastrointest Endosc* 2004, **59**, 163–171.

Raijman I, Ben-Menachem T, Reddy G, Weiland S. Symptomatic response to endoluminal gastroplication (ELGP) in patients with gastroesophageal reflux disease (GERD): a multicentre experience. *Gastrointest Endosc* 2001, **53**, AB74.

Repici A, Fumagalli U, Malesci A, Barbera R, Gambaro C, Rosati R. Endoluminal fundoplication (ELF) for GERD using EsophyX: a 12-month follow-up in a single-center experience. *J Gastrointest Surg* 2010, **14**, 1–6.

Richards WO, Scholz S, Khaitan L, Sharp KW, Holzman MD. Initial experience with the stretta procedure for the treatment of gastroesophageal reflux disease. *J Laparoendosc Adv Surg Tech A* 2001, **11**, 267–273.

Richards WO, Houston HL, Torquati A, *et al.* Paradigm shift in the management of gastroesophageal reflux disease. *Ann Surg* 2003, **237**, 638–647.

Rudolph CD, Mazur LJ, Liptak GS, *et al.* Guidelines for evaluation and treatment of gastroesophageal reflux in infants and children: recommendations of the North American Society for Pediatric Gastroenterology and Nutrition. *J Pediatr Gastroenterol Nutr* 2001, **32**, S1–S31.

Shepherd RW, Wren J, Evans S, Lander M, Ong TH. Gastroesophageal reflux in children. Clinical profile, course and outcome with active therapy in 126 cases. *Clin Pediatr* 1987, **26**, 55–60.

Swain CP, Kadirkamanathan SS, Gong F, *et al.* Knot tying at flexible endoscopy. *Gastrointest Endosc* 1994, **40**, 722–729.

Swain P, Park PO, Mills T. Bard EndoCinch: the device, the technique, and pre-clinical studies. *Gastrointest Endosc Clin North Am* 2003, **13**, 75–88.

Swain P, Park PO. Endoscopic suturing. *Best Pract Res Clin Gastroenterol* 2004, **18**, 37–47.

Thiny MT, Shaheen NJ. Is Stretta ready for primetime? *Gastroenterology* 2002, **123**, 643–644.

Thomson, M. Disorders of the oesophagus and stomach in infants. *Baillière's Clin Gastroenterol* 1997, **11**, 547–571.

Thomson M, Frischer-Ravens A, Hall S, Afzal N, Ashwood P, Swain CP. Endoluminal gastroplication in children with significant gastro-oesophageal reflux disease. *Gut* 2004, **53**, 1745–1750.

Thomson M, Antao B, Hall S, *et al.* Medium-term outcome of endoluminal gastroplication with the Endocinch device in children. *J Pediatr Gastroenterol Nutr* 2008, **46**, 172–177.

Torquati A, Houston HL, Kaiser J, Holzman MD, Richards WO. Long-term follow-up study of the Stretta procedure for the treatment of gastroesophageal reflux disease. *Surg Endosc* 2004, **18**, 1475–1479.

Veit F, Schwagten K, Auldist AW, Beasley SW. Trends in the use of fundoplication in children with gastro-oesophageal reflux. *J Paediatr Child Health* 1995, **31**, 121–126.

Velanovich V, Ben-Menachem T, Goel S. Case-control comparison of endoscopic gastroplication with laparoscopic fundoplication in the management of gastroesophageal reflux disease: early symptomatic outcomes. *Surg Laparosc Endosc Percutan Tech* 2002, **12**, 219–223.

Watson DI. Endoscopic antireflux surgery: are we there yet? *World J Surg* 2008, **32**, 1578–1580.

29

Foreign body ingestion

Raoul Furlano, George Gershman, and Jenifer R. Lightdale

 KEY POINTS

- Button battery ingestion is an endoscopic emergency and work-up includes a chest X-ray.
- Management of ingestion of more than one magnet includes endoscopic removal if possible within 24 hours of diagnosis.
- Once an object has cleared the esophagus, indications for its removal will depend upon its size, as well as whether it is blunt or sharp.
- Large or long objects that do not pass the pylorus and become trapped in the stomach will need to be removed, i.e., if wider than 2.5 cm in diameter or >6 cm in length.
- Esophageal food bolus impaction in a symptomatic patient with drooling or neck

pain is an indication for emergent endoscopic removal.
- If the child tolerates their secretions, endoscopic removal of a food bolus in the esophagus may be postponed to alalow an elective procedure and provide additional time for spontaneous clearance.
- The best grasping tools for sharp objects include retrieval forceps, retrieval nets, and polypectomy snares. It is good practice for a pediatric endoscopy unit to maintain a "foreign body retrieval box" that holds a variety of instruments.

Introduction

Endoscopy is a common and useful means of accessing the upper gastrointestinal tract for the purpose of retrieving ingested foreign bodies in children. The majority of foreign body ingestions occur in younger ages, with a peak incidence between the ages of 6 months and 6 years [1]. In contrast to adults, the great majority of children accidentally ingest common objects found in the home, including coins, toys, jewelry, magnets, and batteries. At least 80% pass through the gastrointestinal tract without the need for any intervention [2,3].

Indications for removal depend upon a patient's age and size, the type and form of the swallowed item, its location as well as the clinical symptoms and time since ingestion. Coins are the most common ingested objects among children around the world [4,5]. Usually, coins larger than 2.5 cm are more likely to become impacted, especially in children less than 5 years old. Spontaneous clearance of coins occurs in about 30% of patients [6] while coins in the distal esophagus may clear before endoscopic removal in as many as 60% of patients [7,8].

It is critical to distinguish coins from button batteries, as the latter are highly associated

Practical Pediatric Gastrointestinal Endoscopy, Third Edition. Edited by George Gershman and Mike Thomson.
© 2021 John Wiley & Sons Ltd. Published 2021 by John Wiley & Sons Ltd.
Companion website: www.wiley.com/go/gershman3e

with mucosal injury and perforation. Modern changes in battery production towards larger diameter, higher voltage lithium cells, as well as their ubiquitous presence in common household items, have increased the urgency with which button battery impaction, particularly in the esophagus, should be approached.

Diagnostic evaluation

A child with witnessed or suspected ingestion of a coin or another foreign body (FB) should always undergo radiography to evaluate for esophageal impaction [1,9]. One should not misinterpret a coin as a disc battery, and lateral films can be helpful to distinguish one from the other. When radiologically evaluating a suspected coin, it is essential to have a good look at the object's edges to exclude a "double halo sign" which would be more suggestive of a button battery.

For the purpose of initial diagnosis, radiographs can confirm the location, size, shape, and number of ingested FB and can help to exclude aspirated objects [1,9]. Radiographs identify most radiopaque FB, but may not be of much use in delineating commonly ingested radiolucent foreign bodies, including fish bones, wood, plastic and thin metal objects [1,9].

In addition to localization of objects, the presence of free mediastinal or peritoneal air should be assessed. A contrast examination should not be performed routinely as this increases the risk of aspiration. Although magnetic resonance imaging (MRI) can be used to delineate a foreign body, it may be variably helpful. Therefore, most guidelines suggest a computed tomography (CT) scan as a secondary study, particularly if an object is radiolucent and an understanding of location of the object is necessary to consider potential for endoscopic removal [10–12].

Of course, many sharp-pointed objects – particularly very thin ones like fish bones — are not visible by any radiographs, so endoscopy should still follow a radiological examination with negative findings when a high index of suspicion is present. If observation rather than removal is chosen in the asymptomatic patient, then close monitoring with serial abdominal X-rays may be considered. Patients who are discharged without endoscopic examination or if a foreign body is not found should be instructed to immediately report abdominal pain, vomiting, persistent temperature elevations, hematemesis, or melena [6,13].

The average transit time for an ingested foreign object in children has been described as 3.6 days, while the mean time from ingestion of a sharp object to perforation has been reported at 10.4 days [14]. Surgical removal may be appropriate if a radiopaque foreign body is found on serial X-rays not to progress for three days, or if a patient becomes symptomatic [14,15].

Esophageal impaction of a foreign body

Esophageal impaction of a foreign body – whether it is blunt or sharp – requires more urgent intervention compared to more distally located foreign bodies. Symptoms associated with all foreign body ingestions include vomiting, drooling, dysphagia, odynophagia, globus sensation, as well as respiratory symptoms of coughing, stridor, and choking [16]. Any of these may suggest impaction of the ingested object in the esophagus, place a patient at higher risk for aspiration, and necessitate urgent removal. While most patients will be completely asymptomatic, all esophageal foreign bodies, including esophageal food impactions, should be removed urgently (within two hours for a lithium button battery or a sharp pointed object; within 24 hours from presentation otherwise), to avoid significant esophageal injury or erosion into the mediastinum [10–12].

Foreign bodies in the stomach and small bowel

The frequency and type of ingested sharp objects are highly dependent on cultural factors. Esophageal fish bones are most frequently encountered in patients living in Asian and Mediterranean areas, where it is customary to introduce fish into the diet at a young age [17].

Although safety pin ingestions have decreased greatly around the world with the advent of modern diapers [14], pin ingestions more generally remain prevalent in ethnic groups that use pins to fasten clothing or religious garments [18,19].

Toothpick ingestions are more prevalent among older age groups, but can occur not infrequently in young children as well [20,21].

If a sharp object becomes impacted in the esophagus, the patient may have overt symptoms, including pain, dysphagia, odynophagia, and drooling. However, delayed intestinal perforation, extraluminal migration, abscess, peritonitis, fistula formation, appendicitis, liver, bladder, heart, and lung penetration, and rupture of the common carotid artery have all been described in patients who have remained asymptomatic for weeks after ingesting a sharp foreign body [12,19,20,22–27].

Severe complications of swallowing a sharp object – including need for urgent surgery or death – are higher in patients who become symptomatic 48 hours after ingestion occurred [28] or who have swallowed a radio-lucent foreign body, which can delay diagnosis of impaction [21,29]. Maintaining a high index of suspicion and performing timely endoscopic removal prior to passage beyond the distal duodenum remain the best ways to avoid these tragic outcomes.

Once an object has cleared the esophagus, indications for its removal will depend upon its size, as well as whether it is blunt or sharp. Large or long objects that do not pass the pylorus and become trapped in the stomach will need to be removed. Recent consensus guidelines suggest removal of blunt foreign bodies from the stomach or duodenum if the child is symptomatic or if the object is wider than 2.5 cm in diameter or >6 cm in length. Otherwise, blunt foreign bodies that have been localized in the stomach can be followed expectantly and retrieved only if they produce symptoms or do not pass spontaneously after four weeks. In contrast, sharp-pointed objects in the stomach or proximal duodenum should be removed urgently (within two hours) to minimize their chance of passing out of endoscopic reach and perforating the distal small bowel 10–12].

Batteries

A number of foreign body ingestions should be recognized to represent a special circumstance. For example, cylindrical batteries do not typically discharge electrical current as button (disc) batteries do, but nevertheless have the potential to leak caustic fluid, particularly if the outer casing is compromised [30]. Urgent endoscopic removal (<24 hours) of cylindrical batteries is generally recommended when they are impacted in the esophagus. If a single battery is located in the stomach, it may be appropriate to monitor the patient expectantly in the outpatient setting [10–12]. Multiple battery ingestions have also been described, often in the context of suicidal attempts by adolescents, and may be more appropriately managed with elective endoscopic removal [31].

Magnets

Another special circumstance involves ingestion of multiple magnets of any strength, or ingestion of a magnet and another metal object. This type of ingestion can pose a particular risk of injury when the two items attract themselves and trap a portion of bowel wall between them. The resulting pressure between the two can lead to bowel wall necrosis with fistula formation, perforation, obstruction, volvulus or peritonitis [32–35]. The concern with ingesting magnets has been amplified in recent years with increasing prevalence of neodymium, or rare earth, magnets in toys and other small objects. These magnets have more than five times the attractive force of conventional magnets and have demonstrated the tendency to cause gastrointestinal injury much more readily than their conventional counterparts. Though the same potential for injury and principles for management apply to nonneodymium magnets, the relative risk is significantly less due to their decreased magnetic pull.

Urgent removal of all magnets within endoscopic reach should be pursued. For those beyond endoscopic reach, close observation and surgical consultation for nonprogression through the GI tract is advised [10–12].

Drug packets

In regions of high drug trafficking, so-called "body packing" can also involve teenagers. Illegal drugs are packed into latex condoms, balloons or plastic and swallowed for transportation [36]. Leakage or rupture of these packets can be fatal, therefore endoscopic removal should not be attempted [10,11].

Food bolus impaction

Food bolus impaction in children may indicate underlying esophageal pathology, such as eosinophilic esophagitis, peptic or other strictures, achalasia, and other motility disorders [37–41]. Hence, in contrast to other foreign body ingestions, it may be appropriate for the endoscopist to obtain biopsies after the food bolus has been removed [10–12]. On the other hand, dilation of any underlying stricture is best deferred for another date, after the biopsies have been reviewed and appropriate treatment instituted as needed. Dilation at the initial presentation is particularly best avoided if the impaction has been in place for a prolonged period of time, as acutely inflamed mucosa may increase risks of perforation [12].

Esophageal food bolus impaction in a symptomatic patient with drooling or neck pain is an indication for emergent endoscopic removal. If the child tolerates their secretions, endoscopic removal may be postponed and an urgent (<24 hours) endoscopic removal may be considered, allowing an elective procedure and providing additional time for spontaneous clearance [10–12].

The technique of removal can include piecemeal extraction, suction, and/or gentle pushing of the bolus down into the stomach, though visualization of the distal esophagus is necessary to ensure that there is no stricture distal to the bolus [10–12]. Use of glucagon to relax the lower esophageal sphincter to hasten spontaneous clearance may not be effective, particularly in children with underlying eosinophilic esophagitis [12,42,43].

Equipment and management approaches for foreign body removal

Optimal endoscopic management of foreign bodies depends on their location and type. Success rates of retrieval depend on the experience level of the endoscopist and device choice [1]. The best grasping tools for sharp objects include retrieval forceps, retrieval nets, and polypectomy snares [44]. It is good practice for a pediatric endoscopy unit to maintain a "foreign body retrieval box" that holds a variety of instruments and can be carried easily into a procedure room. Indeed, given the variety of objects that children may ingest, it is not uncommon for an endoscopist to switch to a different instrument after attempting with a first. When possible, the endoscopist should trial a chosen instrument's effectiveness at grasping a foreign body similar to the one that has been ingested at the bedside, prior to inserting the instrument through the endoscope.

Of course, to some extent, size of the child will limit access to some devices, especially if a smaller endoscope is employed. For example, a 6 mm gastroscope has a 2 mm channel and will only accommodate small polypectomy retrieval nets (diameter of 20 mm), polypectomy snares, or Dormia basket devices [45,46]. A number of instruments have been developed specifically for foreign body removal. In particular, baskets or nets are very useful and come in different sizes. Generally speaking, removal of long, thin, and/or sharp objects using rat-tooth forceps can be accomplished easily [46]. Polypectomy snares may also provide a good option, particuarly for longer sharp objects such as toothpicks, and can be used to close open safety pins in the stomach prior to withdrawal. If the sharp end of an object is facing cephalad, it may be safest to push the object into the stomach with rat-tooth forceps and rotate the sharp end caudally prior to removal.

Table 29.1 Equipment compatible with a pediatric endoscope (2 mm channel)

Small biopsy forceps
Small polyp snare
Pediatric Roth net
Small alligator forceps
Small rat-tooth forceps
Small injection needle
Small APC probe
Two-pronged grasper

Table 29.1 lists equipment that can fit in the single small working channel of most pediatric endoscopes.

 • See companion website for videos relating to this chapter topic: www.wiley.com/go/gershman3e

REFERENCES

1 Ikenberry SO, Jue TL, Anderson MA, *et al.* Management of ingested foreign bodies and food impactions. *Gastrointest Endosc* 2011, **73**, 1085–1091.

2 Chu KM, Choi HK, Tuen HH, Law SY, Branicki FJ, Wong J. A prospective randomized trial comparing the use of the flexible gastroscope versus the bronchoscope in the management of foreign body ingestion. *Gastrointest Endosc* 1998, **47**, 23–27.

3 Kim JK, Kim SS, Kim JI, *et al.* Management of foreign bodies in the gastrointestinal tract: an analysis of 104 cases in children. *Endoscopy* 1999, **31**, 302–304.

4 Denney W, Ahmad N, Dillard B, Nowicki MJ. Children will eat the strangest things: a 10-year retrospective analysis of foreign body and caustic ingestions from a single academic center. *Pediatr Emerg Care* 2012, **28**, 731–734.

5 Chen X, Milkovich S, Stool D, van As AB, Reilly J, Rider G. Pediatric coin ingestion and aspiration. *Int J Pediatr Otorhinolaryngol* 2006, **70**, 325–329.

6 Gregori D, Scarinzi C, Morra B, *et al.* Ingested foreign bodies causing complications and requiring hospitalization in European children: results from the ESFBI study. *Pediatr Int* 2010, **52**, 26–32.

7 Farmakakis T, Dessypris N, Alexe DM, *et al.* Magnitude and object-specific hazards of aspiration and ingestion injuries among children in Greece. *Int J Pediatr Otorhinolaryngol* 2007, **71**, 317–324.

8 Braumann C, Goette O, Menenakos C, Ordemann J, Jacobi CA. Laparoscopic removal of ingested pin penetrating the gastric wall in an immunosuppressed patient. *Surg Endosc* 2004, **18**, 870.

9 Guelfguat M, Kaplinskiy V, Reddy SH, DiPoce J. Clinical guidelines for imaging and reporting ingested foreign bodies. *Am J Roentgenol* 2014, **203**, 37–53.

10 Thomson M, Tringali A, Dumonceau JM, *et al.* Paediatric gastrointestinal endoscopy: European Society for Paediatric Gastroenterolgy Hepatology and Nutrition and European Society of Gastrointestinal Endoscopy Guidelines. *J Pediatr Gastroenterol Nutr* 2017, **64**, 133–153.

11 Tringali A, Thomson M, Dumonceau JM, *et al.* Pediatric gastrointestinal endoscopy: European Society of Gastrointestinal Endoscopy (ESGE) and European Society for Paediatric Gastroenterology Hepatology and Nutrition (ESPGHAN) guideline executive summary. *Endoscopy* 2017, **49**, 83–91.

12 Kramer RE, Lerner DG, Lin T, *et al.* Management of ingested foreign bodies in children: a clinical report of the NASPGHAN Endoscopy Committee. *J Pediatr Gastroenterol Nutr* 2015, **60**, 562–574.

13 Ingraham CR, Mannelli L, Robinson JD, Linnau KF. Radiology of foreign bodies: how do we image them? *Emerg Radiol* 2015, **22**, 425–430.

14 Paul RI, Christoffel KK, Binns HJ, Jaffe DM. Foreign body ingestions in children: risk of complication varies with site of initial health care contact. *Pediatric Practice Research Group. Pediatrics* 1993, **91**, 121–127.

15 Rodríguez-Hermosa JI, Codina-Cazador A, Sirvent JM, Martín A, Gironès J, Garsot E. Surgically treated perforations of the gastrointestinal tract caused by ingested foreign bodies. *Colorectal Dis* 2008, **10**, 701–707.

16 Jayachandra S, Eslick GD. A systematic review of paediatric foreign body ingestion: presentation, complications, and management. *Int J Pediatr Otorhinolaryngol* 2013, **77**, 311–317.

17 Reilly BK, Stool D, Chen X, Rider G, Stool SE, Reilly JS. Foreign body injury in children in the twentieth century: a modern comparison to the Jackson collection. *Int J Pediatr Otorhinolaryngol* 2003, **67**, S171–S174.

18 Aydogdu S, Arikan C, Cakir M, *et al.* Foreign body ingestion in Turkish children. *Turk J Pediatri* 2009, **51**, 127–312.

19 Türkyilmaz Z, Karabulut R, Sönmez K, Basaklar AC, Kale N. A new method for the removal of safety pins ingested by children. *Ann Acad Med Singapore* 2007, **36**, 206–207.

20 Akcam M, Kockar C, Tola HT, Duman L, Gündüz M. Endoscopic removal of an ingested pin migrated into the liver and affixed by its head to the duodenum. *Gastrointest Endosc* 2009, **69**, 82–84.

21 Hameed K HM, Rehman S. Management of foreign bodies in the upper gastrointestinal tract with flexible endoscope. *J Postgrad Med Institute (Peshwar-Pakistan)* 2011, **25**, 433–435.

22 Braumann C, Goette O, Menenakos C, Ordemann J, Jacobi CA. Laparoscopic removal of ingested pin penetrating the gastric wall in an immunosuppressed patient. *Surg Endosc* 2004, **18**, 870.

23 Mehran A, Podkameni D, Rosenthal R, Szomstein S. Gastric perforation secondary to ingestion of a sharp foreign body. *J Soc Laparoendosc Surgeons* 2005, **9**, 91–93.

24 Goh BK, Chow PK, Quah HM, *et al.* Perforation of the gastrointestinal tract secondary to ingestion of foreign bodies. *World J Surg* 2006, **30**, 372–377.

25 Garcia-Segui A, Bercowsky E, Gómez-Fernández I, Gibernau R, Gascón Mir M. Late migration of a toothpick into the bladder: initial presentation with urosepsis and hydronephrosis. *Arch Esp Urol* 2012, **65**, 626–629.

26 Karadayi S, Sahin E, Nadir A, Kaptanoglu M. Wandering pins: case report. *Cumhuriyet Med J* 2009, **31**, 300–302.

27 Sai Prasad TR, Low Y, Tan CE, Jacobsen AS. Swallowed foreign bodies in children: report of four unusual cases. *Ann Acad Med Singapore* 2006, **35**, 49–53.

28 Palta R, Sahota A, Bemarki A, Salama P, Simpson N, Laine L. Foreign-body ingestion: characteristics and outcomes in a lower socioeconomic population with predominantly intentional ingestion. *Gastrointest Endosc* 2009, **69**, 426–433.

29 Tokar B, Cevik AA, Ilhan H. Ingested gastrointestinal foreign bodies: predisposing factors for complications in children having surgical or endoscopic removal. *Pediatr Surg Int* 2007, **23**, 135–139.

30 Litovitz T, Schmitz BF. Ingestion of cylindrical and button batteries. an analysis of 2382 cases. *Pediatrics* 1992, **89**, 747–757.

31 Sahn B, Mamula P, Ford CA. Review of foreign body ingestion and esophageal food impaction management in adolescents. *J Adolesc Health* 2014, **55**, 260–266.

32 McCormick S, Brennan P, Yassa J, Shawis R. Children and mini-magnets: an almost fatal attraction. *Emerg Med J* 2002, **19**, 71–73.

33 Dutta S, Barzin A. Multiple magnet ingestion as a source of severe gastrointestinal complications requiring surgical intervention. *Arch Pedatr Adolesc Med* 2008, **162**, 123–125.

34 Centers for Disease C and Prevention. Gastrointestinal injuries from magnet ingestion in children – United States, 2003–2006. *Morb Mortal Wkly Rep* 2006, **55**, 1296–1300.

35 Kay M, Wyllie R. Pediatric foreign bodies and their management. *Curr Gastroenterol Rep* 2005, **7**, 212–218.

36 Beno S, Calello D, Baluffi A, Henretig FM. Pediatric body packing: drug smuggling reaches a new low. *Pediatr Emerg Care* 2005, **21**, 744–746.

37 Longstreth GF, Longstreth KJ, Yao JF. Esophageal food impaction: epidemiology and therapy. A retrospective, observational study. *Gastrointest Endosc* 2001, **3**, 193–198.

38 Byrne KR, Panagiotakis PH, Hilden K, Thomas KL, Peterson KA, Fang JC. Retrospective analysis of esophageal food impaction: differences in etiology by age and gender. *Dig Dis Sci* 2007, **52**, 717–721.

39 Cheung KM, Oliver MR, Cameron DJ, Catto-Smith AG, Chow CW. Esophageal eosinophilia in children with dysphagia. *J Pediatr Gastroenterol Nutr* 2003, **37**, 498–503.

40 Lao J, Bostwick HE, Berezin S, Halata MS, Newman LJ, Medow MS. Esophageal food impaction in children. *Pediatr Emerg Care* 2003, **19**, 402–407.

41 Hurtado CW, Furuta GT, Kramer RE. Etiology of esophageal food impactions in children. *J Pediatr Gastroenterol Nutr* 2011, **52**, 43–46.

42 Weant KA, Weant MP. Safety and efficacy of glucagon for the relief of acute esophageal food impaction. *Am J Health Syst Pharm* 2012, **69**, 573–577.

43 Thimmapuram J, Oosterveen S, Grim R. Use of glucagon in relieving esophageal food bolus impaction in the era of eosinophilic esophageal infiltration. *Dysphagia* 2013, **28**, 12–16.

44 Chaves DM, Ishioka S, Félix VN, Sakai P, Gama-Rodrigues JJ. Removal of a foreign body from the upper gastrointestinal tract with a flexible endoscope: a prospective study. *Endoscopy* 2004, **36**, 887–892.

45 Chu KM, Choi HK, Tuen HH, Law SY, Branicki FJ, Wong J. A prospective randomized trial comparing the use of the flexible gastroscope versus the bronchoscope in the management of foreign body ingestion. *Gastrointest Endosc* 1998, **47**, 23–27.

46 Kim JK, Kim SS, Kim JI, *et al.* Management of foreign bodies in the gastrointestinal tract: an analysis of 104 cases in children. *Endoscopy* 1999, **31**, 302–304.

30

Non-variceal endoscopic hemostasis

George Gershman, Jorge H. Vargas, and Mike Thomson

 KEY POINTS

- Key components of successful management of acute gastrointestinal bleeding in children are correct estimation of the severity of bleeding, proper selection of children for an urgent endoscopy, and
- highquality training of the performing pediatric endoscopist.
- A variety of endoscopic tools and techniques are available for endoscopic hemostasis of non-variceal bleeding.

Introduction

Acute gastrointestinal bleeding (AGIB) in children is a true medical emergency associated with significant morbidity and mortality even in developed countries. Recent retrospective analysis of AGIB in patients admitted to the 47 pediatric tertiary centers in the US (data extracted from Pediatric Hospital Information System) revealed mortality of almost 0.4% and 3% in children with the primary and secondary diagnosis of AGIB respectively. The key preventable reasons why children are still dying from AGIB are underestimation of severity of bleeding on admission, delayed endoscopy, lack of specialists trained in therapeutic endoscopy, and miscalculation of risk of recurrent bleeding.

To address the first pair of issues, the Sheffield scoring system has been developed to select children who will benefit from urgent endoscopy and endoscopic hemostasis. The

score is computed by adding the numerical value for clinically relevant characteristics in four categories:

- history (melena – 1, large hematemesis – 1)
- clinical assessment (heart rate of >20 bpm above the mean for age – 1, capillary refill time >2 seconds – 4)
- laboratory findings (fall of hemoglobin of >20 g/L – 3)
- management and resuscitation (need for fluid bolus 3, need for blood transfusion: fall of hemoglobin of >20 g/L – 6, need for other blood products – 4).

A cut-off of 8 for intervention from a maximal score of 24 has a positive predictive value and negative predictive value of about 91% and 89% respectively. The Sheffield scoring system stratifies children with AGIB in three categories: 1 immediate intervention for children with uncontrolled bleeding who require volume control; 2 endoscopic intervention within 12 hours for children in whom the threshold score is reached, but who are stable; 3 elective or no endoscopy for children whose clinical bleeding risk score does not reach the intervention threshold and in whom AGIB would appear to have ceased.

The next challenge is a lack of equipment and specialists in endoscopic hemostasis in children. One answer to this could be development of AGIB "super-centers" or collaboration with adult gastroenterologists skilled in endoscopic hemostasis. Each approach has pros and cons based on differences in hospital policies, type of medical systems (social versus private), and lack of enthusiasm on the part of our adult colleagues to get involved in the pediatric field.

It has been proved that early endoscopy within 24 hours is associated with reduction in transfusions, rebleeding (RB) and need for surgery compared to later endoscopy. Furthermore, endoscopic stigmata of active or resent bleeding organized by Forrest classification (F) defines indications for endoscopic hemostasis and hospitalization based on the probability of rebleeding risk:

- 50–100% in patients with spurting (F 1a) or oozing blood (F 1b) (Figure 30.1)
- under 50% if visible nonbleeding vessel (F 2a) or adherent clot (F 2b) (Figure 30.2) is found
- less than 10% in cases of ulcer with a flat pigmented spot (F 2c) (Figure 30.3) or clear base (F 3) (Figure 30.4).

In addition to the Forrest classification, there are other endoscopic features of peptic ulcers that can predict adverse outcomes and/or endoscopic treatment failure. These include large ulcer (>2 cm), large nonbleeding visible vessel, presence of blood in the gastric lumen, and ulcer location on the posterior duodenal wall or proximal lesser curvature of the stomach. Further research is needed to prove the same concept in children.

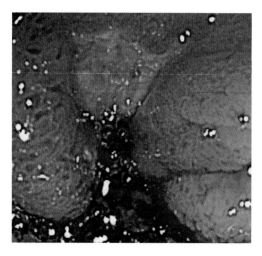

Figure 30.1 Active bleeding F 1b from a duodenal ulcer.

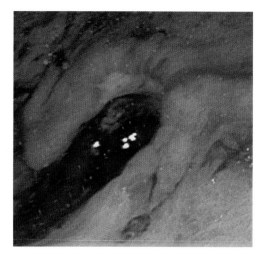

Figure 30.2 Adherent clot (F 2b) at the base of a gastric ulcer.

General considerations

Low incidence of non-variceal AGIB in children and lack of pediatric research are the reasons why pediatric gastroenterologists rely on recommendations derived from the practice of our adult colleagues.

The main source for diagnosis and management of non-variceal AGIB is the guidelines from the American College of Gastroenterology and European Society of Gastrointestinal Endoscopy.

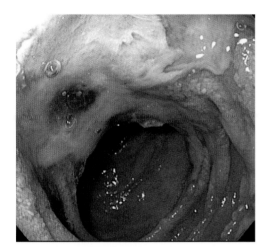

Figure 30.3 A flat pigmented spot (F 2c) at the base of a duodenal ulcer.

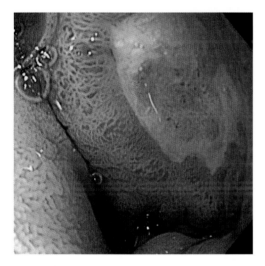

Figure 30.4 Clear base of a duodenal ulcer (F 3).

The key elements of these recommendations acceptable to pediatric practice are:

- immediate assessment of hemodynamic status in patients who present with acute AGIB with prompt intravascular volume replacement initially using crystalloid fluids if hemodynamic instability exists
- restrictive red blood cell transfusion strategy that aims for a target hemoglobin between 7 g/dL and 9 g/dL
- high-dose intravenous proton pump inhibitors for 72 hours for patients treated

endoscopically or patients with Forrest 2b ulcers who did not receive endoscopic hemostasis

- avoidance of routine use of nasogastric or orogastric aspiration/lavage
- intravenous dose of erythromycin 3 mg/kg to a maximum of 250 mg 30–120 minutes before upper endoscopy in patients with clinically severe or ongoing bleeding
- endoscopic treatment for Forrest 1a, 1b and 2a ulcers
- consideration for endoscopic clot removal for Forrest 2b ulcers
- avoidance of endoscopic treatment for Forrest 2c and 3 ulcers
- avoidance of using epinephrine injection as an endoscopic monotherapy
- avoidance of routine second-look endoscopy except in patients with clinical evidence of rebleeding following initial endoscopic hemostasis.

Choice of endoscope

Endoscopy during active bleeding is challenging due to poor visibility and the need to remove large amounts of blood and manipulate with a hemostatic device and flushing water on the target simultaneously. Therefore, a double-channel therapeutic endoscope is preferable if it is appropriate to the patient size. If this is not feasible, an adult-size upper GI endoscope can be used in children more than 10 kg. Pediatric-size upper GI endoscopes have limited suction capacity and are reserved for toddlers. Slim endoscopes ≤6 mm are kept for neonates and infants.

Techniques of endoscopic hemostasis

Methods of endoscopic hemostasis can be classified into three categories:

- nonthermal hemostasis
- constrictive, mechanical devices
- thermal coagulation.

Epinephrine injection therapy

Epinephrine in saline (1:10000) is a vasoconstrictive agent routinely used for hemostasis in children with non-variceal bleeding. It is injected into the bleeding site through the 23 or 25 gauge needle (both are available for endoscopes with 2.8mm and 2mm biopsy channels). The needle should be primed (filled with epinephrine) before insertion into the biopsy channel to prevent air embolism.

Currently, injection of epinephrine is recommended in combination with thermal or constrictive endoscopic devices, particularly in patients with bleeding ulcer (Forrest 1a, 1b, and 2a).

Limited pediatric data reveal a high rate of rebleeding after epinephrine monotherapy (40%) in children with acute non-variceal upper gastrointestinal bleeding, supporting a concept of combination endoscopic hemostasis.

Indications for epinephrine injections are:

- bleeding ulcer
- bleeding arteriovenous malformation
- bleeding after polypectomy.

The injection technique should be adjusted to the specific cause of bleeding; for example, a bleeding ulcer with a visible vessel requires peripheral four quadrants injections, typically 0.5–1 mL per site, followed by direct injection into the bleeding vessel. In contrast, target injection into the bleeding spot is an initial step of endoscopic hemostasis caused by ateriovenous malformations or bleeding from the base of the polyp after polypectomy. The amount of epinephrine solution should not exceed 16 mL (recommended adult dose). In our practice, we rarely inject more than 4 mL of epinephrine solution per session to avoid local ischemia or perforation.

Endoscopic hemostatic powder and gel

Topical application of hemostatic agents is a new, nontraumatic, and very effective type of endoscopic hemostasis which has been rapidly gaining ground in adult gastroenterology over the last decade. It can be used for localized or diffuse lesions as primary or salvage treatment, when bleeding persists despite application of conventional methods of endoscopic hemostasis.

Three agents are commercially available in the United States.

- Hemospray® (Cook Medical, Bloomington, IN, USA) is an inorganic, nonabsorbable nanocompound sprayed through a catheter inserted into the working channel of an endoscope. The powder is delivered with the aid of a pressurized CO_2 canister to a bleeding area. It absorbs water, forming an adhesive barrier that creates a hemostatic plug. Hemospray is delivered through a standard 10 French catheter. Each burst release 1–5g of powder. To prevent clotting the catheter, it is recommended to keep the catheter 2–3cm away from the bleeding source. Available data showed immediate hemostasis of 92%, with a seven-day rebleeding rate of close to 21%.
- The EndoClot® (EndoClot Plus Inc., Santa Clara, CA, USA) polysaccharide hemostatic system is another noncontact endoscopic device that delivers hemostatic powder. It is composed of modified polymer particles, which absorb water from blood. This dehydration process increases the concentration of platelets, red blood cells, and coagulation proteins (thrombin, fibrinogen, etc.), resulting in the rapid formation of a hemostatic layer.
- Ankaferd Blood Stopper (Ankaferd Health Products, Istanbul, Turkey) is a 100mL herbal extract composed of five different plant species. It works presumably by formation of an encapsulated web of erythrocyte aggregation.
- Purastat (This is a fourth more recent admission) is a gel and is good for point bleeders and has the advantage of allowing good vision with no spray obscuring the field.

Hemostatic clips

Metal clips are very effective in controlling active hemorrhage from bleeding vessels in a peptic ulcer base, Dieulafoy lesion, Mallory–Weiss tears, and polypectomy site. Single-use preloaded rotatable two-pronged clips, which can be reopened and repositioned up to five times, are commercially available (Figure 30.5).

The endoscope with 2.8 mm biopsy channels is necessary to accommodate a standard clipping device, which consists of a metal cable within a metal coil sheath covered by a 2.2 mm Teflon® catheter. However, application of a Resolution Clip® (Boston Scientific) without a Teflon catheter allows it to adapt to an endoscope with a smaller 2.2 mm working channel.

The keys for successful application of a clipping device are:

- good visibility of bleeding point
- precise positioning of the clip on the target lesion
- full opening of the clip before deployment
- minimal extension of the clipping device beyond the tip of the endoscope
- avoidance of excessive force while embedding the clip into the tissue before deployment
- application of an additional clip if necessary.

The most challenging scenario for hemostatic clip therapy is bleeding from a large ulcer on the posterior wall of the duodenal bulb or superior duodenal angle. Rotating the patient into prone or supine and use of a double-channel therapeutic endoscope may improve visibility and navigation of the scope in front of the bleeding vessel to secure the optimal conditions for clip deployment.

Primary hemostasis of a bleeding ulcer or Dieulafoy lesion can be achieved in 84–100% of cases respectively.

Complications associated with clipping hemostasis are quite rare.

Over-the-scope clip

Since 2007, over-the-scope clips (OTSC) have been successfully used by adult gastroenterologists for endoscopic hemostasis and closure of perforations (Figures 30.6 and 30.7).

In conjunction with its sister device, it allows for full-thickness biopsies of the low GI tract. It is available in three different sizes: 11, 12, and 14 mm with 3 or 6 mm depths of caps for

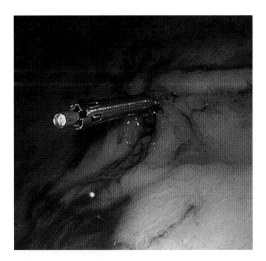

Figure 30.5 Single-use preloaded rotatable two-pronged clips: a single clip.

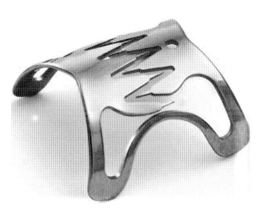

Figure 30.6 Over-the-scope clip.

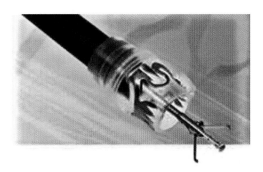

Figure 30.7 Delivery system.

grasping more or less tissue during approximation. The OTSC is mounted over the tip of the endoscope with an applicator similar to a cup for an esophageal varices ligature. It may be used in combination with an additional tool such as a "twin grasper" to approximate edges before deployment of the clip.

The device is controlled by an extraendoscopic channel which is attached to the outside of the scope. The central grasping forceps are deployed to stabilize the tissue of choice and then suction is applied for five seconds until vision is obliterated, similar to variceal banding, and then the jaws of the capture clip are released to oppose each other for closure when the handle is turned outside the patient.

Thermal coagulation

Thermal hemostasis embraces different methods which target non-variceal causes of bleeding, such as:

- ulcers with bleeding or nonbleeding visible vessels
- ulcers with an adherent clot
- Mallory–Weiss tear with active bleeding
- vascular malformations, e.g., Dieulafoy lesions
- bleeding after polypectomy.

Three types of thermal devices are currently used in pediatric practice.

Bipolar or multipolar thermal devices

The heating unit of these devices consists of two (bipolar – bipolar probe is also called the 'gold' probe and can have a needle within it in order to inject epinephrine quadrantically around a point bleeder in order to achieve hemostasis before application of the gold probe to the visible vessel) or 4–6 (multipolar) active electrodes incorporated into a thermal probe. Advantages of the system are:

- elimination of the need for a grounding plate
- mechanical compression of the bleeding vessel
- large contact area

- low risk of tissue adherence to the probe and rebleeding after pulling the probe back into the biopsy channel
- less depth of thermal coagulation
- effective coagulation with tangential position of the probe, essential for hemostasis of a bleeding duodenal ulcer
- ability to irrigate through the thermal probe.
- Small (2.2 mm) and large (3.2 mm) bipolar or multipolar probes are commercially available. Large probes allow for application of stronger pressure on a bleeding vessel and depth of coagulation.

The depth of coagulation is related to the power setting. Low-to-mid range of setting (15–25 W) is preferable for deep coagulation. Escalating the power setting increases water evaporation leading to a diminished degree of coagulation.

Computer-controlled thermal probes (heater probes)

The device generates and controls heat up to 250 °C by pulses of energy delivered to a silicon clip surrounded by a low heat capacity metal envelope without any electric current in the tissue. The probe is supplemented by a three-jet water system.

The metal envelope warms up to the designated temperature in less than 0.2 seconds and cools off in less than 0.5 seconds. The computer controls the temperature and total energy delivered to the tissue. The endoscopist adjusts the energy delivery to the source of bleeding in the range of 5–30 J.

Advantages of the heater probe include:

- elimination of direct contact of the probe with the tissue
- no adherence to the tissue
- automatic control of energy delivered to the tissue
- adjustable depth of coagulation.

Bipolar/multipolar and heater probes have been used more often in pediatric patients than any other type of thermal hemostatic devices.

Commercially available bipolar/multipolar and heater probes fit easily into the 2.8 mm biopsy channel endoscopes. Both methods provide enough heat for coagulation of mesenteric arteries up to 2 mm in experimental models.

Argon plasma coagulation (APC)

Plasma coagulation is the result of ionization of a noble gas (argon is the cheapest), which fills a small gap between the electrical electrode and the target tissue. Ionization of argon occurs when a high-frequency current creates sufficient electric field strength.

Ionized argon conducts an electrical current and flows along the same pathway. The released energy induces desiccation and coagulation without carbonization and evaporation, which prevents deep tissue destruction. The depth of coagulation is proportional to the power setting and application time but almost never exceeds 3 mm. Holding a probe in one site for five seconds produces coagulation depth of 2–3 mm with a power setting of 30–60 W.

The advantages of APC coagulation are:

- larger area of coagulation compared with bipolar or multipolar probes
- decreased depth of tissue destruction.

The procedure carries a risk of perforation due to direct contact between tissue and probe, and stretching of the stomach and bowel wall due to the accumulation of argon. Thin (1.5 mm) probes are commercially available and suitable for small-caliber pediatric endoscopes. This makes it possible to apply APC even in neonates and infants.

Two types of complications have been described in adults: perforation or submucosal emphysema due to direct contact of the probe with mucosa and flow of argon gas through the damaged mucosa.

Technique of thermal coagulation

A detailed description of endoscopic hemostasis with different thermal devices is beyond the scope of the chapter.

Before the procedure, the pediatric gastroenterologist should become familiar with the available equipment, the proper setting of the coagulator, and optimal treatment requirements for different types of bleeding lesions.

Bleeding from a non-variceal lesion in the stomach or duodenum can be arterial from a visible vessel or venous/parenchymal. During endoscopy, a visible nonbleeding vessel appears as a pyramid-like protuberance in the ulcer base. Observation of a forceful pulsating eruption of blood from the ulcer leaves no doubt about the arterial nature of the bleeding. Immediate endoscopic intervention is required, creating pressure by forcing a bipolar or heater probe up against the bleeding vessel, followed by four pulses of 30 J using the heater probe or 8–10-second pulses with a power setting of 15–20 W on a 50 W generator for bipolar or multipolar probe before repositioning the probe.

Coagulation is repeated until the visible vessel becomes flat and bleeding is stopped. The procedure is complicated by poor visibility, especially when the source of bleeding is located in the duodenum. Forceful irrigation and suction is more effective with therapeutic endoscopy.

Finding a large blood clot at the site of bleeding is another challenging situation. The risk of worsening bleeding has to be weighed against the potential benefits before an attempt to remove an adherent clot to expose a bleeding vessel. Treatment requires careful washing out of blood and loose fibrin until the edge of the ulcer becomes visible. The next step is injection of epinephrine under the clot in a circular fashion, to decrease the risk of bleeding during dislodgment of the clot from the ulcer and expose the underlying vessel for endoscopic hemostasis. Once again, this is a challenging procedure, which requires a highly skillful endoscopist and supportive team.

Presence of a nonbleeding vessel permits better assessment of the lesion and more precise positioning of the hemostatic device.

The power setting and force application should be adjusted in patients with angiodysplasia to avoid perforation. The APC technique is preferable in such circumstances.

 • See companion website for videos relating to this chapter topic: www.wiley.com/go/gershman3e

REFERENCES

1 Attard TM, Miller M, Pant C, Kumar A, Thomson M. Mortality associated with gastrointestinal bleeding in children: a retrospective cohort study. *World J Gastroenterol* 2017, **23**, 1608–1617.

2 Baracat F, Moura E, Bernardo W, *et al.* Endoscopic hemostasis for peptic ulcer bleeding: systematic review and meta-analyses of randomized control trials. *Surg Endosc* 2016, **30**, 2155–2168.

3 hiu PW. Second-look endoscopy in acute non-variceal gastrointestinal bleeding. *Best Pract Res Clin Gastroenterol* 2013, **27**, 905–911.

4 Emura T, Hosoda K, Harai S, *et al.* Dieulafoy lesion in a two-year-old boy: a case report. *J Med Case Rep* 2016, **10**, 293.

5 Garber A, Jang S. Novel therapeutic strategies in the management of non-variceal upper gastrointestinal bleeding. *Clin Endosc* 2016, **49**, 421–424.

6 Ghassemi KA, Jensen DM. What does lesion blood flow tell us about risk stratification and successful management of non-variceal UGI bleeding? *Curr Gastroenterol Rep* 2017, **19**, 17.

7 Giles H, Lal D, Gerred S, *et al.* Efficacy and safety of TC-325 m (hemospray TM) for non-variceal for upper non-variceal gastrointestinal bleeding in Middlemore hospital: the early New Zealand experience. *N Z Med J* 2016, **129**, 38–43.

8 Goenka MK, Rai VK, Goenka U, *et al.* Endoscopic management of gastrointestinal leaks and bleeding with over-the-scope clip: a prospective study. *Clin Endosc* 2017, **50**, 58–63.

9 Gralneck IM, Dumonceau J-M, Kuipers EJ, *et al.* Diagnosis and management of nonvariceal upper gastrointestinal hemorrhage: European Society of Gastrointestinal Endoscopy (ESGE) Guideline. *Endoscopy* 2015, **47**, a1–a46.

10 Grassia R, Campone P, Iiritano E, *et al.* Non-variceal upper gastrointestinal bleeding: rescue treatment with a modified cyanoacrylate. *World J Gastroenterol* 2016, **22**, 10609–10616.

11 Guo SB, Gong AX, Leng J, *et al.* Application of endoscopic hemoclips for non-variceal bleeding in the upper gastrointestinal tract. *World J Gastroenterol* 2009, **15**, 4322–4326.

12 Kay MH, Wyllie R. Therapeutic endoscopy for nonvaricial gastrointestinal bleeding. *J Pediatr Gastroenterol Nutr* 2007, **45**, 157–171.

13 Kawamura T, Yasuda K, Morikawa S. Current status of endoscopic management for non-variceal upper gastrointestinal bleeding. *Dig Endosc* 2010, **22**, S26–S30.

14 Kim SY, Hyun JJ, Jung SW, Lee SW. Management of non-variceal upper gastrointestinal bleeding. *Clin Endosc* 2012, **45**, 220–223.

15 Krishnan A, Velayutham V, Satyanesan J, *et al.* Role of endoscopic band ligation in non-variceal upper gastrointestinal bleeding. *Trop Gastroenterol* 2013, **34**, 91–94.

16 Laine L, Jensen DM. Management of patients with ulcer bleeding. *Am J Gastroenterol* 2012, **107**, 345–360.

17 Nojkov B, Cappell MS. Distinctive aspects of peptic ulcer disease, Dieulafoy's lesion and Mallory–Weiss syndrome in patients with advanced alcoholic liver disease or cirrhosis. *World J Gastroenterol* 2016, **22**, 446–466.

18 Pagnelli M, Alvarez F, Halac U. Use of hemospray for non-variceal esophageal bleeding in an infant. *J Hepatol* 2014, **61**, 712–713.

19 Thomson M, Belsha D. Endoscopic management of acute gastrointestinal bleeding in children: time for a radical re-think. *J Pediatr Surg* 2016, **51**, 206–210.

20 Thomson MA, Leton N, Belsha D. Acute upper gastrointestinal bleeding in childhood: development of the Sheffield scoring system to predict need for endoscopic therapy. *J Pediatr Gastroenterol Nutr* 2015, **60**, 632–636.

21 Ünal F, Cakir F, Baran M, *et al.* Application of endoscopic hemoclips for non-variceal upper gastrointestinal bleeding in children. *Turk J Gastroenterol* 2014, **25**, 147–151.

22 Wedi E, Fischer A, Hochberger J, *et al.* Multicenter evaluation of first line endoscopic treatment with the OTSC in acute non-variceal gastrointestinal bleeding and comparison with the Rockall cohort: the FLETRock study. *Surg Endosc* 2018, **32**, 307–314.

23 Wedi E, Gonzalez S, Menke D, *et al.* One hundred and one over-the-scope-clip applications, for severe gastrointestinal bleeding, leaks and fistulas. *World J Gastroenterol* 2016, **22**, 1844–1853.

31

Variceal endoscopic hemostasis

Patrick McKiernan, Lauren Johanson, and Mike Thomson

 KEY POINTS

- Currently, a three-grade classification system is used in the UK and Europe, and has been shown to have reasonable interobserver repeatability.
- High-risk varices in children can be considered as one of the following patterns: grade 3 esophageal varices, grade 2 esophageal varices with red color changes and/or gastric varices along the cardia/fundus.
- Banding is preferable to sclerotherapy.
- ESGE-ESPGHAN guidance is that endoscopy should occur within 12 hours of an acute upper gastrointestinal bleed if the child requires ongoing circulatory support, if they

- have known esophageal varices, or if a large hematemesis or melena has occurred.
- Repeat endoscopy before discharge, following an acute variceal bleed treated successfully, is recommended.
- Endoscopic ultrasound (EUS) may help to target sclerotherapy with histoacryl glue in the gastric fundus.
- The major limitation of injecting this glue is not embolization or local complications for the child, but damage to the biopsy channel of the endoscope itself.
- Primary prophylactic variceal treatment is not proven but is probably sensible in children.

Portal hypertension and variceal formation

Portal hypertension is defined as a hepatic venous pressure gradient (HVPG) of >5 mmHg. It is caused by increased portal blood flow and/or increased portal resistance. In children, portal hypertension is predominantly caused by intrahepatic disease, but important presinusoidal causes include extrahepatic portal vein obstruction (EHPVO) or congenital hepatic fibrosis [1]. Where HVPG is >10 mmHg esophageal varices may form, and bleeding may occur when the HVPG is >12 mmHg. Although mortality following the first bleed is low when

specialist medical care is available (<1%) [2], recurrent variceal hemorrhage has a mortality of up to 8% [3]. Variceal bleeding may precipitate the need for earlier liver transplantation.

Diagnosis, classification, and risk stratification of varices

Upper gastrointestinal endoscopy remains the reference for diagnosis of esophageal varices (Figure 31.1). There are no evidence-based pediatric guidelines for the management of portal hypertension and hence the timing of

---

Practical Pediatric Gastrointestinal Endoscopy, Third Edition. Edited by George Gershman and Mike Thomson.
© 2021 John Wiley & Sons Ltd. Published 2021 by John Wiley & Sons Ltd.
Companion website: www.wiley.com/go/gershman3e

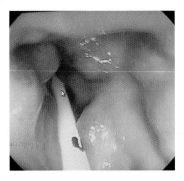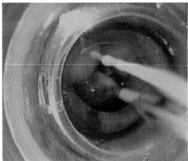

Figure 31.1 Large esophageal varices before and after band ligation.

Table 31.1 Classification system for esophageal varices

Grade I	Small and nontortuous varices
Grade II	Tortuous varices but occupying <1/3 of the distal esophageal radius
Grade III	Large and tortuous varices covering >1/3 of the distal esophageal radius

the first endoscopy is debatable. In our unit, the development of splenomegaly is an indication of clinically significant portal hypertension. At endoscopy, the size and distribution of varices in addition to red color changes should be recorded.

Currently, a three-grade classification system (Table 31.1) is used in the UK and Europe. This has been shown to have reasonable interobserver repeatability [4].

A retrospective study has shown that high-risk varices in children can be considered as one of the following patterns: grade 3 esophageal varices, grade 2 esophageal varices with red color changes and/or gastric varices along the cardia [5].

Primary prophylaxis

There are limited studies addressing primary prophylaxis of variceal hemorrhage in children. There has been one randomized controlled trial to date, which used sclerotherapy [6]. Duché *et al.* demonstrated that primary prophylaxis by a skilled operator was safe in 36 children with high-risk varices due to biliary atresia [7], and a number of uncontrolled studies have shown that endoscopic variceal ligation (EVL) is safe and effective. In 2015, a group of experts could not recommend routine primary prophylaxis in children because of a lack of definitive proof of efficacy and safety of current techniques [8].

Acute bleeding

Initial management should be according to an institutional protocol and usually involves treatment with octreotide and antibiotics. Therapeutic endoscopy should be performed under general anesthetic, as soon as possible once the patient is hemodynamically stable. ESGE-ESPGHAN guidance is that endoscopy should occur within 12 hours of an acute upper gastrointestinal bleed if the child requires ongoing circulatory support, if they have known esophageal varices, or if a large hematemesis or melena has occurred [9]. If bleeding continues, the procedure should be carried out immediately. If a bleeding varix is identified, this should be treated first. Where no bleeding point is found, treatment should usually be commenced, so long as no other potential site for bleeding exists and varices are high risk.

Endoscopic sclerotherapy is well established and the choice of sclerosant appears unimportant, with 5% ethanolamine oleate used widely. The injection is carried out via the endoscopic operating channel using single-use injectors. Endoscopes with working channels down to 2.2 mm may be used. Injections are started just above the gastroesophageal junction and may be intra- or paravariceal. All varices at this level should be treated, with 1–3 mL of sclerosant being used per injection, then repeated if necessary to all varices 3–5 cm caudally. No more than 10–15 mL of sclerosant should be used per session, depending on patient size. Varices more than 5 cm from the gastroesophageal junction should not be treated unless actively bleeding.

Endoscopic ultrasound (EUS) may help to target sclerotherapy with histoacryl glue in the gastric fundus (Figure 31.2). It affords a real-time image of the gastrointestinal wall and feeding blood vessels, treatment of which may reduce variceal recurrence. After sclerotherapy, Doppler may be used to confirm variceal ablation.

Sclerotherapy is very effective, with control of acute bleeding in 90% of cases. Complications are more likely following emergency sclerotherapy, occurring in approximately 18% [10], and include esophageal ulceration, bleeding, mediastinitis, esophageal perforation, chylothorax, pneumothorax, and stricture formation.

There is a procedural mortality of approximately 1%.

Band ligation (EVL) was first reported in humans in 1989. In this technique, a hollow cylinder with prestretched rubber rings is attached to the front of an endoscope. The variceal column is directly sucked into the hollow cylinder and the band is released around the base of the varix (Figure 31.3). Strangulation of the varix stops acute bleeding. Over the next few days, ischemic necrosis of the mucosa and submucosa develops and the rings are sloughed, leaving shallow mucosal ulceration. Epithelialization occurs within 2–3 weeks and the submucosal vascular layers are replaced by maturing scar tissue by eight weeks [11].

An initial control endoscopy is carried out to recognize bleeding points and document the distance to the gastroesophageal junction to prevent inadvertent gastric banding. The apparatus is loaded onto the endoscope, ensuring a secure fit, and then repassed as far as the gastroesophageal junction. The bander is maneuvered to the most distal variceal column and suction applied (see Figure 31.3). When the varix fills the cylinder, the tripwire is pulled and the endoscope pulled back. Care must be taken, especially in small children, that the esophageal wall is not aspirated into the cylinder. Subsequent bands are applied in a proximal direction to variceal columns in the lower

(a)   (b)

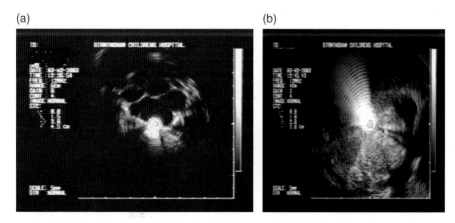

Figure 31.2 (a) EUS varices preinjection. (b) EUS varices with needle.

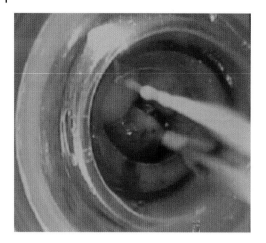

Figure 31.3 Varices being banded.

5–6 cm of the esophagus. Up to 10 bands can be used per session but we usually restrict this to four, as more is often uncomfortable. Some manufacturers insert a colured band to remind the operator when a single band remains. EVL is much better tolerated than sclerotherapy [12]; 10–15% of children complain of transient retrosternal pain but esophageal stricture has not been reported in the pediatric literature.

Where feasible, EVL is the preferred technique for managing acute bleeding. A major advantage is that once the bleeding point is ligated, bleeding control with improved visibility is immediate. EVL can be used in children <10 kg so long as the loaded bander can be passed through the cricopharynx. However, it is not possible to pass the banding equipment in all children, so sclerotherapy should continue to be available.

Following endoscopic therapy, patients should fast for at least two hours and solid feeding should be withheld until liquids are tolerated. Sucralfate should be given for five days as this appears to decrease the risk of early rebleeding [13]. Proton pump inhibitors and antibiotics probably do not affect rebleeding rate. Clipping may be used occasionally but is not routinely recommended [14]. Post-Kasai variceal banding is reported [15].

Hemospray®

Hemostatic spray is a simple technique in which powder is sprayed through the endoscope onto actively bleeding lesions where it forms a mechanical hemostatic barrier. This has been effective in the treatment of diffuse portal hypertensive gastropathy. It has also been applied directly to actively bleeding varices with good short-term effect. While not a definitive treatment, this appears safe and easy to administer, particularly if experienced interventional endoscopists are not immediately available [16] (see Chapter 30).

Self-expanding metal stents

This technique has recently been described in adult practice for resistant bleeding. The stent is deployed in the lower esophagus with or without direct endoscopic visualization and provides immediate hemostasis while allowing oral intake [17]. The stent can be left in place for 14 days, to facilitate definitive treatment, and subsequently removed endoscopically. There is no reported pediatric experience with the technique yet, but it would appear to be a useful addition to our therapeutic options.

Secondary prophylaxis

Following a variceal bleed in children, rebleeding rates are as high as 80% [18,19], hence all should receive secondary prophylaxis. Where the underlying liver disease is compensated, this will often be endoscopic but many techniques are available.

Where feasible, EVL is the preferred endoscopic method and is safer and more effective than sclerotherapy [12,20,22]. EVL should be undertaken every 2–4 weeks until varices are ablated. Subsequent follow-up endoscopies are recommended at 6–12-monthly intervals with recurrent varices being ablated where possible. EVL can safely be undertaken as a day case.

Gastric varices

The Sarin classification is used to describe the location of gastric varices [23]. Type 1 gastroesophageal (GEV) varices are continuous with esophageal varices, extending for 2–5 cm below the gastroesophageal junction along the lesser curve; type 2 varices extend beyond the gastroesophageal junction towards the greater curve into the fundus (Figure 31.4). Type 1 isolated gastric varices (IGV) are gastric fundal varices, whereas type 2 IGV are ectopic varices occurring elsewhere in the stomach or the first part of the duodenum.

Although gastric varices are less likely to bleed than esophageal varices, the mortality and rebleeding rates are higher where they do [24]. Type 2 GEV bleed most frequently and the risk of death is greatest from IGV bleeds [25].

Conventional endoscopic treatment with banding or sclerotherapy is not effective. In adults, endoscopic cyanoacrylate (CYA) injection is first-line treatment for the acute and chronic management of bleeding gastric varices [26,27]. CYA is a tissue adhesive agent that rapidly hardens upon contact with blood and intravariceal injection causes rapid variceal occlusion (see Figure 31.2).

Prior to the procedure, the endoscopic tip is coated with silicone oil and the instrument channel flushed with oil to reduce the risk of glue adherence and endoscope damage. The injection needle is primed with either sterile water or saline, depending on the product. CYA is injected directly into the varix in 0.5–1 mL aliquots. The injection time depends on the agent used and whether it has been diluted. Traditionally, probing with a blunt-tipped instrument was used to confirm variceal obliteration. EUS, where available, is now the preferred method (see Figure 31.2). A case study of 21 children with active gastric variceal bleeding showed primary hemostasis of 96% [28]. CYA may be successfully used in infants weighing less than 10 kg [29].

The major limitation of injecting this glue is not embolization or local complications for the child, but damage to the biopsy channel of the endoscope itself. If *any* glue leaks from the injecting endoscopic needle (which is the same as a standard injecting needle) then this will be blocked, thus rendering the endoscope totally unusable. This dictates that the operator must employ great care when performing this procedure. Hence the tip of the catheter is not removed through the biopsy channel and is cut with scissors before removal to prevent the glue accidentally being extruded into the channel on catheter removal (Figure 31.5).

Acute injection of thrombin into gastric varices is described in small series but is generally not common practice. In adult patients who have undergone thrombin injections, hemostasis in the acute setting has been successful in up to 92% of cases. Patients usually receive 1–4 sessions of thrombin, with a mean

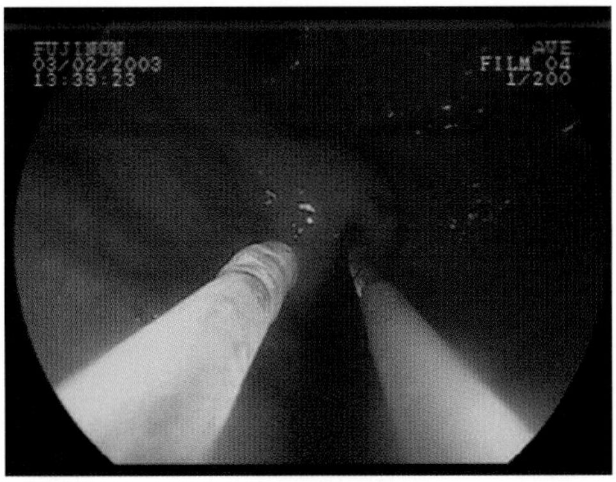

Figure 31.4 Varices with EUS probe.

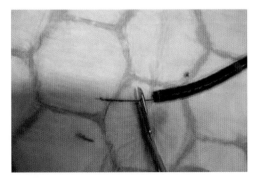

Figure 31.5 Cutting the catheter after glue injection prior to removal to protect the endoscope biopsy channel.

total dose of approximately 10 mL for variceal eradication. Dry thrombin for reconstitution can be kept in the endoscopy unit fridge for acute use and technique is identical to other injection techniques.

 • See companion website for videos relating to this chapter topic: www.wiley.com/go/gershman3e

REFERENCES

1 Grammatikopoulos T, McKiernan PJ, Dhawan A. Portal hypertension and its management in children. *Arch Dis Child* 2018, **103**, 186–191.

2 Shneider BL, de Ville de Goyet JV, Leung DH, *et al.* Primary prophylaxis of variceal bleeding in children and the role of mesorex bypass: summary of the Baveno VI Pediatric Satellite Symposium. *Hepatology* 2016, **63**, 1368–1380.

3 Molleston JP. Variceal bleeding in children. *J Pediatr Gastroenterol Nutr* 2003, **37**, 538–545.

4 D'Antiga L, Betalli P, De AP, *et al.* Interobserver agreement on endoscopic classification of oesophageal varices in children. *J Pediatr Gastroenterol Nutr* 2015, **61**, 176–181.

5 Duché M, Ducot B, Ackermann O, *et al.* Experience with endoscopic management of high-risk gastroesophageal varices, with and without bleeding, in children with biliary atresia. *Gastroenterology* 2013, **145**, 801–807.

6 Gonçalves M, Cardoso S, Maksoud J. Prophylactic sclerotherapy in children with eosophageal varices: long-term results of a controlled prospective randomized trial. *J Paediatr Surg* 2000, **35**, 401–405.

7 Duché M, Ducot B, Ackermann O, Guerin F, Jacquemin E, Bernard O. Portal hypertension in children: high-risk varices, primary prophylaxis and consequences of bleeding. *J Hepatol* 2017, **66**, 320–327.

8 Shneider BL, de Ville de Goyet J, Leung DH, *et al.* Primary prophylaxis of variceal bleeding in children and the role of MesoRex Bypass: summary of the Baveno VI Pediatric Satellite Symposium. *Hepatology* 2016, **63**, 1368–1380.

9 Tringali A, Thomson M, Dumonceau J-M, *et al.* Pediatric gastrointestinal endoscopy: European Society of Gastrointestinal Endoscopy (ESGE) and European Society for Paediatric Gastroenterology Hepatology and Nutrition (ESPGHAN) Guideline executive summary. *Endoscopy* 2017, **49**, 83–91.

10 Kim SJ, Seak Hee O, Jin Min J, Kyung Mo K. Experiences with endoscopic interventions for variceal bleeding in children with portal hypertension: a single center study. *Paediatr Gastroenterol Hepatol Nutr* 2013, **16**, 248–253.

11 Stiegmann GV, Sun JH, Hammond WS. Results of experimental endoscopic eosphageal varix ligation. *Am Surg* 1988, **4**, 10–108.

12 de Franchis R, Primignani M. Endoscopic treatments for portal hypertension. *Seminar Liv Dis* 1999, **19**, 439–455.

13 Burroughs AK, McCormick PA. Prevention of variceal rebleeding. *Gastroenterol Clin North Am* 1992, **21**, 119–147.

14 Ohnuma N, Takahashi H, Tanabe M, Yoshida H, Iwai J, Muramatsu T. Endoscopic variceal ligation using a clipping apparatus in children with portal hypertension. *Endoscopy* 1997, **29**, 86–90.

15 Sasaki T, Hasegawa T, Nakajima K, *et al.* Endoscopic variceal ligation in the management of gastroesophageal varices in postoperative biliary atresia. *J Pediatr Surg* 1998, **33**, 1628–1632.

16 Ibrahim M, El-Mikkawy A, Abdalla H, Mostafa I, Deviere J. Management of acute variceal bleeding using hemostatic powder. *United European Gastroenterol J* 2015, **3**, 277–283.

17 Hogan BJ, O'Beirne JP. Role of self-expanding metal stents in the management of variceal haemorrhage: hype or hope? *World J Gastrointest Endosc* 2016, **8**, 23–29.

18 Alvarez F, Bernard O, Brunelle F, Hadchouel P, Odievre, Alagille D. Portal obstruction in children. I. Clinical investigation and hemorrhage risk. *J Pediatr* 1983, **103**, 696–702.

19 Howard ER, Stringer MD, Mowat AP. Assessment of injection sclerotherapy in the management of 152 children with oesophageal varices. *Br J Surg* 1988, **75**, 404–408.

20 Gimson AE, Ramage JK, Panos MZ, *et al.* Randomised trial of variceal banding ligation versus injection sclerotherapy for bleeding oesophageal varices. *Lancet* 1993, **342**, 391–394.

21 Jalan R, Hayes PC. UK guidelines on the management of variceal haemorrhage in cirrhotic patients. *Gut* 2000, **46**, III1–III15.

22 Laine L, Cook D. Endoscopic ligation compared with sclerotherapy for treatment of esophageal variceal bleeding. A meta-analysis. *Ann Intern Med* 1995, **123**, 280–287.

23 Sarin SK, Lahoti D, Saxena SP, Murthy NS, Makwana UK. Prevalence, classification and natural history of gastric varices: a long term follow-up study in 568 portal hypertension patients. *Hepatology* 1992, **16**, 1343–1349.

24 Sarin SK, Kumar A. Gastric varices: profile, classification, *and management. Am J Gastroenterol* 1989, **84**, 1244–1249.

25 Gimson AES, Westaby D, Williams R. Endoscopic sclerotherapy in the management of gastric variceal haemorrhage. *J Hepatol* 1991, **13**, 274–278.

26 Rengstoff D, Binmoeller K. A pilot study of 2-octyl cyanoacrylate injection for treatment of gastric fundal varices in humans. *Gastrointest Endosc* 2004, **59**, 553–558.

27 Weilert, F, Binmoellar, K. Endoscopic management of gastric variceal bleeding. *Gastroenterol Clin North Am* 2014, **43**, 807–818.

28 Oh SH, Kim SJ, Rhee WK, Kim KM. Endoscopic cyanoacrylate injection for the treatment of gastric varices in children. *World J Gastroenterol* 2015, **21**, 2719–2724.

29 Rivet C, Robles-Medrandra C, Dumortier J, Le Gall C, Ponchon T, Lachaux A. Endoscopic treatment of gastroesophageal varices in young infants with cyanoacrylate glue: a pilot study. *Gastrointest Endosc* 2009, **69**, 1034–1038.

32

Endoscopic approach to obscure gastrointestinal bleeding lesions

Natalia Nedelkopoulou, Sara Isoldi, Dalia Belsha, and Mike Thomson

---

 KEY POINTS

- The mid-small bowel is now amenable to exploration by video wireless capsule endoscopy.
- Endotherapy of occult/obscure small bowel bleeding is now possible with enteroscopy.

- Imaging modalities such as plain CT, CT angiography, magnetic resonance angiography, and standard vascular angiography may help in diagnosis.

Introduction

Advances in imaging, anesthesia, and endoscopies have enabled pediatric gastroenterologists to perform diagnostic and therapeutic endoscopies in children safely and effectively, so they are nowadays considered routine clinical procedures [1]. This undoubtedly has led to the better understanding and management of pediatric gastrointestinal pathologies and brought to light new diseases, like eosinophilic esophagitis. Over the past years, the pediatric gastroenterology societies and endoscopy training centers worldwide have been joining their forces to introduce a standardized curriculum for trainers and trainees [2,3].

Despite these advances, if the pathology that the endoscopy is aimed to identify is located between the ampulla of Vater and the ileocecal valve, this can pose challenges even to experienced pediatric gastroenterologists and significant utilization of healthcare resources. The detection of the underlying source of obscure gastrointestinal (GI) bleeding in children warrants a cost-effective approach based upon patient presentation and clinical expertise [4].

Classification

Failure to identify the source of GI bleeding after endoscopic evaluation with EGD, ileocolonoscopy, and small bowel radiography is defined as obscure gastrointestinal bleeding (OGIB) [5]. Pediatric patients may present with overt GI bleeding, manifested as hematemesis, coffee-ground emesis, hematochezia or melena. Overt GI bleeding is further classified as ongoing and prior bleeding, with the first having the highest diagnostic yield [4,6]. The American Gastroenterological Association defines occult GI bleeding as the initial presentation of a positive occult blood test (FOBT) result and/or iron deficiency anemia when there is no evidence of visible blood loss to the patient or clinician [7]. Heraclitus of Ephesus

---

Practical Pediatric Gastrointestinal Endoscopy, Third Edition. Edited by George Gershman and Mike Thomson.
© 2021 John Wiley & Sons Ltd. Published 2021 by John Wiley & Sons Ltd.
Companion website: www.wiley.com/go/gershman3e

said "If you do not expect the unexpected, you will not recognize it when it arrives." Table 32.1 shows the differential diagnosis of OGIB in children.

Evaluation and management of obscure gastrointestinal bleeding

The American Society of Gastrointestinal Endoscopy (ASGE) and the American Gastroenterology Association (AGA) have recommended that EGD and ileocolonoscopy should be repeated when evaluating a patient with OGIB. Missed lesions at the first endoscopy can frequently occur because of various reasons, like suboptimal bowel preparation, the presence of blood or if the lesion is not actively bleeding. The diagnostic yield for repeat EGD has been reported to be up to 29%, whereas for repeat colonoscopy it is up to 6% [8,9]. It is of the utmost importance that a child with active GI bleeding is stabilized first, before any endoscopic evaluation or intervention is performed.

Capsule endoscopy (CE)

Capsule endoscopy was first described in 2000 (see Chapter 15) and since then it has gained wide acceptance as a minimally invasive and safe tool for the evaluation of the small intestine. A systemic review of 22 840 capsule endoscopies revealed that OGIB is the most common indication [10] and the diagnostic yield in detection of the source of OGIB has been reported up to 80%, with a higher diagnostic yield in overt compared to occult bleeding [11–13]. It is also proposed that the diagnostic yield is enhanced when the CE is performed in the early stage of OGIB [14].

There are five different capsules available (Medtronic PillCam, Olympus EndoCapsule, IntroMedic Mirocam, Capsovision CapsoCam, Jinshan Science OMOM capsule), but most studies in OGIB have been performed with the PillCam [4,15].

In 2009, the FDA approved the use of CE for children 2 years of age or older but in our unit, and in the literature, CE has been used safely in selected cases even in younger children [16–18]. Older children are asked to swallow the capsule, whereas in young children it is placed in the duodenum endoscopically.

Capsule endoscopy is superior to other diagnostic modalities and the American College of Gastroenterology clinical guideline recommended that CE should be considered first to determine the source of OGIB [19]. However, it has some limitations, with the main one being the inability to obtain biopsies and perform endoscopic therapies. The rate of capsule retention has been reported as 1.4% for adults with OGIB and the risk of retention is higher post abdominal surgery, abdominal radiation therapy or Crohn's disease with small bowel involvement [10]. A dissolvable test capsule is available but of limited value in children [20].

To date, there is no consensus as to which agents and bowel preparation improve the visualization quality, diagnostic yield, and completion rate, but one systematic review and metaanalysis showed that the combination of polyethylene glycol and simethicone appears to be the best approach for small bowel preparation before CE [21].

Several adult studies have compared the outcomes of CE with enteroscopies (push, single-balloon, double-balloon) (see Chapter 15) in OGIB and the recommended approach is to perform CE first prior to enteroscopy and if CE reveals findings that require biopsy or endoscopic intervention, to proceed with enteroscopy [22–26]. A retrospective study in 36 children comparing the diagnostic accuracy and concordance of CE and double-balloon endoscopy (DBE) showed that CE has excellent negative predictive value for DBE and histological findings but is limited by its low specificity, whereas both sensitivity and specificity of DBE are good [27]. Overall, CE and enteroscopy should be considered to have complementary roles in the diagnostic and therapeutic management of OGIB.

Table 32.1 Principal causes of obscure gastrointestinal bleeding in children

Esophagus	Esophagitis
	Esophageal erosions
	Varices
Stomach	Angiodysplasia/vascular abnormalities
	Dieulafoy lesion
	Gastric antral vascular ectasia (GAVE)
	Gastric duplication cyst
	Cameron lesions
	Portal hypertensive gastropathy
Duodenum	Celiac disease
	Angiodysplasia/vascular abnormalities
	Hemobilia (stone, trauma)
	Duodenal/ampullary neoplasm
	Aortoenteric fistula
	Pancreatic aneurysm
Jejunum/ileum	Polyposis syndromes
	Crohn's disease
	Nonsteroidal antiinflammatory drug enteropathy
	Meckel diverticulum
	Intestinal duplication
	Angiodysplasia/vascular abnormalities
	Primary neoplasias/metastasis
	Portal hypertensive intestinal vasculopathy
	Infections (i.e., tuberculosis)
Colon	Angiodysplasia/vascular abnormalities
	Portal hypertensive colonopathy
Miscellaneous	Von Willebrand's disease
	Hereditary telangiectasia
	Blue rubber bleb nevus syndrome
	Amyloidosis
	Pseudoxanthoma elasticum
	Ehlers–Danlos syndrome
	Diverticula
	Ectopic gastric mucosa
	Radiations
	Osler–Weber–Rendu syndrome
	Kaposi's sarcoma with AIDS
	Plummer–Vinson syndrome
	Malignant atrophic papulosi

Diagnostic and therapeutic approach with enteroscopy

Double-balloon enteroscopy

Since the first description of DBE by Yamamoto *et al.* in 2001 [28], it has become a valuable addition to endoscopic techniques when the GI pathology is beyond the reach of conventional endoscopy both in adult and pediatric populations. DBE requires a longer endoscope that offers the advantage of visualization of the entire small bowel with the combination of an oral and anal approach. Its utility is enhanced by the ability to obtain tissue and undertake endotherapeutic procedures. DBE is performed with a 200 cm long enteroscope and a 145 cm long overtube [28].

Over the past decade, the body of evidence on the safety and efficacy of DBE in pediatric patients has gradually increased [29–32]. In Japan, 10 pediatric patients with OGIB were investigated with DBE, with a diagnostic yield of 70% [33]. We have previously published our experience in 16 pediatric patients with OGIB who underwent 30 DBE procedures that revealed ulcers, polyps, varices, strictures, and angiodysplasias. The endotherapeutic interventions included application of argon plasma coagulation and endoclips, injection of epinephrine, and banding using conventional endoscope. The examination time was 45–275 minutes (median 92.5) based on technical difficulties and therapeutic interventions. The diagnostic yield in OGIB was 50%, with therapeutic utility of 43% [34].

The group of Luo *et al.* reported the safety and efficacy of single-balloon endoscopy (SBE) in children with small bowel bleeding. The endoscopic findings in the small bowel included nonspecific inflammation, allergic purpura, Crohn's disease, Meckel's diverticulum, and Peutz–Jeghers syndrome [35]. In another study, 22 children with OGIB were investigated with CE followed by SBE that led to a diagnostic yield of 95%, with 82% of the cases achieving complete resolution of the bleeding after therapy [36].

To date, only adult studies have compared SBE versus DBE with contradicting results; some studies favor SBE based on the diagnostic yield and significantly shorter average examination time via an anterograde approach through the mouth for SBE [37,38]; however, a recent metaanalysis has not shown statistically significant differences between the two endoscopic approaches [39].

Push enteroscopy

The depth of insertion into the small bowel can be maximized with the use of an enteroscope with an overtube or a variable stiffness colonoscopy. The existing evidence on the safety and efficacy of push enteroscopy in pediatric patients is limited.

Intraoperative enteroscopy

This endoscopic approach achieves the evaluation of the entire small bowel with a mid small bowel enterotomy through which the scope is advanced anterograde and retrograde. We have reported the case of a 5-year-old girl with OGIB who was diagnosed with idiopathic small bowel diaphragm disease who had a successful definitive therapeutic DBE and minimally invasive bowel surgery for her small bowel pathology. She was noted to have multiple strictures throughout the mid-distal small bowel on wireless CE and the diaphragm-like strictures in the distal ileum were divided with an endoknife transmurally with the enteroscope and a segment of the terminal ileum was resected surgically. Laparoscopic-assisted enteroscopy in a pediatric patient has also been successfully performed for endotherapeutic treatment of small bowel lesions in blue rubber bleb nevus syndrome with APC.

Bleeding scans and other modalities

In cases of active GI bleeding, additional imaging modalities can be considered to detect the source of GI bleeding. The use of gastrointestinal bleeding scintigraphy with technetium 99m-labeled red blood cells has been reported in infants as young as 8 months old [40]. It is preferred in children because of the lower absorbed radiation dose [41], providing that the rate of hemorrhage is greater than 0.1–0.4 mL/min. For nonactively bleeding lesions, angiography can add to the diagnostic work-up and several studies have shown that CT angiography can be a valuable tool in children with OGIB to decide on an appropriate treatment plan and the need for endovascular interventions [42–44]. Even though MR enterography has been largely replaced by CE in the assessment of the small bowel in OGIB in children, a recent prospective study in 25 children with

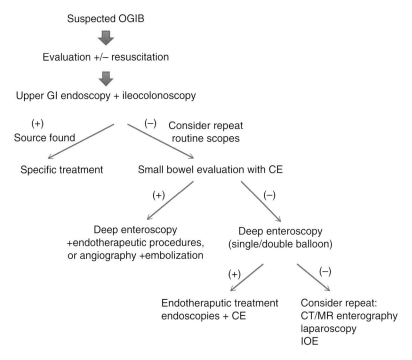

Figure 32.1 Algorithm for the management of OGIB in children. CE, capsule endoscopy; CT, computed tomography; GI, gastrointestinal; IOE, intraoperative enteroscopy; MR, magnetic resonance.

OGIB showed that CT angiography remains a safe and accurate imaging modality with a sensitivity and specificity of 86% and 100% respectively [45] and should be included in the diagnostic work-up, especially in centers in which CE is not available. Plain CT may also be useful in detection of lesions such as gastric duplication cysts.

and requires a stepwise and cost-effective approach based on the patient's presentation and the expertise of the pediatric gastroenterology team. Figure 32.1 shows a proposed algorithm for the management of OGIB in children. It is vital that pediatric gastroenterologists are familiar with the diagnostic yields and limitations of each diagnostic endoscopic and imaging modality when managing children with OGIB.

Conclusion

In conclusion, OGIB in children carries the potential of significant morbidity and mortality

 • See companion website for videos relating to this chapter topic: www.wiley.com/go/gershman3e

REFERENCES

1 Friedt M, Welsch S. An update on pediatric endoscopy. *Eur J Med Res* 2013, **18**, 24.

2 Thomson M, Elawad M, Barth B, *et al.* Worldwide strategy for implementation of paediatric endoscopy: report of the FISPGHAN Working Group. *J Pediatr Gastroenterol Nutr* 2012 **55**, 636–639.

3 Thomson M, Heuschkel R, Donaldson N, *et al.* Acquisition of competence in paediatric ileocolonoscopy with virtual endoscopy training. *J Pediatr Gastroenterol Nutr* 2006, **43**, 699–701.

4 Pasha SF, Leighton JA. Detection of suspected small bowel bleeding: challenges and controversies. *Expert Rev Gastroenterol Hepatol* 2016, **10**, 1235–1244.

5 Raju GS, Gerson L, Das A, *et al*. American Gastroenterological Association (AGA) Institute technical review on obscure gastrointestinal bleeding. *Gastroenterology* 2007, **133**, 1697–1717.

6 Singh V, Alexander JA. The evaluation and management of obscure and occult gastrointestinal bleeding. *Abdom Imaging* 2009, **34**, 311–319.

7 Raju GS, Gerson L, Das A, *et al*. American Gastroenterological Association (AGA) Institute medical position statement on obscure gastrointestinal bleeding. *Gastroenterology* 2007, **133**, 1694–1696.

8 Zuckerman GR, Prakash C, Askin MP, Lewis BS. AGA technical review on the evaluation and management of occult and obscure gastrointestinal bleeding. *Gastroenterology* 2000, **118**, 201–221.

9 Leighton JA, Goldstein J, Hirota W, *et al*. Obscure gastrointestinal bleeding. *Gastrointest Endosc* 2003, **58**, 650–655.

10 Liao Z, Gao R, Xu C, *et al*. Indications and detection, completion, and retention rates of small-bowel capsule endoscopy: a systematic review. *Gastrointest Endosc* 2010, **71**, 280–286.

11 Carey EJ, Leighton JA, Heigh RI, *et al*. A single-center experience of 260 consecutive patients undergoing capsule endoscopy for obscure gastrointestinal bleeding. *Am J Gastroenterol* 2007, **102**, 89–95.

12 Flemming J, Cameron S. Small bowel capsule endoscopy: indications, results, and clinical benefit in a University environment. *Medicine* 2018, **97**, e0148.

13 Hadithi M, Heine GD, Jacobs MAJ, *et al*. A prospective study comparing video capsule endoscopy with double-balloon enteroscopy in patients with obscure gastrointestinal bleeding. *Am J Gastroenterol* 2006, **101**, 52–57.

14 Pennazio M, Santucci R, Rondonotti E, *et al*. Outcome of patients with obscure gastrointestinal bleeding after capsule endoscopy: report of 100 consecutive cases. *Gastroenterology* 2004, **126**, 643–653.

15 Bandorski D, Kurniawan N, Baltes P, *et al*. Contraindications for video capsule endoscopy. *World J Gastroenterol* 2016, **22**, 9898–9908.

16 Nuutinen H, Kolho KL, Salminen P, *et al*. Capsule endoscopy in pediatric patients: technique and results in our first 100 consecutive children. *Scand J Gastroenterol* 2011, **46**, 1138–1143.

17 Oikawa-Kawamoto M, Sogo T, Yamaguchi T, *et al*. Safety and utility of capsule endoscopy for infants and young children. *World J Gastroenterol* 2013, **19**, 8342–8348.

18 van der Reijden SM, van Wijk MP, Jacobs MAJ, *et al*. Video capsule endoscopy to diagnose primary intestinal lymphangiectasia in a 14-month-old child. *J Pediatr Gastroenterol Nutr* 2017, **64**, e161.

19 Gerson LB, Fidler JL, Cave DR, *et al*. ACG Clinical guideline: diagnosis and management of small bowel bleeding. *Am J Gastroenterol* 2015, **110**, 1265–1287.

20 Tokuhara D, Watanabe K, Cho Y, *et al*. Patency capsule tolerability in school-aged children. *Digestion* 2017, **96**, 46–51.

21 Kotwal VS, Attar BM, Gupta S, *et al*. Should bowel preparation, antifoaming agents, or prokinetics be used before video capsule endoscopy? A systematic review and meta-analysis. *Eur J Gastroenterol Hepatol* 2014, **26**, 137–145.

22 Nakamura M, Niwa Y, Ohmiya N, *et al*. Preliminary comparison of capsule endoscopy and double-balloon enteroscopy in patients with suspected small-bowel bleeding. *Endoscopy* 2006, **38**, 59–66.

23 Otani K, Watanabe T, Shimada S, *et al*. Clinical utility of capsule endoscopy and double-balloon enteroscopy in the management of obscure gastrointestinal bleeding. *Digestion* 2018, **97**, 52–58.

24 Teshima CW, Kuipers EJ, van Zanten SV, *et al*. Double balloon enteroscopy and capsule

endoscopy for obscure gastrointestinal bleeding: an updated meta-analysis. *J Gastroenterol Hepatol* 2011, **26**, 796–801.

25 Okamoto J, Tominaga K, Sugimori S, *et al.* Comparison of risk factors between small intestinal ulcerative and vascular lesions in occult versus overt obscure gastrointestinal bleeding. *Dig Dis Sci* 2016, **61**, 533–541.

26 Segarajasingam DS, Hanley SC, Barkun AN, *et al.* Randomized controlled trial comparing outcomes of video capsule endoscopy with push enteroscopy in obscure gastrointestinal bleeding. *Can J Gastroenterol Hepatol* 2015, **29**, 85–90.

27 Danialifar TF, Naon H, Liu QY. Comparison of diagnostic accuracy and concordance of video capsule endoscopy and double balloon enteroscopy in children. *J Pediatr Gastroenterol Nutr* 2016, **62**, 824–827.

28 Yamamoto H, Sekine Y, Sato Y, *et al.* Total enteroscopy with a nonsurgical steerable double-balloon method. *Gastrointest Endosc* 2001, **53**, 216–220.

29 Blanco-Velasco G, Hernandez-Mondragon OV, Blancas-Valencia JM, *et al.* Safety and efficacy of small bowel polypectomy using a balloon-assisted enteroscope in pediatric patients with Peutz–Jeghers syndrome. *Rev Gastroenterol Mex* 2018, **83**, 234–237.

30 Geng LL, Chen PY, Wu Q, *et al.* Bleeding Meckel's diverticulum in children: the diagnostic value of double-balloon enteroscopy. *Gastroenterol Res Pract* 2017, **2017**, 7940851.

31 Yokoyama K, Yano T, Kumagai H, *et al.* Double-balloon enteroscopy for pediatric patients: evaluation of safety and efficacy in 257 cases. *J Pediatr Gastroenterol Nutr* 2016, **63**, 34–40.

32 Leung YK. Double balloon endoscopy in pediatric patients. *Gastrointest Endosc* 2007, **66**, S54–S56.

33 Nishimura N, Yamamoto H, Yano T, *et al.* Safety and efficacy of double-balloon enteroscopy in pediatric patients. *Gastrointest Endosc* 2010, **71**, 287–294.

34 Urs AN, Martinelli M, Rao P, *et al.* Diagnostic and therapeutic utility of double-balloon enteroscopy in children. *J Pediatr Gastroenterol Nutr* 2014, **58**, 204–212.

35 Luo YH, You JY, Liu L, *et al.* [Clinical application of single-balloon enteroscopy in children with small intestinal bleeding]. *Zhongguo Dang Dai Er Ke Za Zhi* 2013, **15**, 546–549.

36 Oliva S, Pennazio M, Cohen SA, *et al.* Capsule endoscopy followed by single balloon enteroscopy in children with obscure gastrointestinal bleeding: a combined approach. *Dig Liver Dis* 2015, **47**, 125–130.

37 Lu Z, Qi Y, Weng J, et al. Efficacy and safety of single-balloon versus double-balloon enteroscopy: a single-center retrospective analysis. *Med Sci Monit* 2017, **23**, 1933–1939.

38 Lenz P, Roggel M, Domagk D. Double- vs. single-balloon enteroscopy: single center experience with emphasis on procedural performance. *Int J Colorectal Dis* 2013, **28**, 1239–4126.

39 Lipka S, Rabbanifard R, Kumar A, *et al.* Single versus double balloon enteroscopy for small bowel diagnostics: a systematic review and meta-analysis. *J Clin Gastroenterol* 2015, **49**, 177–184.

40 Hsiao YH, Wei CH, Chang SW, *et al.* Juvenile polyposis syndrome: an unusual case report of anemia and gastrointestinal bleeding in young infant. *Medicine* 2016, **95**, e4550.

41 Fahey FH, Treves ST, Adelstein SJ. Minimizing and communicating radiation risk in pediatric nuclear medicine. *J Nucl Med Technol* 2012, **40**, 13–24.

42 Parra DA, Chavhan GB, Shammas A, *et al.* Computed tomography angiography in acute gastrointestinal and intra-abdominal bleeding in children: preliminary experience. *Can Assoc Radiol J* 2013, **64**, 345–350.

43 Ninomiya IS, Steimberg C, Udaquiola J, *et al.* [Intestinal venous vascular malformation: unusual etiology of gastrointestinal bleeding in pediatrics. Case report]. *Arch Argent Pediatr* 2016, **114**, e159–e162.

44 Komarnicka J, Brzewski M, Banaszkiewicz A, *et al.* Computed tomography (CT) angiography in pre-embolization assessment of location of gastrointestinal bleeding in paediatric patient with granulomatosis with polyangiitis (Wegener's Granulomatosis) – case report. *Pol J Radiol* 2017, **82**, 589–592.

45 Casciani E, Nardo GD, Chin S, *et al.* MR enterography in paediatric patients with obscuregastrointestinal bleeding. *Eur J Radiol* 2017, **93**, 209–216.

33

Percutaneous endoscopic gastrostomy

Natalie Bhesania, Mike Thomson, and Marsha Kay

 KEY POINT

- PEG insertion does not increase gastroesophageal reflux.

Introduction

The first reported percutaneous endoscopic gastrostomy (PEG) tube placement was in 1980 by Ponsky, Gauderer, and Izant in a pediatric patient. PEG tube insertion was initially reported in pediatric patients, was subsequently popularized in adults, and was later reintroduced for use in children by pediatric gastroenterologists. Although initially developed by surgeons, it is now performed at an equal or greater frequency by adult and pediatric gastroenterologists. Despite many similarities in the indications and some technical aspects of the procedure between children and adults, there are also significant differences in the indications, limitations, and technical aspects of the procedure.

Indications

In the pediatric population, PEG is appropriate in children who require a gastrostomy tube and do not require a simultaneous open abdominal procedure. PEG tubes can be considered in very young pediatric patients, including neonates, and have been successfully utilized in patients as small as 2.5 kg. PEGs can be placed for a variety of indications which include medication administration, nutritional support, gastric decompression or a combination of these reasons. It is important to recognize that PEG insertion does not predispose to development of gastroesophageal reflux. Patients who are, however, undergoing a simultaneous fundoplication, pyloroplasty or pyloromyotomy would likely not derive additional benefit from placement of a PEG tube compared to a surgical gastrostomy. PEG tube placement does not interfere with subsequent fundoplication, pyloroplasty or pyloromyotomy.

Benefits of PEG tube insertion compared to a surgical gastrostomy include reduced procedure time and cost, smaller incision, shorter length of stay, and decreased incidence of postoperative complications including wound infection, wound dehiscence, bowel obstruction, pain, atelectasis, and impaired mobility.

Practical Pediatric Gastrointestinal Endoscopy, Third Edition. Edited by George Gershman and Mike Thomson.
© 2021 John Wiley & Sons Ltd. Published 2021 by John Wiley & Sons Ltd.
Companion website: www.wiley.com/go/gershman3e

The decision regarding placement should be individualized based on the patient's medical needs and requires a multidisciplinary approach.

Contraindications

There are only a few absolute contraindications to PEG tube placement. It should not be attempted in the setting of an unstable patient, uncorrectable coagulopathy, existing bleeding disorders with an INR >1.5 (normal range 0.9–1.3), elevated PTT >50 sec (normal range 23–32.4 sec) and/or platelet count $<50 \times 10^9$/L (normal range 150–450 10^9/L), abdominal ascites, peritonitis, portal hypertension with gastric varices, and in a patient with a pharyngeal or esophageal obstruction. If there is any factor that interferes with successful transillumination of the gastric wall, failure to identify finger indentation performed during the procedure or if there is a suspicion that the anterior gastric wall is not opposed to the abdominal wall such as in the case of an intervening colon or other abdominal organ, PEG tube insertion should not be attempted.

Certain medical conditions require more attention and PEGs should be considered only with significantly increased caution in patients with the following clinical aspects: patients on peritoneal dialysis, scoliosis or spine abnormalities, small size, ventriculoperitoneal (VP) shunts, prior abdominal surgery, especially gastric surgery, congenital abnormalities such as situs inversus, hepatomegaly, splenomegaly or other abdominal masses, small laryngeal or tracheal size, tracheal compromise or ventilatory issues. The presence of a VP shunt or use of peritoneal dialysis prior to PEG placement is associated with a particularly poor outcome and high complication rate following placement, especially infectious complications including fungal peritonitis. As with any endoscopic procedure, the patient should be medically stable, airway protection and management are imperative, and the endoscopist should be willing to abort the procedure if the procedure is not progressing as anticipated.

Decision to proceed with PEG and preprocedure evaluation

The preprocedure evaluation varies between centers, but a thorough history and physical exam is the first step in the assessment. It is important to carefully evaluate and identify the need for an accompanying antireflux procedure and to ensure tolerance of gastric feeds prior to the procedure. Depending on the clinical scenario, additional studies including pH or impedance probe testing, modified barium swallow, and motility testing may be indicated preoperatively to determine if a simultaneous antireflux procedure is indicated.

It is a common misconception that PEG tube placement results in gastroesophageal reflux (GER). However, open gastrostomy is associated with a significantly increased risk of severe postoperative GER compared to PEG insertion (odds ratio 6–7:1). Potential contributing factors include alteration of the angle of His and reduced lower esophageal sphincter (LES) pressure by an open gastrostomy.

In our center, the standard evaluation prior to PEG includes an upper GI X-ray to exclude malrotation and to identify if part of the stomach is located below the ribcage and therefore amenable to PEG placement. In addition, a 10-day trial of outpatient nasogastric (NG) feeds is preferred when medically possible prior to PEG placement. If patients are unable to tolerate NG feeds this would also warrant further evaluation and consideration for an accompanying antireflux procedure.

When comparing different techniques for gastrostomy tube placement, a recent retrospective study performed in pediatric patients less than 18 years found that the open Stamm gastrostomy technique was associated with a higher rate of minor complications, including unintentional tube dislodgment, frequent emergency room visits, and need for reoperation within 30 days, compared to other techniques including PEG, fluoroscopy-guided, laparoscopic and laparoscopic-assisted PEG tube placement.

Three important considerations when deciding to proceed with PEG are:

- PEG tubes do not prevent aspiration in a patient with oral pharyngeal dysphagia who continues oral feedings
- if the stomach is completely under the ribcage, a PEG is unlikely to be successfully placed
- PEG tubes can be pulled out.

Technique

Personnel

In most pediatric centers, two physicians perform PEGs; one is in charge of all manipulations with the endoscope, the other is responsible for delivering the loop-insertion wire through the abdominal wall into the stomach. In our center, two pediatric gastroenterologists or pediatric surgeons perform PEG. In some centers, the procedure may be done by the interventional radiologist. Insertion of a PEG tube is an advanced endoscopic procedure, with a higher rate of associated complications, and the performing physicians must be able to recognize if the procedure is progressing in a nonstandard fashion and make rapid adjustments or terminate the procedure if necessary.

Patient preparation

PEG tube insertion can be performed in the operating room, endoscopy suite or at the bedside. Given the requirement for patient cooperation and to prevent discomfort in this vulnerable patient population, PEG placement is performed in the operating room with general anesthesia at our institution, with sedation provided by a pediatric anesthesiologist. Some centers use conscious or "deep" sedation. Deep sedation has been reported to be successful even in children with underlying congenital heart disease.

The patient is NPO prior to the procedure and receives a single dose of a broad-spectrum cephalosporin or an alternative antibiotic based on allergy profile, as this has been shown to reduce wound infections. The patient is placed in the supine position with the head of the bed flat or slightly elevated to reduce the risk of aspiration if the patient is not intubated. The abdomen should be prepped and draped as for a standard operative procedure.

PEG insertion procedure

The PEG insertion is started with a thorough endoscopic inspection of the oral, esophageal, and gastric mucosa without intubation of the pylorus. Any retained secretions are suctioned to avoid intraoperative and/or postoperative aspiration. Next, the stomach is filled with air to move it up toward the abdominal wall. Excessive air insufflation which significantly flattens the gastric folds or results in visible abdominal distension should be avoided as this may distend the small bowel loops and interfere with gastric indentation. The light from a properly oriented endoscope should be directed toward the abdominal wall and clearly visible, especially in a dimmed room. At the brightest point of transillumination, finger pressure is applied. The indentation at the abdominal wall produced by palpation is seen endoscopically and the site is marked by the second physician (Figure 33.1). It should be at least 2 cm away from the costal margin as tubes placed too close to the ribs can cause significant pain. See Table 33.1 for some "tricks of the trade."

The site is then prepped using standard technique. A snare is advanced through the biopsy channel and positioned at the proposed entry site. After the sterile prep is completed, local anesthesia is administered.

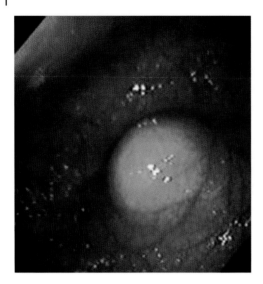

Figure 33.1 Finger indentation of the anterior gastric wall.

The 25 G or 22 G needle attached to a syringe is advanced through the gastric wall while pulling back slightly on the syringe plunger. Safe site selection is confirmed when endoscopic visualization of the needle tip entry corresponds with air entry into the syringe. This is known as the "safe tract" technique (Figure 33.2).

Lidocaine 1% is injected while the needle is withdrawing. A 0.5–1 cm incision is made at the entry site. This incision should be sized to accommodate the diameter of PEG tube that has to be inserted. Too tight an incision increases the risk of postoperative wound infection due to compromised tissue around the PEG tube by the dilator forcefully pulled through the abdominal wall.

The needle–cannula assembly is inserted into the stomach through the incision under direct endoscopic visualization. The snare is closed around the cannula and the needle is removed. The loop-insertion wire is passed through the cannula into the stomach. The snare is loosened from the cannula and tightened around the wire (Figure 33.3).

The wire, snare, and endoscope are removed together from the patient and the wire is

Table 33.1 Tricks of the trade

- This is a procedure that is best done quickly. Once the endoscopic portion of the procedure starts, it is usually accomplished by an experienced team within approximately 10 minutes. Longer procedures are associated with excessive air insufflation which makes identifying the gastric impression more difficult and may increase the risk of distending the small bowel or colon with air and therefore interposing a loop of bowel between the stomach and the anterior gastric wall, with its resultant complications.

- If things aren't going well in terms of positioning, the PEG tube should not be placed. There may be something – liver, bowel, mesentery, etc. – between the trocar and the anterior gastric wall. Unless the liver has been punctured, these complications are usually self-limiting if the angiocatheter/trocar is removed and the PEG is not placed.

- If significant bleeding occurs or stool is visualized at any point, surgical consultation is appropriate.

- When faced with a patient with atypical anatomy (cardiac surgery patients, patients with a scoliosis, etc.), the PEG may require placement in a nonstandard position (i.e., right side of the abdomen in a patient with situs inversus). The endoscopic technique should be similar to standard procedure. Avoid location selection by formula (i.e., one-third of the distance between. . .). Pick the location that is best based on the individual patient's anatomy.

removed from the snare and the scope. The insertion wire exiting the patient mouth is attached to the tapered dilated segment of the PEG tube. This is accomplished by insertion of the big loop of the insertion wire through the small loop on the PEG tube. The PEG tube is threaded through the big loop, internal bolster end first, and pulled to tighten in place. The tube is lubricated and the insertion segment of the wire at the abdominal wall is continuously pulled until, first, the dilating segment and then the tube itself exit the incision. The tube is pulled until the internal bolster sits snugly against the gastric mucosa (Figure 33.4).

There may be some resistance when the guidewire catheter knot reaches the

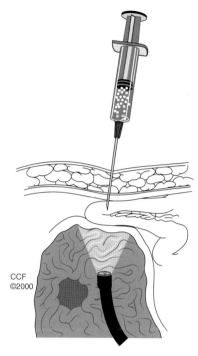

CCF
©2000

Figure 33.2 Schematic representation of the safe tract technique. In this case, a loop of bowel is present between the anterior gastric wall and the anterior abdominal wall. On occasion, this can be identified during the procedure by noting air bubbles in the syringe, *without* the endoscopist seeing the cannula in the gastric lumen. The needle–cannula assembly should be removed and repositioned to an alternate site, or the procedure should be converted to an open gastrostomy.

abdominal wall. In this case, circular rotation of the guidewire with steady traction will facilitate removal of the tube. Excessive traction should be avoided especially in small, malnourished or immunocompromised patients, as there have been reports of catheters being pulled entirely through the abdominal wall.

The insertion wire is cut and external bolster is advanced over the PEG tube to a point where it is loosely touching the skin. The PEG tube is cut to a comfortable length for the caretaker. The endoscope is reinserted to confirm the proper positioning of the internal bolster against the gastric wall. The external bolster is adjusted as necessary so that proper tension is

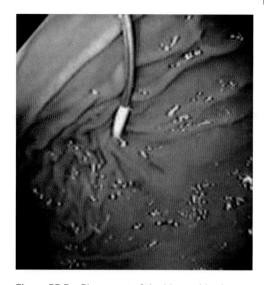

Figure 33.3 Placement of the blue guidewire through the catheter. A sufficient length of guidewire should be passed through the catheter to grasp with the endoscopic forceps or the snare.

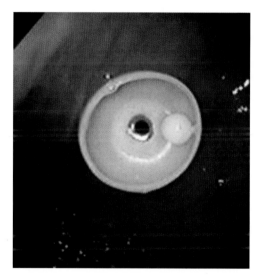

Figure 33.4 Internal view of a PEG tube alongside the anterior gastric wall. This particular tube has a nondeflatable internal disc, which acts as the internal bolster.

achieved. It is prudent to leave a small space between the external bolster and the skin to accommodate tissue swelling within the immediate postoperative period. A sterile dressing with betadine ointment is applied to the abdominal entry site.

The tubes can be used within 6–24 hours. Early initiation of post-PEG insertion feedings is not associated with an increased complication rate but may be associated with higher gastric residual volumes. We typically initiate feedings with a clear liquid such as a balanced electrolyte solution prior to initiation of formula feedings. Feedings are advanced based on the individual patient's tolerance.

Consideration should be given to aborting the procedure if any of the following are identified or occur: failure to identify good gastric impression, excess angiocatheter length without seeing the tip in the stomach, air bubbling in the needle syringe without seeing the tip in the stomach, gastric varices or significant ulceration, identification of fecal matter at any point during the procedure.

Postprocedure management

Once the tract has healed, the PEG tube can be replaced by a regular gastrostomy tube or button. We usually wait at least two months to allow the tract to mature completely, although replacement of PEG tubes following accidental dislodgment has been reported within two weeks.

There are two methods of PEG replacement: by traction or endoscopy. A traction removal is stressful for the patient and associated with some degree of pain and small risk of complications, including gastric tear and extravasation. If this method is chosen, oral midazolam with Tylenol® and good lubrication of the gastrostomy tract are very useful. In our practice, we prefer an endoscopic technique. Once the PEG tube is cut externally just above the skin, the internal bumper with the stump is retrieved using alligator forceps or a small snare. We do not cut the bumper and allow it to pass, as intestinal obstruction, impaction, perforation, and migration into the esophagus with subsequent tracheoesophageal fistula and other complications have been reported with cut and unretrieved bumpers.

The procedure is finished by confirmation of the replacement tube in the stomach. Absence of the replacement tube within the stomach is alarming for possible penetration into the abdominal cavity or the intestinal loop between the abdominal wall and stomach. Surgical consultation is warranted at this point.

If a low-profile gastrostomy device has been chosen for PEG tube replacement, the length of the tract is measured. Gastrostomy buttons are available in a variety of lengths (0.8–6.5 cm) and diameters (12–24 Fr), depending on the brand. Once a gastrostomy button is in place, it requires replacement every 4–6 months. With time, the size of the device, especially the length, should be adjusted according to the patient weight and corresponding lengthening of the gastrostomy track to avoid gastric ulcerations and/or buried bumper syndrome. This is especially important if there is rapid early weight gain in patients undergoing PEGs for malnourishment.

Complications

Complications of PEG can be minor, major, early or late. Rates in the literature vary greatly in the range of 4–44%, but generally in the lower portion of the range, between 10% and 15%. Major complications can occur in 1–10% of cases within 6–12 months of PEG placement. Many are preventable with appropriate antibiotic prophylaxis, good endoscopic/percutaneous technique, and recognition by the performing physicians that things are not going well with a decision to abort the procedure and proceed with an open gastrostomy. Sometimes complications are unavoidable due to patient anatomy or underlying disease and this should be discussed with parents prior to the endoscopic procedure.

Reported minor complications which can become major complications include cellulitis, uncomplicated pneumoperitoneum, tube defects/disconnection, GER, granulation tissue at the insertion site, and pain at the insertion site. Reported major complications include gastrocolic fistula, gastroileal fistula, gastrocoloileal cutaneous fistula, intrahepatic placement, duodenal hematoma, complicated pneumoperitoneum, aspiration, peritonitis, catheter complications including migration, buried bumper syndrome (Figure 33.5), partial gastric separation, catheter/bumper impaction if not retrieved, intussusception secondary to catheter migration, VP shunt infection, gastric or bowel perforation, gastric or bowel volvulus, and death.

Late complications include gastrocolic fistula, gastroileal fistula, catheter migration/buried bumper syndrome/partial gastric separation, gastric ulceration, cellulitis, fasciitis, gastric or bowel perforation, catheter migration or other catheter-related complications, bronchoesophageal fistula (following catheter removal), and aortic perforation (following cut-and-pass technique). PEG tubes in children are not associated with a higher rate of subsequent revision when compared to surgically placed open gastrostomy tubes if tube revisions due to unrecognized bowel perforation at initial PEG placement are excluded.

When comparing minor versus major complication rates in pediatric patients following PEG placement, Fortunato *et al.* reported minor complications in 4% of children prior to hospital discharge and 20% after hospital discharge. The most common minor postoperative complication reported was wound infection. Major complications occurred in less than 1% of subjects which include gastric separation and gastrocolonic fistula.

A recent "in press" article reporting NICU bedside placement of PEG in 106 neonates reported a total complication rate of 8.4%, of which 1.8% were major complications. The major complications in that study included one case of migration of the PEG tube bumper and one case of dislodgment. This review concluded that bedside PEG placement was safe in appropriately selected neonates.

Once enteral access is no longer required, the gastrostomy tube or button can be removed and the gastrostomy site can be allowed to close on its own over a period of several weeks. In 5–30% of cases a chronic gastrocutaneous fistula remains patent, particularly in patients with longer duration of gastrostomy tube use. In this circumstance we have utilized either endoscopic clipping, fibrin glue injection or surgical closure to close the tube site.

(a)   (b)   (c)

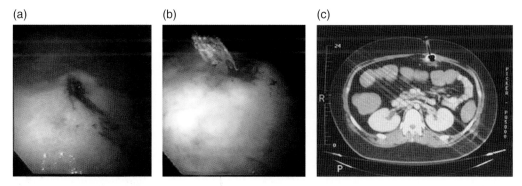

Figure 33.5   (a) Buried bumper syndrome. The gastrostomy bumper is no longer in the stomach, but the impression of the bumper is seen within the abdominal wall. (b) The gastrostomy tube is buried in the abdominal wall, although the stoma remains open. This was confirmed by injection of a small amount of saline. (c) CT scan of the abdomen showing the extragastric location of a gastrostomy tube in a patient with buried bumper syndrome. *Source:* Courtesy of George Gershman, MD.

New uses of the PEG technique

Innovative pediatric and adult gastroenterologists and surgeons have further modified the techniques of PEG. Utilizing modifications of the PEG technique, tubes can be placed directly in the jejunum (DPEJ or PEJ) for feeding and decompression in the setting of malignant small bowel obstruction in the adult literature. In addition, PEGs can be placed in the cecum (PEC) for antegrade colonic enemas. The DPEJ technique currently has limited applicability in young children due to equipment and size limitations but has been reported in a small series of pediatric patients. If larger series confirm earlier reported success with PECs, this is likely to become an increasingly reported technique in children with neurological abnormalities and developmental abnormalities resulting in chronic constipation.

Conclusion

PEGs are being increasingly utilized in pediatric patients. Placement of a PEG tube does not increase the incidence of postoperative gastroesophageal reflux or interfere with subsequent gastric surgery. PEG placement is an advanced endoscopic procedure associated with a higher rate of complications than standard EGD. Placement of PEGs in children requires modification of the technique used in adults due to size and anatomical considerations and also due to different anticipated duration of use.

- See companion website for videos relating to this chapter topic: www.wiley.com/go/gershman3e

 FURTHER READING

Avitsland TL, Kristensen C, Emblem R, Veenstra M, Mala T, Bjornland K. Percutaneous endoscopic gastrostomy in children: a safe technique with major symptom relief and high parental satisfaction. *J Pediatr Gastroenterol Nutr* 2006, **43**, 624–628.

Belsha D, Thomson M, Dass D, Lindley R, Marven S. Assessment of the safety and efficacy of percutaneous laparoscopic endoscopic jejunostomy. *J Pediatr Surg* 2016, **51**, 513–518.

Chaer RA, Rekkas D, Trevino J, Brown R, Espat J. Intrahepatic placement of a PEG tube. *Gastrointest Endosc* 2003, **57**, 763–765.

Chang WK, McClave SA, Yu CY, Huang HH, Chao YC. Positioning a safe gastric puncture point before percutaneous endoscopic gastrostomy. *Int J Clin Pract* 2007, **61**, 1121–1125.

DeLegge MH. Percutaneous endoscopic gastrostomy. *Am J Gastroenterol* 2007, **102**, 2620.

Ebina K, Kato S, Abukawa D, Nakagawa H. Endoscopic hemostasis of bleeding duodenal ulcer in a child with Henoch–Schonlein purpura. *J Pediatr* 1997, **131**, 934–936.

El-Matary W. Percutaneous endoscopic gastrostomy in children. *Can J Gastroenterol* 2008, **22**, 993–998.

Fortunato JE, Troy AL, Cuffari C, *et al.* Outcome after percutaneous endoscopic gastrostomy in children and young adults. *J Pediatr Gastroenterol Nutr* 2010, **50**, 390–393.

Fröhlich T, Richter M, Carbon R, Barth B, Köhler H. Review article: percutaneous endoscopic gastrostomy in infants and children. *Aliment Pharmacol Ther* 2010, **31**, 788–801.

Gauderer MWL, Ponsky JL, Izant RJ. Gastrostomy without laparotomy: a percutaneous endoscopic technique. *J Pediatr Surg* 1980, **15**, 872–875.

George DE, Dokler M. Percutaneous endoscopic gastrostomy in children. *Tech Gastrointest Endosc* 2002, **4**, 201–206.

Heuschkel RB, Gottrand F, Devarajan K, *et al.* ESPGHAN position paper on management of percutaneous endoscopic gastrostomy in children and adolescents. *J Pediatr Gastroenterol Nutr* 2015, **60**, 131–141

Lalanne A, Gottrand F, Salleron J, *et al.* Long-term outcome of children receiving percutaneous endoscopic gastrostomy feeding. *J Pediatr Gastroenterol Nutr* 2014, **59**, 172–176.

McCarter TL, Condon SC, Aguilar RC, Gibson DJ, Chen YK. Randomized prospective trial of early versus delayed feeding after percutaneous endoscopic gastrostomy placement. *Am J Gastroenterol* 1998, **93**, 419–421.

McSweeney ME, Jiang H, Deutsch AJ, Atmadja M, Lightdale JR. Long-term outcomes of infants and children undergoing percutaneous endoscopy gastrostomy tube placement. *J Pediatr Gastroenterol Nutr* 2013, **57**, 663–667.

McSweeney ME, Smithers CJ. Advances in pediatric gastrostomy placement. *Gastrointest Endosc Clin North Am* 2016, **26**, 169–185.

Minar P, Garland J, Martinez A, Werlin S. Safety of percutaneous endoscopic gastrostomy in medically complicated infants. *J Pediatr Gastroenterol Nutr* 2011, **53**, 293–295.

Panigrahi H, Shreeve DR, Tan WC, Prudham R, Kaufman R. Role of antibiotic prophylaxis for wound infection in percutaneous endoscopic gastrostomy (PEG): result of a prospective double-blind randomized trial. *J Hosp Infect* 2002, **50**, 312–315.

Schrag SP, Sharma R, Jaik NP, *et al.* Complications related to percutaneous endoscopic gastrostomy (PEG) tubes. A comprehensive clinical review. *J Gastrointestin Liver Dis* 2007, **16**, 407–418.

Segal D, Michaud L, Guimber D, Ganga-Zandzou PS, Turck D, Gottrand F. Late-onset complications of percutaneous endoscopic gastrostomy in children. *J Pediatr Gastroenterol Nutr* 2001, **33**, 495–500.

Srinivasan R, Fisher RS. Early initiation of post-PEG feeding: do published recommendations affect clinical practice? *Dig Dis Sci* 2000, **45**, 2065–2068.

Sulkowski JP, de Roo AC, Nielsen J, *et al.* A comparison of pediatric gastrostomy tube placement techniques. *Pediatr Surg Int* 2016, **32**, 269–275.

Taylor AL, Carroll TA, Jakubowski J, O'Reilly G. Percutaneous endoscopic gastrostomy in patients with ventriculoperitoneal shunts. *Br J Surg* 2001, **88**, 724–727.

Valusek PA, St. Peter SD, Keckler SJ, *et al.* Does an upper gastrointestinal study change operative management for gastroesophageal reflux? *J Pediatr Surg* 2010, **45**, 1169–1172.

Vervloessem D, van Leersum F, Boer D, *et al.* Percutaneous endoscopic gastrostomy (PEG) in children is not a minor procedure: risk factors for major complications. *Semin Pediatr Surg* 2009, **18**, 93–97.

Virnig DJ, Frech EJ, DeLegge MH, Fang JC. Direct percutaneous endoscopic jejunostomy: a case series in pediatric patients. *Gastrointest Endosc* 2008, **67**, 984–987.

Wollman B, d'Agostino HB. Percutaneous radiologic and endoscopic gastrostomy: a 3-year institutional analysis of procedure performance. *Am J Roentgenol* 1997, **169**, 1551–1553.

Wyllie R. Changing the tube: a pediatrician's guide. *Curr Opin Pediatr* 2004, **16**, 542–544.

34

Single-stage percutaneous endoscopic gastrostomy

Andreia Nita, Jorge Amil-Dias, Arun Urs, Mike Thomson, and Prithviraj Rao

---

 KEY POINTS

- Primary placement of a balloon gastrostomy allows only one procedure.
- Carbon dioxide insufflation is probably preferable to air. Single-stage PEG and classic PEG share a similar safety profile and

complication rate. Single-stage PEGs have a lower rate of peristomal infection, as the PEG catheter is not passed through the oropharynx, less common postoperative feeding intolerance, and fewer concerns for dislodgment.

Introduction

Single-stage PEG is a novel adaptation of the preexisting technique. The standard procedure for gastrostomy is performed in two steps, with a change from a PEG tube to a PEG button 6–8 weeks after PEG tube placement, a necessary time frame for the stoma to mature.

The new alternative to classic PEG is coming forward as a superior method in selected cases: one-step endoscopic procedure for inserting a low-profile tube button that permits initial placement of a balloon-retained device.

Indications

Single-stage PEG is used in patients who are at high anesthetic risk and experience chronic problems with feeding, requiring long-term or lifetime enteral nutritional support, such as neurologically impaired children.

Contraindications

These are the same as for standard PEG placement (see Chapter 33). Relative contraindication: small child (10 kg) due to potential reduced surface area for triangulation around the stoma site with gastropexy needles.

Advantages of single-stage PEG

A single-stage PEG button allows the button to be placed without requiring a second procedure. There are several advantages for the patient: no additional anesthetic session or hospitalization, cosmetically better than a long tube (facilitating social integration), durable device with a significantly longer interval between device changes [1]. The procedure is of particular advantage to patients with a high anesthetic risk as it incorporates just one session of anesthesia and one interventional

---

Practical Pediatric Gastrointestinal Endoscopy, Third Edition. Edited by George Gershman and Mike Thomson.
© 2021 John Wiley & Sons Ltd. Published 2021 by John Wiley & Sons Ltd.
Companion website: www.wiley.com/go/gershman3e

endoscopy and associated health costs are thus reduced [2].

Studies have shown that single-stage PEG and classic PEG share a similar safety profile and complication rate [1–5], with more benefits derived from a single-stage PEG button: a lower rate of peristomal infection [2], as the PEG catheter is not passed through the oropharynx, less common postoperative feeding intolerance [1], and fewer concerns for dislodgment [3] (Table 34.1).

The single-stage PEG can also be performed in instances where gastro-jejunal feeding is needed [4].

Drawbacks

Although the recent ESPGHAN position paper on management of PEG in children welcomes the advantages of single-stage PEG, it acknowledges that published experience in children is limited [6].

Technique

Personnel

Two physicians are needed to perform single-stage PEG. One performs the endoscopy and the other performs the abdominal portion under aseptic conditions.

Procedure

1. Site identification

The patient is in the supine position. The endoscopist introduces the endoscope in the stomach and insufflates the stomach with air. Transillumination and indentation are used to identify the site of PEG placement which should be one-third of the distance from the umbilicus to the left costal margin at the midclavicular midline. The endoscopist should see the depression caused by indentation on the anterior surface of the gastric wall (Figure 34.1) and the physician performing the intervention should clearly see the transillumination on the same spot (Figure 34.2).

2. Marking the site

Three marks should be made in a triangular shape that surrounds the PEG site, being equidistant – approximately 2 cm from each mark to the site of PEG (Figure 34.3).

3. Placing of gastropexy

1) Attach a syringe with saline to the preloaded gastropexy needle (Figure 34.4) and insert the needle in one of the corners of the triangle (Figure 34.5). Correct position is

Table 34.1 Advantages of single-stage PEG

For the patient	For the medical system
1) One procedure, one anesthetic session	1) Cost-effective
2) Fewer tube changes	2) Safe
3) Longer interval between changes	3) Rapid technique
4) Cosmetically better	
5) Fewer peristomal infections	
6) Fewer dislodgments	
7) Less postoperative feeding intolerance	
Patients in need of long-term to lifetime enteral nutrition	
Patients with high anesthetic risk	
Published experience in children is limited	

confirmed by air noted only while entering the stomach.

2) Remove the suture thread (Figure 34.6). Detach the syringe.

3) Bend the strip on the needle (Figure 34.7). Dislodge the T-bar by pushing the inner hub into the outer hub.

4) Withdraw the needle and pull the T-bar until it is positioned on the gastric mucosa (Figure 34.8).

5) Slide and close the suture lock on the abdominal surface (Figure 34.9).

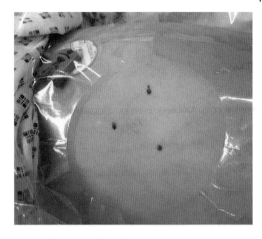

Figure 34.3 Marking the site.

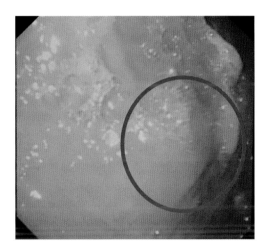

Figure 34.1 Indentation.

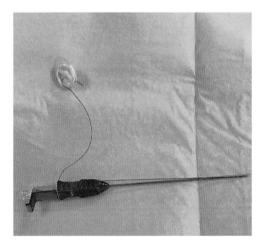

Figure 34.4 T-fastener device.

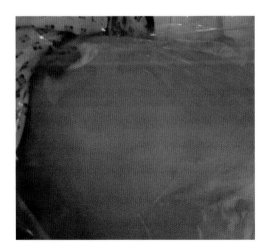

Figure 34.2 Transillumination.

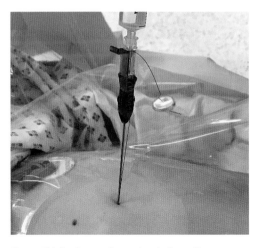

Figure 34.5 Insert the preloaded needle.

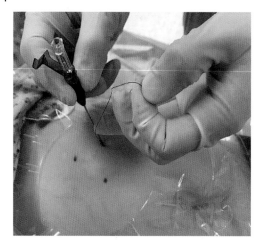

Figure 34.6 Release the suture thread.

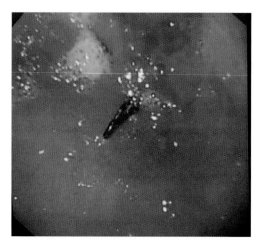

Figure 34.8 Pull the T-bar against the mucosa.

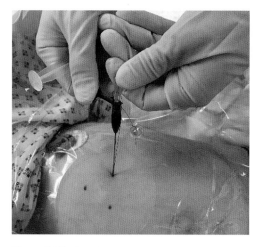

Figure 34.7 Bend the locking strip and push the inner hub.

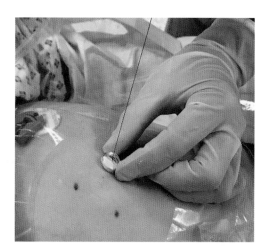

Figure 34.9 Slide and close suture lock.

6) Repeat the procedure for the other two marked sites. At the end of it, the anchor set should be placed on the corners of the triangle (Figures 34.10 and 34.11). The gastric wall is now fixed to the anterior abdominal wall.

4. Creating the stoma tract
1) Identify the PEG placement site at the center of the gastropexy triangle.
2) Anesthetize the site of PEG placement (Figure 34.12).
3) Make a small (<0.5 cm) but deep incision (Figure 34.13).

4) Insert the safety introducer needle (Figure 34.14).
5) Advance the guidewire and remove the safety introducer needle, keeping the safety collar (Figures 34.15–34.17).

5. Dilation of the stoma tract and measuring the stoma length
1) Advance the dilator over the guidewire in order to dilate the stoma tract to the desired size using clockwise and anticlockwise movements while endoscopically maintaining visualization of its inner part throughout the entire procedure (Figures 34.18 and 34.19).

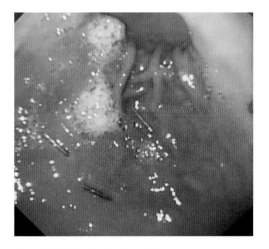

Figure 34.10 Gastric view of gastropexy.

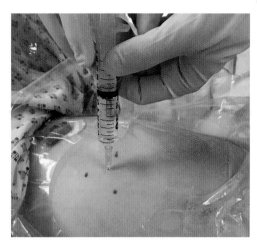

Figure 34.12 Local anesthesia injection.

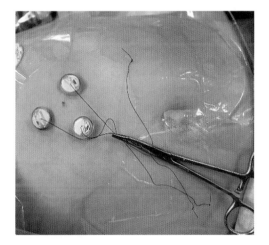

Figure 34.11 Abdominal view of gastropexy.

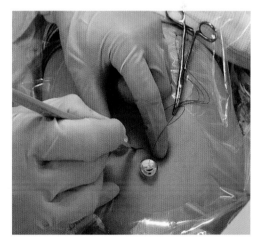

Figure 34.13 Make the incision.

2) With the guidewire in place, remove the dilator and advance the measuring device over the guidewire (Figure 34.20).
3) Inflate the balloon of the measuring device and slide the disc to the abdominal wall while pulling. Measure the length. Deflate the balloon and remove the measuring device but keep the guidewire (Figure 34.21).
4) Continue dilation by advancing the dilator over the guidewire again and using the same movements as above until the appropriate diameter is reached (12–16 French) (Figures 34.22 and 34.23).

5) Rotate the dilator central part to release the peel-away sheath from the dilator (Figures 34.24 and 34.25).
6) Remove the dilator and the guidewire, leaving the peel-away sheath in the stoma tract (Figure 34.26).

6. Button placement
1) Advance the appropriate-sized button through the peel-away sheath while peeling the sheath down to the skin level (Figures 34.27–34.29).
2) When the button is in the stomach, peel the sheath completely and remove it (Figure 34.30–34.35).

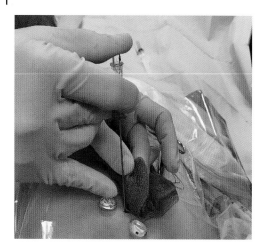

Figure 34.14   Introduce the safety needle.

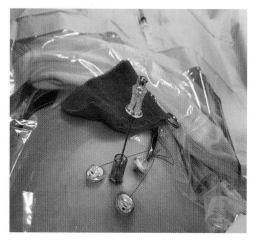

Figure 34.15   Activate safety collar.

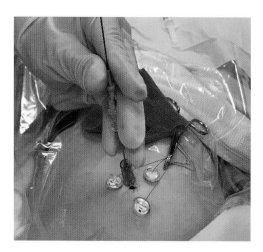

Figure 34.16   Remove the safety needle while introducing the guidewire.

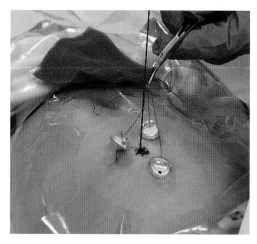

Figure 34.17   Remove the safety needle while introducing the guidewire.

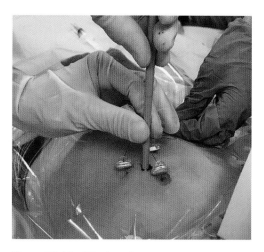

Figure 34.18   Dilation of stoma tract.

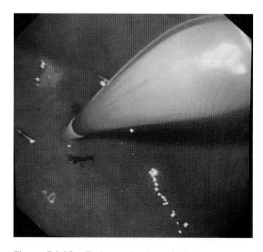

Figure 34.19   Endoscopic view of dilator.

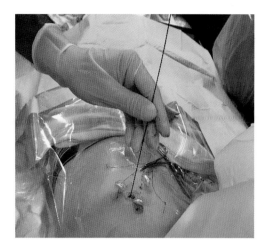

Figure 34.20   Remove the dilator.

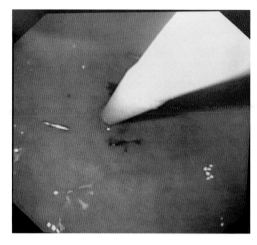

Figure 34.23   Keep the endoscopic view.

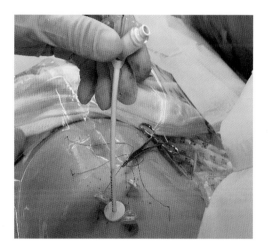

Figure 34.21   Measure the length.

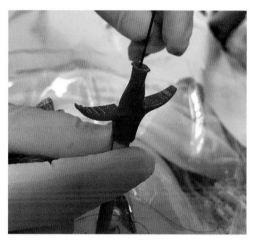

Figure 34.24   Rotate the dilator central part to release the peel-away sheath from the dilator.

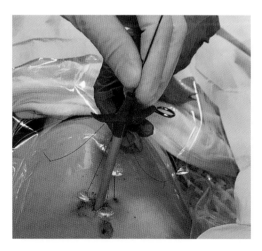

Figure 34.22   Continue dilation.

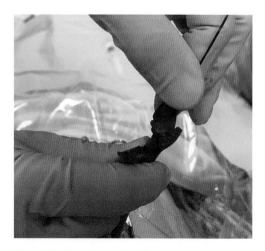

Figure 34.25   Rotate the dilator central part to release the peel-away sheath from the dilator.

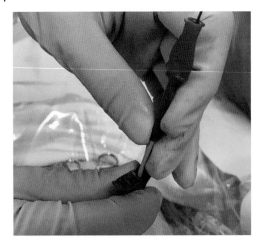

Figure 34.26 Remove the dilator and the guidewire, leaving the peel-away sheath in the stoma tract.

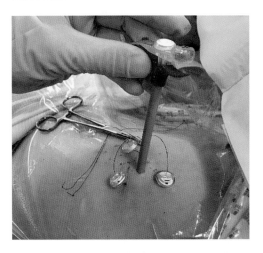

Figure 34.27 Advance the button while peeling the sheath.

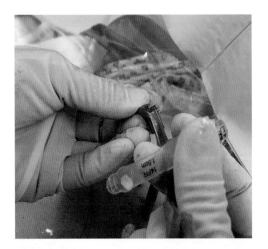

Figure 34.28

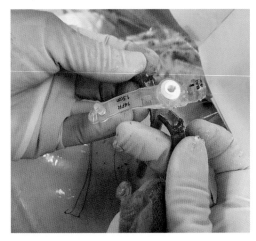

Figure 34.29

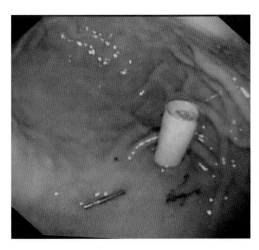

Figure 34.30 Endoscopic view of the button revealed as the sheath is peeled away.

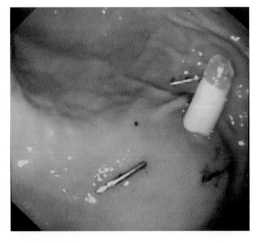

Figure 34.31

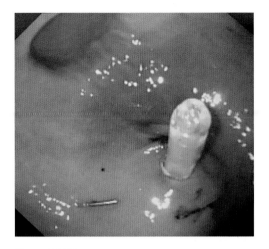

Figure 34.32

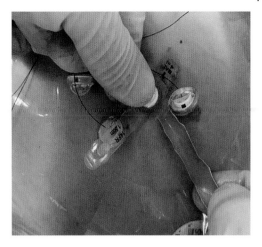

Figure 34.34

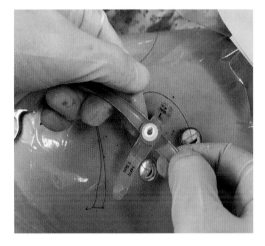

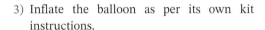

Figure 34.33 Peel the sheath down to the skin and remove it.

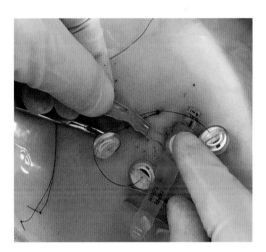

Figure 34.35

3) Inflate the balloon as per its own kit instructions.

After completion of all steps, the balloon should be placed in the center of the triangle delimited by the three gastropexy T-bars (from the gastric view) and the button in the center of the triangle delimited by the three suture locks (from abdominal view) (Figures 34.36 and 34.37).

Postprocedure management

- Both the stoma and gastropexy areas should be inspected daily for signs of infection.

- Enteral feeding can be started as per classic PEG insertion protocols.
- The sutures may be left to be absorbed or may be cut but no earlier than two weeks post procedure.

Complications

Complications are the same as the standard PEG although pneumoperitoneum has a slightly higher incidence (see Chapter 33).

Once enteral access is no longer required, the button can be removed in an outpatient

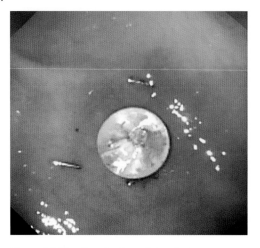

Figure 34.36 Gastric view of the single-stage PEG.

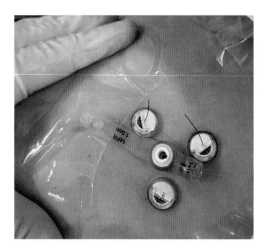

Figure 34.37 Abdominal view.

setting or at home and the gastrostomy site can be allowed to close by itself.

Useful tips

- Pick the location that is best based on individual anatomy.
- Ensure at least 1 cm distance between triangulation sites and in addition 1 cm distance from the gastrostomy site to the gastropexy needle site.
- Ensure the position of the gastrostomy site is correct with the aid of a local anesthetic needle. The risk of colonic interposition between the abdominal wall and stomach can be minimized by using the local anesthetic syringe. Whilst introducing this syringe into the stomach, if air bubbles are noticed in the syringe only before visualization of needle in stomach, then this raises the possibility of colonic interposition.
- "Pull" the gastropexy sutures up (i.e., pull the stomach against the abdominal wall) gently and only when the dilator is being introduced into the stomach. Excess pulling force may risk snapping of the suture or eroding of the T-bars into the gastric mucosal wall.

- Use CO_2 instead of air as it is absorbed more easily following escape into the peritoneal cavity after stomal opening in the stomach.
- Secure the gastrostomy button using Tegaderm® or similar sheaths in the first 72 hours of inpatient stay to minimize movement of the gastrocutaneous fistula and reduce the risk of leak by the formation of a "Y" tract.

Materials

The procedure described in this chapter was performed using a Halyard® introducer kit for gastrostomy feeding tube.

Consent

The mother of the patient shown in the images consented for the procedure to be performed and for photos to be taken and used for educational purposes.

 • See companion website for videos relating to this chapter topic: www.wiley.com/go/gershman3e

REFERENCES

1 Jacob A, Delesalle D, Coopman S, *et al*. Safety of the one-step percutaneous endoscopic gastrostomy button in children. *J Pediatr* 2015, **166**, 1526–1528.

2 Novotny NM, Vegeler RC, Breckler FD, Rescorla FJ. Percutaneous endoscopic gastrostomy buttons in children: superior to tubes. *J Pediatr Surg* 2009, **44**, 1193–1196.

3 Michaud L, Robert-Dehault A, Coopman S, Guimber D, Turck D, Gottrand F. One-step percutaneous gastrojejunostomy in early infancy. *J Pediatr Gastroenterol Nutr* 2012, **54**, 20–21.

4 Gothberg G, Bjornsson S. One-step insertion of low-profile gastrostomy in pediatric patients vs pull percutaneous endoscopic gastrostomy: retrospective analysis of outcomes. *J Parenter Enteral Nutr* 2016, **40**, 423–430.

5 Evans JS, Thorne M, Taufiq S, George DE. Should single-stage PEG buttons become the procedure of choice for PEG placement in children? *Gastrointest Endosc* 2006, **64**, 320–324.

6 Heuschkel RB, Gottrand F, Devarajan K, *et al*. ESPGHAN position paper on management of percutaneous endoscopic gastrostomy in children and adolescents. *J Pediatr Gastroenterol Nutr* 2015, **60**, 131–141.

35

Pediatric laparoscopic-assisted direct percutaneous jejunostomy

Mike Thomson, Jonathan Goring, Richard Lindley, and Sean Marven

---

 KEY POINTS

- Close teamwork between endoscopist and laparoscopic surgeon is key to success.
- Malrotation is a contraindication which may lead to volvulus.
- Standard pull gastrostomy technique is used beyond the duodenojejunal flexure.
- The laparoscopist clamps the proximal jejunum and the endoscopist ideally uses

carbon dioxide insufflation – both prevent excess small bowel inflation which can obscure the laparoscopic view.

- As with a PEG, the PEJ may be changed by endoscopy for a balloon at around three months after the original insertion.

Introduction

Artificial enteric nutritional support is vital in the management of patients who are unable to maintain oral nutrition such as those with upper GI motility disorders, gastroesophageal reflux disease (GERD), faltering growth (FG), recurrent pneumonia, and oral feeding difficulties. Enteral nutrition via a percutaneous gastrostomy (PEG) tube may not be indicated because of severe GERD and/or delayed gastric emptying and/or antro-pyloric dysmotility.

In some of these circumstances and mainly in the neurologically impaired child, postpyloric feeding can be crucial, thereby avoiding the need for parenteral nutrition. For delivery of long-term postpyloric feeding, a direct jejunostomy tube provides more stable and secure jejunal access compared with a percutaneous gastrostomy with jejunal extension (PEGJ), with fewer reported complications of blockage/displacement and consequently a decrease in the need for radiological/endoscopic replacement/intervention. Naso-jejunal tubes often migrate and/or are inadvertently pulled out. PEGJ tubes regularly require replacement with necessary X-ray exposure – which can be lessened by the endo-clip maneuver attached to their tip as previously described.

Direct jejunostomy has been attempted before by using, variously, a Roux-en-Y loop or a direct surgical jejunostomy. Both have been associated with significant complications and have generally fallen out of favor.

A new approach has recently been advanced which involves a similar technique to PEG but involves the laparoscopist and endoscopist working in tandem.

Practical Pediatric Gastrointestinal Endoscopy, Third Edition. Edited by George Gershman and Mike Thomson.
© 2021 John Wiley & Sons Ltd. Published 2021 by John Wiley & Sons Ltd.
Companion website: www.wiley.com/go/gershman3e

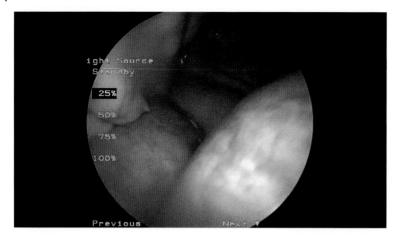

Figure 35.1 Laparoscopic view of endoscopic light source seen through the small bowel wall (note that the brightness of the laparoscope is reduced at this point to facilitate identification).

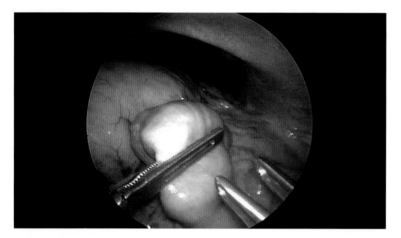

Figure 35.2 A Johan instrument is used to occlude the jejunum distal to the endoscope to facilitate distension and reduce passage of distal gas.

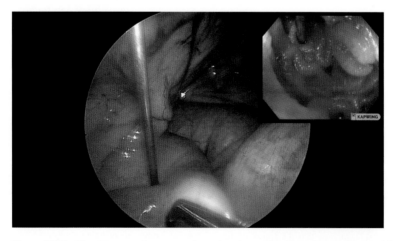

Figure 35.3 Simultaneous laparoscopic and endoscopic view of trocar inserted into the small bowel.

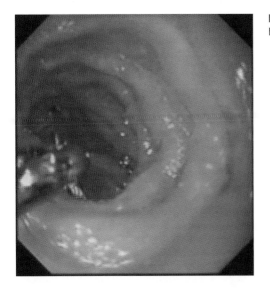

Figure 35.4   Endoscopic view of wire grasped by biopsy forceps.

(a)

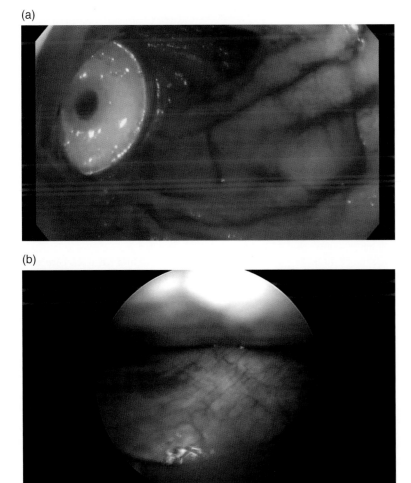

(b)

Figure 35.5   PEJ placed – endoscopic (a) and laparoscopic (b) views showing PEG bumper against jejunal mucosa and loop of jejunum brought up to anterior abdominal wall.

The endoscope is inserted (often either a dual-channel therapeutic gastroscope or a variable stiffness pediatric colonoscope is preferred as they allow deep jejunal penetration). Once the surgeon has identified the DJ flexure then the laparoscopic lights can be dimmed – this allows for visualization of the light at the tip of the endoscope (Figure 35.1) A soft clamp (laparoscopic Johan instrument) has already been applied distal to this area (Figure 35.2) which prevents distal small bowel distension and resultant obscuring of the view from the laparoscopic angle. A trocar is inserted through the anterior abdominal wall and the endoscope can immobilize the small bowel loop in question (Figure 35.3). As with the PEG technique, a wire is passed through the trocar and grasped by the biopsy forceps (Figure 35.4). Then as for a standard PEG technique, the PEJ is attached

outside the patient's mouth then pulled through to anchor the small bowel to the anterior abdominal wall (Figure 35.5). As for a standard PEG, after three months or so the PEJ can be changed by endoscopy for a low-profile balloon jejunostomy.

Conclusion

This is an ideal example of the surgical–endoscopy interface and is a significant advance on previous iterations which were mainly surgical alone. Further experience will refine this technique.

- See companion website for videos relating to this chapter topic: www.wiley.com/go/gershman3e

 FURTHER READING

Allen JW, Ali A, Wo J, *et al.* Totally laparoscopic feeding jejunostomy. *Surg Endosc* 2002, **16**, 1802–1805.

Belsha D, Thomson M, Dass D. Assessment of the safety and efficacy of percutaneous laparoscopic endoscopic jejunostomy (PLEJ). *J Pediatr Surg* 2016, **1**, 513–518.

Bobowicz M, Makarewicz W, Polec T, *et al.* Totally laparoscopic feeding jejunostomy – a technique modification. *Videosurg Miniinvas Tech (Wideochir Inne Tech Maloinwazyjne)* 2011, **6**, 256–620.

Bueno JT, Schattner MA, Barrera R, *et al.* Endoscopic placement of direct percutaneous jejunostomy tubes in patients with complications after esophagectomy. *Gastrointest Endosc* 2003, **57**, 536–540.

Denzer U, Lohse AW, Kanzler S, *et al.* Mini-laparoscopically guided percutaneous gastrostomy and jejunostomy. *Gastrointest Endosc* 2003, **58**, 434–438.

Egnell C, Eksborg S, Grahnquist L. Jejunostromy enteral feeding in children:

outcome and safety. *J Parenter Enteral Nutr* 2014, **38**, 631–636.

Freeman C, Delegge MH. Small bowel endoscopic enteral access. *Curr Opin Gastroenterol* 2009, **25**, 155–159.

Gilchrist BF, Luks FI, DeLuca FG, *et al.* A modified feeding Roux-en-Y jejunostomy in the neurologically damaged child. *J Pediatr Surg* 1997, **32**, 588–589.

Mellert J, Naruhn MB, Grund KE, *et al.* Direct endoscopic percutaneous jejunostomy (EPJ). Clinical results. *Surg Endosc* 1994, **8**, 867–869.

Michaud L, Robert-Dehault A, Coopman S, *et al.* One-step percutaneous gastrojejunostomy in early infancy. *J Pediatr Gastroenterol Nutr* 2012, **54**, 820–821.

Mohiuddin SS, Anderson CE. A novel application for single-incision laparoscopic surgery (SILS): SIL jejunostomy feeding tube placement. *Surg Endosc* 2011, **25**, 323–327.

Moran GW, Fisher NC. Direct percutaneous endoscopic jejunostomy: high completion rates with selective use of a long drainage access needle. *Diagn Ther Endosc* 2009, **2009**, 520879.

Neuman HB, Phillips JD. Laparoscopic Roux-en-Y feeding jejunostomy: a new minimally invasive surgical procedure for permanent feeding access in children with gastric dysfunction. *J Laparoendosc Adv Surg Tech A* 2005, **15**, 71–74.

Rumalla A, Baron TH. Results of direct percutaneous endoscopic jejunostomy, an alternative method for providing jejunal feeding. *Mayo Clin Proc* 2000, **75**, 807–810.

Shike M, Latkany L, Gerdes H, *et al*. Direct percutaneous endoscopic jejunostomies for enteral feeding. *Gastrointest Endosc* 1996, **44**, 536–540.

Smith D, Souc P. Complications of long-term jejunostomy in children. *J Pediatr Surg* 1996, **3**, 787–790.

Taylor JA, Ryckman FC. Management of small bowel volvulus around feeding Roux-en-Y limbs. *Pediatr Surg Int* 2010, **26**, 439–442.

Varadarajulu S, Delegge MH. Use of a 19-gauge injection needle as a guide for direct percutaneous endoscopic jejunostomy tube placement. *Gastrointest Endosc* 2003, **57**, 942–945.

Virnig DJ, Frech EJ, Delegge MH, *et al*. Direct percutaneous endoscopic jejunostomy: a case series in pediatric patients. *Gastrointest Endosc* 2008, **67**, 984–987.

Wolfsen H, Kozarek R, Ball TJ, *et al*. Tube dysfunction following percutaneous endoscopic gastrostomy and jejunostomy. *Gastrointest Endosc* 1990, **36**, 261–263.

Zhu Y, Shi L, Tang H, *et al*. Current considerations in direct percutaneous endoscopic jejunostomy. *Can J Gastroenterol* 2012, **26**, 92–96.

36

Naso-jejunal and Gastro-jejunal tube placement

George Gershman

KEY POINTS

- Naso-jejunal (NJ) or gastro-jejunal (GJ) tubes may offer safe feeding in children who have severe reflux and/or gastroparesis.
- Radiological and endoscopic placement are equally effective.
- The tip of the tube has a thread which can be attached by the endoscopist to the appropriate part of the small bowel using an endo-clip.

Nasoduodenal or naso-jejunal tube feeding is commonly used as a short-term option in children with risk of pulmonary regurgitation due to severe gastroesophageal reflux, gastroparesis, acute pancreatitis or as a bridge to nutritional therapy before surgery or nutritional support for critically ill children with various conditions in intensive care units.

An enteral tube may be placed endoscopically if other options such as spontaneous passage or installation under fluoroscopy with the use of a radiopaque guidewire have failed.

After the appropriate tube is chosen, a small loop at the tip of the tube should be created using a silk suture. The tube is inserted into the stomach via the nose, followed by the endoscope. The tube may be found either conveniently positioned along the greater curvature of the stomach oriented toward the antrum or coiled in the gastric body. In the second scenario, it is pulled back until the tip becomes visible.

The next step is grasping of the silk loop by the single-use preloaded rotatable two-pronged hemostatic clip device and pulling the loop back into the biopsy channel until the end of the tube gets close to the tip of the endoscope. Then, the endoscope is maneuvered through the pylorus into the distal duodenum or proximal jejunum in a standard fashion. The hemostatic clip is advanced forward a few centimeters and attached to the mucosa, preventing accidental ejection of the tube during the withdrawal phase of the procedure (Figure 36.1). Finally, the endoscope is pulled back to the stomach in a twisting fashion to decrease friction between the shaft and the feeding tube. The excess portion of the feeding tube is slowly retracted, leaving a small loop within the stomach. A postprocedure flat abdominal film confirms the appropriate position of the feeding tube.

A similar technique can be used for placement of a gastroduodenal or gastro-jejunal

Practical Pediatric Gastrointestinal Endoscopy, Third Edition. Edited by George Gershman and Mike Thomson.
© 2021 John Wiley & Sons Ltd. Published 2021 by John Wiley & Sons Ltd.
Companion website: www.wiley.com/go/gershman3e

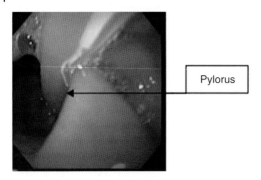

Pylorus

Figure 36.1 Endoscopic view of the feeding tube beyond the pylorus.

feeding tube in children with an established gastrostomy. The only difference is the introduction of the feeding tube into the stomach through the existing gastrostomy.

Alternatively, naso-jejunal intubation can be performed with an over-the-wire method. First, the distal duodenum or proximal jejunum is intubated during an upper endoscopy. Then, a lubricated Teflon®-coated guidewire is fed through the biopsy channel and advanced under direct visualization beyond the tip of the scope until it meets resistance. Using a pull-push or "exchange" technique, the endoscope is slowly withdrawn while the guidewire is simultaneously threaded through, so that it stays in a fixed position in the intestine. A soft lubricated tube is advanced into the oropharynx through the nose and blindly removed from the mouth using the index finger or a plastic grasper. A guidewire is fed into the tube and advanced until it becomes visible. The protective tube is removed. Before insertion of the enteral tube, then the course of the wire is studied under fluoroscopy and adjusted to ensure that there are no coils or loops within the gastric body. A lubricated naso-jejunal tube is advanced along the guidewire into the distal duodenum or proximal jejunum. Once the position of the tube within the distal duodenum or proximal jejunum is confirmed, the guidewire is removed.

For some school-age children and teenagers, a transpyloric insertion of the guidewire can be achieved during transnasal endoscopy with an ultra-slim endoscope.

- See companion website for videos relating to this chapter topic: www.wiley.com/go/gershman3e

 FURTHER READING

O'Keefe SJ, Foody W, Grill S. Transnasal endoscopic placement of feeding tubes in the intensive care unit. *J Parenter Enteral Nutr* 2003, **27**(5), 349–354.

Rafferty GP, Tham TCK. Endoscopic placement of enteral feeding tubes. *World J Gastrointest Endosc* 2010, **2**(5), 155–164.

37

Endoscopic retrograde cholangiopancreatography

Douglas S. Fishman, Paola de Angelis, Luigi Dall'Oglio, and Victor Fox

---

 KEY POINTS

- ERCP in children is probably best undertaken in units which are performing reasonable numbers of pocedures.
- Apart from the infant with cholestasis and diagnostic uncertainty in sclerosing

cholangitis, the majority of pediatric ERCP occurs for therapeutic reasons.
- Pediatric-specific ERCP scopes are usually only required under 10 kg.
- Post-ERCP pancreatitis may occur with an incidence of 2.5–10%.

Introduction

Endoscopic retrograde cholangiopancreatography (ERCP) represents a spectrum of techniques with a shift favoring more therapeutic procedures over diagnostic procedures in recent years. Typically, ERCP is the retrograde opacification of the biliopancreatic tree through endoscopic cannulation of the major or minor papilla.

Each year thousands of ERCPs are performed in adult patients for a range of therapeutic applications. In the past, a relatively low incidence of pancreaticobiliary diseases in children and lack of experience among pediatric surgeons and gastroenterologist in ERCP limited the application in pediatric patients. Significant progress has been made in the diagnosis of pancreaticobiliary disorders in

children, especially chronic pancreatitis. Additionally, the increased incidence of cholelithiasis (particularly in obese children) has increased the demand for therapeutic ERCP.

Indications for ERCP in children vary from region to region. In Western countries, the main indication for ERCP is choledocholithiasis-related conditions (e.g., gallstone pancreatitis) and chronic pancreatitis. In the Middle East, ERCP is commonly performed in children with choledocholithiasis secondary to sickle cell anemia, and in Asia, management of choledochal cysts is a leading indication.

In this chapter, our aim is to describe the critical aspects of pediatric ERCP including indications, preparation, techniques, outcomes, and adverse events related to diagnostic and therapeutic ERCP in infants and children.

Practical Pediatric Gastrointestinal Endoscopy, Third Edition. Edited by George Gershman and Mike Thomson.
© 2021 John Wiley & Sons Ltd. Published 2021 by John Wiley & Sons Ltd.
Companion website: www.wiley.com/go/gershman3e

Duodenoscopes and accessories

Duodenoscopes are the standard endoscopes used for pediatric ERCP. In our practice, the "adult" therapeutic duodenoscope can be used in most children above 10 kg in weight, reserving the smaller endoscopes for children under 10 kg or in some cases less than 12–18 months old. This is due more to necessity and lack of availability of size- and age-appropriate duodenoscopes worldwide. A list of commercially available and secondary market endoscopes is given in Table 37.1. Some experts advocate the use of an 11 mm therapeutic duodenoscope in older children. Newer models with slightly larger working channel diameters relative to

Table 37.1 Duodenoscopes: specification

Manufacturer	Insertion tube (mm)	Working channel (mm)
Fujinon		
ED530XT	13.1	4.2
ED450XL5	12.5	3.2
Olympus		
TJF-Q180V	11.3	4.2
PJF	7.5	2.0
PJF 160	7.5	2.0
JF1T2	11.0	3.2
TJF160VR	12.5	4.2
TJF160F/VF	11.3	4.2
Pentax		
ED-34-i10T	11.6	4.2
ED-3490TK	11.6	4.2
3270/3280K	10.8	3.2
ED 3670TK	12.1	4.8
ED 2330		2.2

Indented products may be available in the secondary market but due to concerns about endoscope reprocessing, manufacturers have either withdrawn endoscopes or discontinued service on these endoscopes.

endoscope size may allow some modfications in these smaller and younger patients.

The smallest duodenoscope has an insertion tube diameter of 7.5 mm, with a 2.0 mm working channel. This endoscope is designed for neonates and infants who weigh less than 10 kg. The major limitation with this endoscope is the relative scarcity of functional tools for the 2 mm channel, triple-lumen or otherwise, and the devices must be 5 Fr or smaller. Other difficulties with the smaller duodenoscopes include increased resistance when passing devices through the distal portion of the endoscope, inability of the elevator to fully angulate, limiting access to the major papilla, and inadequate suction. Risk of accidental thermal injury and perforation of the duodenal wall limit the utility of therapeutic procedures with electrosurgical devices. However, sphincterotomy with a 5 Fr device has been reported.

Unfortunately, many of the smaller caliber endoscopes have become relics. The market for duodenoscopes worldwide has been impacted by the carbapenem-resistant Enterobacteriaceae (CRE) infections noted to affect the elevator of most duodenoscopes. For this reason, the market has been affected in two ways: (i) continual efforts to minimize infection during reprocessing with the introduction of new endoscopes, (ii) discontinuation of production and repairs by the primary manufacturer for the older endoscopes. The result has been a challenge for pediatric ERCP in that the smaller duodenoscopes are now difficult to find and repair, with the caveat that there may be risks in reprocessing. Ultimately, endoscope manufacturers will need to create smaller duodenoscopes with appropriate channel sizes to accommodate the needs of the patients without compromising the issues related to reprocessing and cleaning of the elevator.

Similar to the challenges of the endoscope itself are the tools which can be placed through the working channel. With the trend in therapeutic over diagnostic ERCP, catheters, wires, and other devices should be tailored to the case. The choice of a particular accessory is dictated by the indications, for example, choledocholithiasis or stricture management.

Endoscopic retrograde cholangiopancreatography is a combined endoscopic and radiological technique and requires an optimal set-up of fluoroscopy equipment and the participation of a well-trained radiologist or radiology technician. A percutaneous transhepatic cholangiography (PTC) to establish bile drainage in case of a failed ERCP can be performed by interventional radiologists. Additionally, a PTC and ERCP rendezvous technique is an effective way to treat patients with biliary obstruction. Different types of contrasts media are available. The contrast can be diluted in saline, most commonly in stone disease.

In the 1970s Kawai pioneered the intraductal endoscope for direct visualization of the biliary and pancreatic tree. The initial intraductal endoscopes required a "mother–daughter" system with two endoscopists. Since that time, single-operator fiberoptic and digital endoscopes have become available for use in children and adults. This has been reported in children (as young as 18 months old) for diagnostic and therapeutic indications including stone disease, postsurgical complications, and tumor evaluation. Intraductal endoscopes can also be used percutaneously in conjunction with interventional radiology, via percutaneous catheter.

Performing ERCP in children

Endoscopic retrograde cholangiopancreatography is a combined endoscopic and radiologic technique and requires an optimal set-up of fluoroscopy equipment, endoscopy tower, electrocautery, and other tools. Using a duodenoscope, the procedure is routinely performed with the patient in the prone position, although it can be performed supine. Esophageal intubation with the side-viewing endoscope is different compared to front-viewing instruments. Although it is almost a blind intubation maneuver without direct visualization, it should be done to avoid trauma of the cervical esophagus or perforation of the piriform sinus.

The duodenoscope is inserted into the mouth along the middle of the tongue (with the light source and elevator facing the commissure of the right lip). The endoscope is torqued counterclockwise, with gradual deflection of the distal end of the endoscope towards the posterior wall of the pharynx and advancement into the esophagus. A slight increase in pressure is noted along the cricopharyngeus, with decreased resistance at the moment of esophageal intubation, with the appearance of gliding esophageal mucosa with a clear vascular pattern. Attempts to view the esophageal lumen are counterproductive and may lead to mucosal laceration. The endoscope is advanced without resistance until the vascular pattern disappears. It is usually associated with entrance into the stomach and close contact of the lens with gastric mucosa at the level of the upper gastric body.

For proper orientation, the endoscope should be pulled back and rotated counterclockwise with simultaneous deflection of the distal end to the left. Once the panoramic view of the gastric body is established, the duodenoscope is advanced forward and rotated clockwise. Care should be taken to avoid slipping back into the gastric body. During the transition between the gastric body and the antrum, the lumen of the stomach may disappear. Appearance of the sliding gastric mucosa is reassuring unless significant resistance occurs. The view of the gastric lumen is reestablished by elevating the tip of the duodenoscope and/or pulling the endoscope back gently. In patients with a J-shaped stomach or if there is difficulty in identifying the antrum, the right shoulder of the patient can be rotated towards the midline. Longitudinal prepyloric folds are a good orientation to follow. Transition through the pylorus is accomplished by significant reduction of resistance and changes of mucosal pattern from smooth to the velvety appearance of the villi.

The second portion of the duodenum is reached by upward deflection of the distal tip, clockwise rotation and advancement of the scope. The is the "long" position with the majority of the shaft forming a loop along the gastric wall. To convert it to the "short" position, which is more desirable for cannulation of the major ampulla, the tip of the endoscope should be rotated clockwise and pulled back simultaneously. In infants, it can be difficult to navigate the instrument into the "short" position, often due to the relatively shallow distance from the second portion of the duodenum back to the pylorus. This occasionally leaves no alternative but the "long" position despite the limitations: excessive stretching of the stomach and duodenum, masking of the common bile duct by overlapping duodenoscope (obscuring the image), difficulties with control of the distal tip of the scope, and positioning of the cannula or therapeutic accessories.

As ERCP requires fluoroscopic guidance, it is important to remember that children are at increased risk for exposure to ionizing radiation. We recommend formal or informal fluoroscopy training, as well as additional attempts to limit radiation exposure using pulse fluoroscopy. The ESGE/ESPGHAN also recommends the protection of radiosensitive organs with adjustment of collimation to the smaller size of children. Documentation of fluoroscopic dosage and exposure times should be performed as a quality indicator.

Endoscopic retrograde cholangiopancreatography in children should be performed by an experienced endoscopist in a high-volume center with pediatric involvement. The ASGE suggests a minimum of 200 diagnostic and therapeutic ERCPs prior to assessing competence and NASPGHAN recommends the same number of ERCPs in pediatrics. Data in adults suggest increased adverse events in those performing fewer than 50 endoscopic sphincterotomies per year, highlighting the importance of ongoing assessment. ERCP typically requires general anesthesia (GA), and ESGE/ESPGHAN recommends GA for teenagers, although deep sedation can be considered in older children.

Adverse events in pediatric ERCP

The overall rate of adverse events associated with pediatric ERCP is around 5–8%, compared to the 1–13% reported in adults. Beyond standard endoscopy, each of the technical components during ERCP can be related to an adverse event.

The most commonly reported adverse event is pancreatitis. Based on both adult and pediatric literature, post-ERCP pancreatitis (PEP) is more likely to occur with repeated attempts at wire cannulation, pancreatic sphincterotomy, opacification of secondary and tertiary branches (parenchimography), and acute pancreatitis. Rates of PEP as low as 2.5% have been reported, but typically rates of ~10% are not uncommon and are similar when performed by an adult or pediatric ERCPist. PEP can be mitigated by precise and selective cannulation of the major papilla, and limited injections of the pancreatic duct. NSAIDs (rectal indomethacin) and pancreatic stenting have been shown to decrease rates of PEP in adults. The ESGE/ESPHGAN strongly recommend NSAID prophylaxis in pediatric ERCP >14 years of age. However, there is no consensus regarding these modalities in pediatric ERCP, although they are commonly used. Of note, there is a report in which PEP rates were increased after pancreatic stenting in children. Additionally, the role of octreotide (Sandostatin®) or serine protease inhibitors is unclear. Finally, there is a movement toward increased hydration protocols both before and after ERCP which may be important.

Several adverse events are specifically related to endoscopic biliary or pancreatic sphincterotomy (ES). Bleeding after ES is uncommon and typically can be controlled with injection or spray of 1:10 000 epineph-rine. A needle that can be manipulated by the duodenoscope elevator is necessary. Balloon tamponade with an extraction balloon for 3–5 minutes can be used. Additional tools include hemostatic clips and stents (plastic and fully covered expandable metal), although angiography and surgical therapies could be used if endoscopic treatment was not successful or with persistent or more rapid bleeding.

Also related to sphincterotomy is the risk of retroperitoneal perforation of the duodenum which has been described in children.

Finally, infection, including cholangitis, is a well-known risk of ERCP. The highest risk for infection is in patients with biliary obstruction from tumor, sclerosing cholangitis and liver transplant-related stricture. Prophylactic antibiotics are recommended in these cases as well as patients with biliary obstruction unlikely to be resolved with adequate drainage. Systemic infections have been linked to CRE related to endoscope reprocessing and issues with the duodenoscope elevator. The US Centers for Disease Control and Prevention reported concerns to the FDA in 2013. Although CRE infections have been reported in pediatric patients, to date there have not been any reported cases in children linked to ERCP.

Biliary indications for diagnostic and therapeutic ERCP

Technical success (>90%) for ERCP in children is high. Results and complication rates (2.3–9.7%) of ERCP in children are similar to those in adults, with no procedure-related mortality.

Biliary indications for diagnostic and thera-peutic ERCP are listed in Table 37.2.

Biliary atresia

Biliary atresia (BA) presents in the first few months of life and is defined as segmental or diffuse obliteration of the extrahepatic bile ducts. The extent and site of atresia may be variable. Early diagnosis is critical for success of the Kasai portoenterostomy. In the past 10–20% of infants required surgical exploration and intraoperative cholangiogram to establish a correct diagnosis. ERCP offers superior diagnostic visualization of the biliary tree in infants and neonates, although it is still an invasive procedure. Indications in infants need evaluation in a multidisciplinary setting. Over recent years, ERCP has been shown to be safe and effective in the early diagnosis of BA in challenging cases.

Three types of ERCP findings have been described (Table 37.3). Type 1 findings are

Table 37.2 Biliary indications for diagnostic and therapeutic ERCP

Diagnostic: clinical suspicion or diagnosis	Therapeutic
Biliary atresia	Sphincterotomy
Choledochal cyst	Sphincteroplasty
Choledocholithiasis	Stone extraction
Benign and malignant strictures	Stricture dilation
Primary sclerosing cholangitis	Stent placement (plastic or FCMS)
Pre- and post-operative evaluation	Choledochoscopy
Hepatobiliary tumors	EHL or laser lithotripsy
Hepatic injury (post-surgical or traumatic)	Nasobiliary drainage

EHL, electrohydraulic lithotripsy; FCMS, fully covered metal stent.

Table 37.3 ERCP findings in infants with suspected biliary atresia

Type 1	No visualization of biliary tree; absence of bile in the duodenum, normal pancreaticogram (35% of cases)
Type 2	Opacification of distal common bile duct (CBD) and gallbladder, no bile in duodenum, normal pancreaticogram (35%)
Type 3	3a: Visualization of the gallbladder and CBD. Presence of bile lakes in the porta hepatis
	3b: Visualization of both hepatic ducts bile lakes (30%)

inconclusive, and the diagnosis should be confirmed intraoperatively, while type 2 and 3 findings are diagnostic of BA. Published data from King's College Hospital, London, showed that ERCP allowed avoidance of an exploratory laparotomy in ~40% of infants with cholestatic jaundice and suspected BA. A considerable proportion of these infants had no evidence of hepatic dysfunction during long-term follow-up. The diagnosis established by ERCP was incorrect in only 1.6% of infants with neonatal cholestasis. Two newer approaches, laparoscopic cholangiography and magnetic resonance cholangiopancreatography (MRCP), are available but more data are necessary to validate their diagnostic accuracy. We have also used percutaneous cholecystography to aid in diagnosis.

Choledochal cysts

Choledochal cysts (CC) are anomalies of bile ducts frequently associated with anomalous pancreaticobiliary union (ABPU); the so-called "long common channel" is defined as a confluence of the common bile and pancreatic ducts external to the ampulla and duodenal wall (Figures 37.1 and 37.2). The association is reported in more than 80% of cases. CC are usually identified in infancy or childhood, although cases of delayed diagnosis in older children and adults have been reported. The

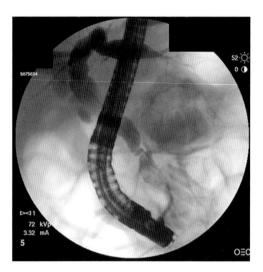

Figure 37.1 Long common channel with choledochal cyst.

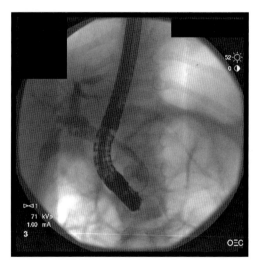

Figure 37.2 Long common channel with choledochal cyst and choledochocele.

Todani classification is the standard nomenclature for CC (Table 37.4). The common presentation includes abdominal pain, jaundice, and acute recurrent pancreatitis. Associated complications include intraductal stones, cholelithiasis, intrahepatic abscess, and biliary neoplasia.

The two most common surgical therapies for CC are complete cyst excision with either hepaticojejunostomy with a Roux-en-Y or duodenoduodenostomy. The diagnostic role of ERCP is to define the anatomy of the pancreaticobiliary junction. This information helps the surgeon estimate the distal level of the CC resection, avoiding complications due to preservation of a long remnant of a choledochal cyst.

In many children with CC complicated by intraductal lithiasis (biliary and/or pancreatic), ERCP with sphincterotomy serves as a bridge before definitive surgical therapy and decompression of the hepatobiliary system. Biliary stents are commonly used, however in ABPU can potentially obstruct the pancreatic duct depending on the angle of the junction.

In cases of small intramural choledochocele, an endoscopic unroofing of the cyst has been described, but there are no reports regarding the long-term outcomes of children managed by this method. On rare occasions, biliary rhabdomyosarcoma can mimic clinical and radiographic findings of CC. ERCP with intraductal endoscopy has also been used for diagnostic purposes and directed biopsies. Endoscopic biopsy can reduce the need for diagnostic laparotomy and tumor spread related to percutaneous biopsy (Figures 37.3 and 37.4).

Choledocholithiasis

Cholelithiasis has become more frequently diagnosed in children. Choledocholithiasis is reported in up to one-third of symptomatic patients. As in adults, obesity and Hispanic background are increasingly recognized as important risk factors for gallstones in children. Sickle cell disease and other hemoglobinopathies remain important pediatric risk factors. Issa *et al.* reported 37% of 125 children who underwent ERCP for obstructive jaundice or biliary colic. All cases were managed endoscopically with ES and balloon stone extraction without the need for surgical CBD exploration.

Therapeutic ERCP with ES and stone extraction is the treatment of choice for children with choledocholithiasis post cholecystectomy. For children with cholelithiasis, there is no consensus on whether suspicion of common bile duct (CBD) stones warrants ERCP before laparoscopic cholecystectomy or routine intraoperative cholangiogram to eliminate the need for pre- or postoperative ERCP. However, there are growing data in children and adults that in patients with choledocholithiasis, cholecystectomy is ideally performed during the same hospital admission.

Table 37.4 Todani classification of choledochal cyst (based on the shape of affected segments)

Type	Description	Occurence
1	1A: Segmental or diffuse saccular dilation of extrahepatic biliary tree	80–90%
	1B: Segmental dilation of CBD (more often in the distal portion), with normal bile duct between the cyst and cystic duct	
	1C: Fusiform dilation of CBD	
2	Choledochal diverticulum: isolated protrusion of the common bile duct wall	2%
3	Choledochocele: isolated involvement of the intraduodenal portion of CBD. The major duodenal papilla is bulging	1.5–5%
4	4a: Multiple dilations of intra- and extrahepatic bile ducts	20%
	4b: Multiple dilation of extrahepatic bile ducts	
5	Caroli disease: Multiple usually small dilations of the intrahepatic bile ducts	

CBD, common bile duct.

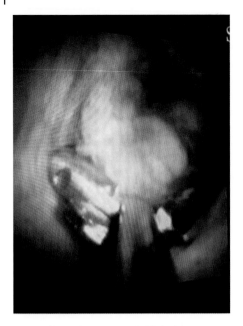

Figure 37.3 Two-year-old child with rhabdomyosarcoma. Cholangioscopic view with forceps biopsy.

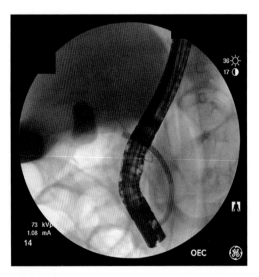

Figure 37.4 Fluoroscopic view of a 4-year-old child with rhabdomyosarcoma during choledochoscopy.

One of the challenges in the management of choledocholithiasis is identifying patients with the highest likelihood of having a stone at the time of endoscopy. The ASGE has previously suggested considering ERCP for patients with (i) stone visualized on imaging, (ii) total bilirubin greater than 4 mg/dL, or (iii) cholangitis. Additional considerations for ERCP are moderate likelihood of stones in patients with a total bilirubin of 1.8 mg/dL and a dilated bile duct above 6 mm. These criteria were unable to predict choledocholithiasis in a small series of pediatric patients, and conjugated bilirubin alone was best at predicting the risk of stone. This has been further evaluated in the multicenter international Pediatric ERCP Database Initiative (PEDI) demonstrating conjugated bilirubin as an important indicator. Of note, more than 35% of patients had a normal bilirubin, highlighting the challenges in these cases. Additionally, more than 50% of patients with gallstone pancreatitis passed their stone prior to ERCP, suggesting the complementary role of MRCP and endoscopic ultrasound (EUS).

In our practice, we perform ERCP prior to cholecystectomy in children with cholelithiasis, visualized stone or dilated CBD on abdominal ultrasound or cross-sectional imaging, gallstone pancreatitis and elevated biochemical markers of obstruction (conjugated bilirubin and gamma-glutamyl transferase). We also perform ERCP postoperatively in patients with persistently elevated or rising aminotransferases or related labs, abdominal pain and imaging suggestive of retained CBD stones.

Primary sclerosing cholangitis

Primary sclerosing cholangitis (PSC) is a chronic progressive liver disorder, commonly associated with inflammatory bowel disease, characterized by ongoing inflammation, obliteration and fibrosis of both intra- and extrahepatic bile ducts. Approximately 50% of symptomatic patients will develop cirrhosis and liver failure and require liver transplantation. PSC is characterized by the development of multiple strictures dividing bile ducts into short segments of normal size or dilated bile ducts of a beaded or pearl necklace pattern

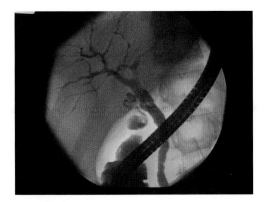

Figure 37.5 Primary sclerosing cholangitis.

(Figure 37.5). The gallbladder and cystic duct are involved in up to 15% of cases. PSC carries an increased risk of malignancy, especially cholangiocarcinoma.

Endoscopic retrograde cholangiopancreatography is indicated in children with suspected PSC, if the results of the MRCP are inconclusive. In some patients, cholestasis is secondary to a dominant stricture defined as a discrete area of narrowing with the extrahepatic biliary tree. Dominant strictures of the extrahepatic bile duct occur in 7–20% of patients with PSC and cholestasis. Patients with CBD stricture are candidates for therapeutic ERCP with the controversy surrounding the use of plastic stents compared to serial balloon dilations without stents. Stenting is associated with more infectious complications and adverse events compared to balloon dilations. A recent randomized controlled trial favors the use of balloon dilation alone, but the ESGE recommendations on PSC leave this decision to the endoscopist as to which method is used. ERCP treatment of dominant strictures can lower morbidity rates in adults compared with percutaneous techniques. Although there is consensus amongst adults, data are lacking on the timing of brushings and biopsies to evaluate for cholangiocarcinoma in pediatric patients. Intraductal endoscopy offers another method with which to investigate indeterminate stricture in these patients.

Postsurgical and posttraumatic biliary disease

A bile leak after laparoscopic cholecystectomy, liver transplantation or traumatic injuries of bile ducts can be successfully treated by ERCP with ES and biliary stent placement or nasobiliary drainage (Figure 37.6). A stricture of the CBD after cholecystectomy can be treated with plastic stents.

The clinical manifestations of a bile leak after blunt abdominal trauma are often insidious and nonspecific. It may delay diagnosis by a few days despite utilization of radioisotope scintigraphy in high-risk injuries such as a laceration greater than 4–cm or extending into the porta hepatis. Early diagnosis reduces morbidity and hospitalization. ERCP with stent placement contributes to prompt discovery of bile leak sources and dramatic recovery by effective reduction of the pressure in the bile ducts even if a stent does not bridge the gap between the damaged ducts.

In patients with suspected strictures post liver transplant, ES with biliary stenting has been used within days of transplant (Figures 37.7–37.10). We prefer plastic stents to FCMS, although they have been used in pediatric liver transplant recipients. Cast syndrome in which sludge and debris form a cast along

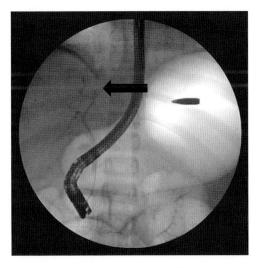

Figure 37.6 Fourteen-year-old child with traumatic bile leak.

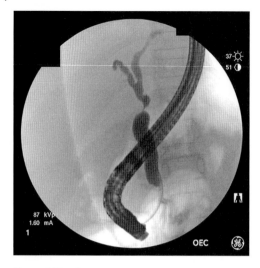

Figure 37.7 Seven-year-old liver transplant recipient with anastomotic stricture.

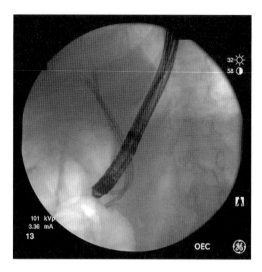

Figure 37.9 Fourteen-year-old liver transplant recipient with two plastic biliary stents.

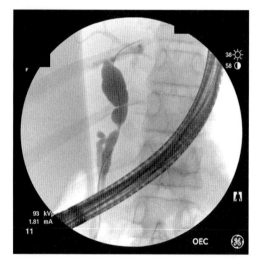

Figure 37.8 Sixteen-year-old liver transplant recipient with acute liver failure with anastomotic stricture.

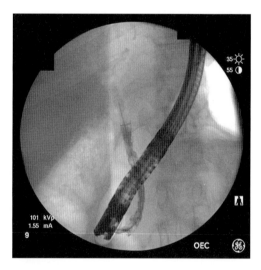

Figure 37.10 Fourteen-year-old liver transplant recipient with fully covered metal stent for biliary stricture.

the length of the duct may require intraductal endoscopy to evaluate and treat.

Pancreatic indications for diagnostic and therapeutic ERCP

Acute recurrent and chronic pancreatitis are the most common indications for ERCP in pediatric patients. A complete list of pancreatic indications is given in Table 37.5.

Acute pancreatitis

Noninvasive imaging such as transabdominal ultrasound (US) (for nonobese patients) is the first-line imaging study for acute pancreatitis in children, specifically in suspected gallstone pancreatitis. Due to risks of ionizing radiation, CT scans are recommended in patients who have clinical deterioration or in whom a diagnosis is unclear. MRCP can be useful for determination of choledocholithiasis, performed

Table 37.5 Pancreatic indications for diagnostic and therapeutic ERCP

Diagnostic	Therapeutic
Recurrent pancreatitis	Biliary pancreatitis
Chronic pancreatitis	Papillary stenosis
Pancreatic mass	Stenosis of the main pancreatic duct
Evaluation of ABPU	
Pancreas divisum	Pancreas divisum
	Pancreatic pseudocyst
	Pancreatic duct leak (posttraumatic or surgical)
	Stricture dilation
	Stent placement (plastic or FCMS)
	Intraductal endoscopy
	EHL or laser lithotripsy
	Nasopancreatic drainage

ABPU, anomalous pancreaticobiliary union; EHL, electrohydraulic lithotripsy; FCMS, fully covered metal stent.

with contrast for pancreatic tumors, and demonstrate loss of enhancement in necrotizing pancreatitis. Both CT and MRCP can determine the extent and severity of acute pancreatitis, as well as sequelae (e.g. acute fluid collection or necrosis). Diagnostic ERCP has largely been replaced by these other imaging modalities (see Table 37.6). A normal diameter of the major pancreatic duct ranges from 1.4 to 2.1 in the head (3–4 mm in adults) of the pancreas to 1.1–1.9 mm in the body.

During the acute phase of pancreatitis, ERCP is only indicated in biliary pancreatitis, pediatric patients with choledochal cysts, or those with associated acute cholangitis secondary to obstruction near the major papilla. Therapeutic ERCP with biliary sphincterotomy is recommended in cases with a high suspicion for an obstructing stone on US, MRCP or EUS. Our recent data suggest patients with gallstone pancreatitis are more likely to have passed a stone than those with suspected choledocholithiasis in the absence of pancreatitis. Finally, there is a role for ERCP in more prolonged bouts of pancreatitis if imaging is

Table 37.6 Role of MRCP and ERCP in children with pancreatic disorders

Type	Diagnostic approach	Therapeutic strategy with ERCP
Acute pancreatitis	MRCP (or CT scan)	Biliary pancreatitis with confirmed dilation of CBD: sphincterotomy, stone extraction, occlusion cholangiogram
Recurrent pancreatitis	MRCP with or without secretin ERCP reserved for children with unresolved diagnostic dilemmas and if MRCP not possible	Biliary and pancreatic sphincterotomy, pancreatic stone extraction, dilation and pancreatic stent • Preoperative management: endoscopic sphincterotomy, dilations, stone removal for children with anomalous pancreaticobiliary junction • Sphincterotomy of the major or minor duodenal papilla • Endoscopic marsupialization of a duplication cyst into the duodenal lumen • Papillary stenosis (formerly SOD type I)
Chronic pancreatitis	Same as recurrent pancreatitis	Endoscopic sphincterotomy, stone/sludge removal, drainage procedures, and intraductal endoscopy

CBD, common bile duct; CT, computed tomography; ERCP, endoscopic retrograde cholangiopancreatography; MRCP, magnetic resonance cholangiopancreatography; SOD, sphincter of Oddi dysfunction.

suggestive of a new stricture or secondary leak. Similarly, ERCP has been utilized effectively in patients with traumatic pancreatitis. In this case pancreatic duct stenting without or without sphincterotomy may be necessary.

Recurrent pancreatitis

There are obstructive and nonobstructive forms of recurrent pancreatitis, with more than 50% of cases having a genetic basis from either PRSS1, CFTR, SPINK1, or CTRC mutations. Limited use of diagnostic ERCP is ideal when MRCP is unrevealing. Endoscopic biopsy and brush cytology can also be used as an adjunct. The role of therapeutic ERCP in acute recurrent pancreatitis remains controversial, but biliary sphincterotomy appears to have utility. In patients with acute recurrent pancreatitis (ARP) after biliary sphincterotomy, pancreatic sphincterotomy with or without stent can be attempted. Studies in children are needed to further evaluate the benefits of sphincterotomy for ARP in children. Therapeutic ERCP is indicated in children with recurrent nonbiliary pancreatitis and severe dilation, strictures, and stones (all findings consistent with chronic pancreatitis) within the main pancreatic duct and congenital anomalies such as pancreas divisum.

Anomalous pancreaticobiliary union

Anomalous pancreaticobiliary union (APBU) or junction is defined as the confluence of the common bile duct and pancreatic duct beyond the sphincter of Oddi. In adults, the distance for anomalous biliopancreatic junction is considered to be 15 mm or greater from the ampulla but a normal junction is considered to be less than 3 mm for children under 1 year old and 5 mm in teenagers. The anomalous junction allows mixing of pancreatic enzymes with bile and it is often associated with a choledochal cyst (CC). APBU is considered an important contributing factor for development of cholangiocarcinoma and protein plugs.

Common clinical manifestations of APBU are chronic abdominal pain, obstructive jaundice, and/or recurrent pancreatitis. Endoscopic sphincterotomy is effective as initial therapy, and surgery in those with CC. There continues to be debate as to the role of definitive surgery in those without CC or whisk shape CC (forme fruste CC).

Pancreas divisum

Pancreas divisum is considered the most common congenital anomaly of the pancreas. It occurs in approximately 5% of the general population. In most cases, it does not produce any symptoms. This malformation occurs during embryogenesis due to lack of fusion between the ventral and dorsal pancreatic buds. The most reliable methods of diagnosis are ERCP or secretin-enhanced MRCP. "Long" position for cannulation is helpful and secretin may also be necessary to identify the orifice. Recent data from the INSPPIRE consortium suggest that pancreas divisum is more common than in the general population and occurred in 14.5% of patients with recurrent and chronic pancreatitis.

The ventral (main) pancreatic duct appears short because it is not connected to the body of the pancreas. The dorsal duct (minor duct of Santorini) drains the body and tail of the pancreas. There is a complete form of pancreas divisum (Figure 37.11) and several incomplete variations, in which a partial communication between the duct exists. Pancreatitis occurs when the minor papilla becomes edematous or stenotic, preventing adequate drainage of pancreatic fluid into the duodenum via the duct of Santorini.

Therapeutic ERCP consists of endoscopic sphincterotomy (Table 37.7) of the minor and also major papilla (in the case of incomplete pancreas divisum) and stone removal, allowing better pancreatic drainage. Temporary placement of a stent into the minor pancreatic duct may contribute to resolution of symptoms in children with recurrent pancreatitis and pancreas divisum. One of the main concerns in performing ES of the minor papilla is the length (and depth) of the incision. Two

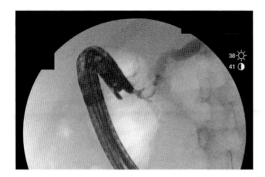

Figure 37.11 Thirteen-year-old child with pancreas divisum and cystic fibrosis. Stone within dorsal pancreatic duct.

Table 37.7 Steps of biliary and pancreatic sphincterotomy technique

Visualization of major papilla

Cannulation and guidewire insertion of biliary and/or pancreatic ducts

Opacification of biliary and/or pancreatic duct

Optimal direction of sphincterotome: 11–12 o'clock for biliary ES and 1–2 o'clock for pancreatic ES

Precut with needle-knife type sphincterotome for unsuccessful standard cannulation technique. Consider pancreatic stent prior to needle-knife to assist in biliary ES. Bleeding is a common early adverse event; papillary stenosis is a late event

ES, endoscopic sphincterotomy.

techniques of minor papilla ES are equally safe and effective: standard pull-type ES for patients with a naïve papilla or a needle-knife cut over an existing plastic stent. The physician's choice of technique is based on the specific endoscopic appearance of the papilla.

Functional biliary sphincter disorder (previously sphincter of Oddi dysfunction; SOD)

Functional biliary sphincter disorder (FBSD), previously referred to as SOD, is a rare cause of abdominal pain in children. It is considered as a motility disorder related to abnormal contractility of the sphincter without anatomical obstruction. The Rome IV Criteria are met for

FBSD if a patient has *all* three: biliary type pain, elevated aminotransferases or dilated bile duct and the absence of bile duct stones or other structural abnormalities. Supportive criteria for FBSD include a normal amylase or lipase, abnormal sphincter of Oddi manometry or findings on hepatobiliary scintigraphy.

The former SOD type I is now thought to be a distinct entity caused by stenosis of the papilla, typically with associated abnormalities including elevated aminotransferases and/or pancreatic enzymes *and* ductal dilation. The treatment of papillary stenosis is typically biliary sphincterotomy. However, contributing to the change not only in name but also in management of SOD type II and III was a recent randomized double-blinded study, EPISOD (Evaluating Predictors and Interventions in Sphincter of Oddi Dysfunction), which evaluated the role of sphincterotomy in SOD. Based on this trial, patients with SOD type III did not respond to sphincterotomy compared to sham treatment. Additionally, manometry findings did not correlate with patient outcomes. Although not the specific aim of the EPISOD trial, patients with SOD type II, with either lab or imaging abnormality, did not have the expected success of sphincterotomy. We do not recommend manometry or sphincterotomy for pediatric patients with FBSD (the former SOD type III). The role of sphincterotomy for pediatric patients with the former SOD II (abnormal imaging or blood tests) requires further study, but is likely to be treated as FBSD. If sphincterotomy is considered in these patients, a more extensive discussion about available evidence in adults may be appropriate. Of note, only limited data are available related to the sphincter pressure in children, in which 65 out of 245 children met criteria for elevated pressure.

Chronic pancreatitis

In at least 70% of pediatric patients with chronic pancreatitis (48% in ARP), mutations in PRSS1, SPINK1, CFTR, and CTRC have been identified. The current treatment typically includes pancreatic sphincterotomy with stent placement. In a large retrospective series from Poland, 223 pancreatic duct stent procedures were performed in 72 children, with a relative decrease in number of annual episodes of pancreatitis per year. Stone removal with balloon or using intraductal endoscopy with electrohydraulic lithotripsy (EIIL) or YAG-holmium laser can also be utilized. The INSPPIRE consortium reported 117 pediatric patients with a physician-rated utility of around 50% for both ARP and chronic pancreatitis (CP). Obstructive symptoms including stones and strictures were more likely to be found if these features were present.

Pancreatic pseudocyst, necrosis, and trauma

Acute fluid collections of the pancreas can develop into pancreatic pseudocysts. If there is pancreatic necrosis, these can become walled-off necrosis (WON). Pancreatic pseudocyst and WON could be suspected based on clinical grounds: persistent abdominal pain, elevated amylase or lipase, or cholestasis due to distal CBD compression four weeks after an initial attack of acute pancreatitis or trauma. Transabdominal ultrasound may identify the collections, but MRCP and CT are the optimal diagnostic tests. Pseudocysts frequently resolve spontaneously.

Common indications for intervention are trauma-related acute pancreatitis with increased risk of main duct disruption, presence of large, well-organized pseudocysts six weeks after the episode of acute pancreatitis, and infected cysts. The endoscopic approach for children with pancreatic fluid collections has evolved, with transgastric drainage by EUS often the primary treatment. ERCP may be necessary but a large cyst may lead to distortion of the duct and also lead to inadequate treatment. In patients with traumatic pancreatitis, treatment includes ERCP with transductal placement with a pancreatic stent over the guidewire. Transgastric drainage (Figure 37.12) with either plastic stents or fully covered metal stents is typically done with EUS to avoid damage to neighboring vessels. The recurrence rate of fluid collections with older methods is approximately 15%. Surgery is indicated if the fluid collection of WON persists.

EUS in pancreatitis

Multiple studies support a high value of EUS as a source of valuable information contributing to the diagnosis and treatment of chronic pancreatitis, pancreatic pseudocyst drainage, choledocholithiasis, pancreas divisum, and duodenal duplication. EUS is complementary

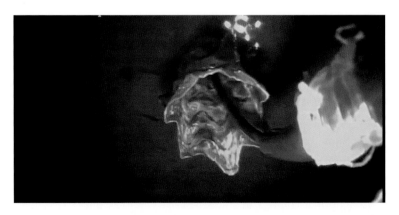

Figure 37.12 Sixteen-year-old child with stent placement cystgastrostomy for pancreatic pseudocyst.

to ERCP in these conditions and can guide therapy.

Duodenal duplication cyst

A duodenal duplication cyst is a known but rare cause of acute recurrent pancreatitis. It represents 4–12% of all intestinal duplications. It is frequently located in the second portion of the duodenum. Duodenal duplications could be connected to or isolated from the biliary tree. Symptoms and signs are vomiting, chronic abdominal pain, and gastrointestinal bleeding due to ulceration of ectopic gastric mucosa.

Diagnosis of the duodenal duplication cyst is made by ultrasound, MRCP, direct endoscopic visualization, and endoscopic ultrasound. EUS provides essential information regarding the relationship between the duodenal duplication, CBD, and pancreas. It helps with decision making for optimal treatment: surgery versus therapeutic endoscopy. Treatment consists of surgical resection or endoscopic opening of the common wall (marsupialization into the duodenal lumen), depending on the location of the duplication, its type, size, and EUS findings. Endoscopic therapy of duplication is summarized in Table 37.8.

Table 37.8 Steps of endoscopic marsupialization of duodenal duplication

Endoscopic visualization
EUS: Assessment of the common wall between the duplication cyst and the duodenum and involvement of the bile ducts
ERCP: Visualization of the extrahepatic bile ducts
Endoscopic dissection of duodenal duplication common wall with needle type or standard sphincterotome
Hemostasis

ERCP, endoscopic retrograde cholangiopancreatography; EUS, endoscopic ultrasound.

Conclusion

Endoscopic retrograde cholangiopancreatography is a very effective diagnostic and therapeutic procedure in children with pancreaticobiliary disorders. It is safe in the hands of an experienced pediatric gastroenterologist. Therapeutic ERCP can be used as a definitive treatment for children with specific pancreaticobiliary disorders and may serve as a bridge therapy to surgery.

 • See companion website for videos relating to this chapter topic: www.wiley.com/go/gershman3e

 FURTHER READING

Antaki F, Tringali A, Deprez P, *et al*. A case series of symptomatic intraluminal duodenal duplication cysts: presentation, endoscopic therapy, and long-term outcome. *Gastrointest Endosc* 2008, **67**, 163–168.

Attwell A, Borak G, Hawes R, *et al*. Endoscopic pancreatic sphincterotomy for pancreas divisum by using a needle-knife or standard pull-type technique: safety and reintervention rates. *Gastrointest Endosc* 2006, **64**, 705–711.

Barange K, Mas E, Railhac N, *et al*. Endoscopic management of biliary and pancreatic diseases in children. *Arch Pediatr* 2009, **16**, 811–813.

Bogue CO, Murphy AJ, Gerstle JT, *et al*. Risk factors complications, and outcomes of gallstones in children: a single-center review. *J Pediatr Gastroenterol Nutr* 2010, **50**, 303–308.

Brown KO, Goldschmiedt M. Endoscopic therapy of biliary and pancreatic disorders in children. *Endoscopy* 1994, **26**, 719–723.

Buscaglia JM, Kallo AN. Pancreatic sphincterotomy: technique, indications and complications. *World J Gastroenterol* 2007, **13**, 4064–4071.

Canty TG Sr, Weinman D. Treatment of pancreatic duct disruption in children by endoscopically placed stent. *J Pediatr Surg* 2001, **36**, 345–348.

Castagnetti M, Houben C, Patel S. Minimally invasive management of bile leaks after blunt liver trauma in children. *J Pediatr Surg* 2006, **41**, 1539–1544.

Chandrasekhara V, Khashab MA, Muthusamy VR, *et al.* Adverse events associated with ERCP. *Gastrointest Endosc* 2017, **85**, 32–47.

Cheng CL, Fogel EL, Sherman S, *et al.* Diagnostic and therapeutic endoscopic retrograde cholangiopancreatography in children: a large series report. *J Pediatr Gastroenterol Nutr* 2005, **41**, 445–453.

Coehen S, Bacon BR, Berlin JA, *et al.* National Institutes of Health State-of-the-Science Conference Statement: ERCP for diagnosis and therapy. Jan 14–16. *Gastrointest Endosc* 2002, **56**, 803–809.

Cohen S, Kalinin M, Yaron A, *et al.* Endoscopic ultrasonography in pediatric patients with gastrointestinal disorders. *J Pediatr Gastroenterol Nutr* 2008, **46**, 551–554.

Costamagna G, Shah SK, Tringali A. Current management of postoperative complications and benign biliary strictures. *Gastrointest Endosc Clin North Am* 2003, **13**, 635–648.

Cotton PB, Laage NJ. Endoscopic retrograde cholangiopancreatography in children. *Arch Dis Child* 1982, **57**, 131–136.

Cotton PB, Durkalski V, Romagnuolo J, *et al.* Effect of endoscopic sphincterotomy for suspected sphincter of Oddi dysfunction on pain-related disability following cholecystectomy: the EPISOD randomized clinical trial. *JAMA* 2014, **311**, 2101–2109.

Etemad B, Whitcomb DC. Chronic pancreatitis: diagnosis, classification, and new genetic developments. *Gastroenterology* 2001, **120**, 682–707.

Fishman DS, Chumpitazi BP, Raijman I, *et al.* Endoscopic retrograde cholangiography for pediatric choledocholithiasis: assessing the need for endoscopic intervention. *World J Gastrointest Endosc* 2016, **8**, 425–432.

Guelrud M. ERCP and endoscopic sphyncterotomy in infants and children with jaundice due to common bile ducts stones. *Gastrointest Endosc* 1992, **38**, 450–453.

Guelrud M. Endoscopic retrograde cholangiopancreatography. *Gastrointest Endosc Clin North Am* 2001, **11**, 585–601.

Guelrud M, Morera C, Rodriguez M, *et al.* Normal and anomalous pancreaticobiliary union in children and adolescents. *Gastrointest Endosc* 1999, **50**, 189–193.

Guelrud M, Jean D, Mendoza S, *et al.* ERCP in the diagnosis of extrahepatic biliary atresia. *Gastrointest Endosc* 1991, **37**, 522–526.

Hand BH. Anatomy and embriology of the biliary tract and pancreas. In: Sivak MV Jr (ed.). Gastroenterologic Endoscopy, 2nd edn. WB Saunders, Philadelphia, 1995, pp. 862–877.

Harpavat S, Raijman I, Hernandez JA, *et al.* Single-center experience of choledochoscopy in pediatric patients. *Gastrointest Endosc* 2012, **76**, 685–688.

Himes RW, Raijman I, Finegold MJ. Diagnostic and therapeutic role of endoscopic retrograde cholangiopancreatography in biliary rhabdomiosarcoma. *World J Gastroenterol* 2008, **14**, 4823–4825.

Holcomb GW III. Gallbladder disease. In: O'Neil JA Jr, Grosfeld JL, Fonkaslrud EW, *et al* (eds). Principles of Pediatric Surgery. Mosby, St Louis, MO, 2003, pp. 645– 646.

Issa H, Al Haddad A, Al Salem AH. Diagnostic and therapeutic ERCP in the pediatric age group. *Pediatr Surg Int* 2007, **23**, 111–116.

Jang JY, Yoon CH, Kim KN. Endoscopic retrograde cholangiopancreatography in pancreatic and biliary tract disease in Korean Children. *World J Gastroenterol* 2010, **16**, 490–495.

Jeffrey GP. Histological and immunohisto-chemical study of the gallbladder lesion in primary sclerosing cholangitis. *Gut* 1991, **32**, 424–429.

Keil R, Snajdauf J, Stuj J, *et al.* Endoscopic retrograde cholangiopancreatography in infants and children. *Indian J Gastroenterol* 2000, **19**, 1757.

Kumar S, Ooi CY, Werlin S, *et al.* Risk factors associated with pediatric acute recurrent and chronic pancreatitis: lessons from INSPPIRE. *JAMA Pediatr* 2016, **170**, 562–569.

Lin TK, Abu-El-Haija M, Nathan JD, *et al.* Pancreas divisum in pediatric acute recurrent and chronic pancreatitis: report from INSPPIRE. *J Clin Gastroenterol* 2019, **53**, 3232–e238.

Lipsett PA, Segev DL, Colombani PM. Biliary atresia and biliary cyst. *Baillière's Clin Gastroenterol* 1997, **11**, 619–641.

Mah D, Wales P, Niere I, *et al.* Management of suspected common bile duct stones in children: role of selective intraoperative cholangiogram and endoscopic retrograde cholangiopancreatography. *J Pediatr Surg* 2004, **39**, 808–812.

Manfredi R, Lucidi V, Gui B, *et al.* Idiopathic chronic pancreatitis in children: MR cholangiopancreatography after secretin administration. *Radiology* 2002, **224**, 675–682.

Maple JT, Ben-Menachem T, Anderson MA, *et al.* The role of endoscopy in the evaluation of suspected choledocholithiasis. *Gastrointest Endosc* 2010, **71**, 1–9.

Mehta S, Lopez ME, Chumpitazi BP, *et al.* Clinical characteristics and risk factors for symptomatic pediatric gallbladder disease. *Pediatrics* 2012, **129**, e82–e88.

Michailidis L, Aslam B, Grigorian A, *et al.* The efficacy of endoscopic therapy for pancreas divisum a meta-analysis. *Ann Gastroenterol* 2017, **30**, 550–558.

Motte S. Risk factors for septicaemia following endoscopic biliary stenting. *Gastroenterology* 1991, **101**, 1374–1381.

Mushin K. Balloon dilation compared to stenting of dominant strictures in primary sclerosing cholangitis. *Am J Gastroenterol* 2001, **96**, 1059–1066.

Nathens AB, Curtis JR, Beale RJ, *et al.* Management of the critically ill patient with severe acute pancreatitis. *Crit Care Med* 2004, **32**, 2524–2536.

Newman KD, Powell DM, Holcom GW III. The management of cholidocholithiasis in children in era of laparoscopic cholecystectomy. *J Pediatr Surg* 1997, **32**, 1116–1119.

Norton KI, Glass RB, Kogan D, *et al.* MR cholangiography in the evaluation of neonatal cholestasis: initial results. *Radiology* 2002, **222**, 687–691.

Nose S, Hasegawa T, Soh H, *et al.* Laparoscopic cholecystocholangiography as an effective alternative exploratory laparotomy for differentiation of biliary atresia. *Surg Today* 2005, **35**, 925–928.

Oracz G, Pertkiewicz J, Kierkus J, *et al.* Efficiency of pancreatic duct stenting therapy in children with chronic pancreatitis. *Gastrointest Endosc* 2014, **80**, 1022–1029.

Ostroff JW. Post-transplant biliary problems. *Gastrointest Endosc Clin North Am* 2001, **11**, 163–183.

Perrelli L, Nanni L, Costamagna G, *et al.* Endoscopic treatment of chronic idiopathic pancreatitis in children. *J Pediatr Surg* 1996, **31**, 1396–1400.

Pfau PR, Chelimsky GG, Kinnard MF, *et al.* Endoscopic retrograde cholangiopancreatography in children and adolescents. *J Pediatr Gastroenterol Nutr* 2002, **35**, 619–623.

Ponsioen CY, Arnelo U, Bergquist A, *et al.* No superiority of stents vs. balloon dilatation for dominant strictures in patients with primary sclerosing cholangitis. *Gastroenterology* 2018, **155**, 752–759.

Rerknimitr R. Biliary tract complications after orthotopic liver transplantation with choledochocholedochostomy anastomosis: endoscopic findings and results of therapy. *Gastrointest Endosc* 2002, **55**, 224–231.

Rocca R, Castellino F, Daperno M, *et al.* Therapeutic ERCP in pediatric patients. *Dig Liver Dis* 2005, **37**, 357–362.

Saeky I, Takahashi Y, Matsuura T. Successful endoscopic unroofing for a pediatric choledo-chocele. *J Pediatr Surg* 2009, **44**, 1643–1645.

Salemis NS, Liatsos C, Kolios M, *et al.* Recurrent acute pancreatitis secondary to a duodenal duplication cyst in an adult. A case report and literature review. *Can J Gastroenterol* 2009, **23**, 749–752.

Saltzman JR. Endoscopic treatment of pancreas divisum: why, when, and how? *Gastrointest Endosc* 2006, **64**, 712–714.

Schaefer JF, Kirschner HJ, Lichy M, *et al.* Highly resolved free-breathing magnetic resonance cholangiopancreatography in the diagnostic workup of pancreaticobiliary diseases in infants and young children-initial experiences. *J Pediatr Surg* 2006, **41**, 1645–1651.

Screiber RA, Barker CC, Roberts EA. Biliary atresia: the Canadian experience. *J Pediatr* 2007, **151**, 659–665.

Shanmugam NP, Harrison PM, Devlin J, *et al.* Selective use of endoscopic retrograde cholangiopancreatography in the diagnosis of biliary atresia in infants younger than 100 days. *J Pediatr Gastroenterol Nutr* 2009, **49**, 435–441.

Sharma SS, Maharshi S. Endoscopic management of pancreatic pseudocyst in children; a long-term follow up. *J Pediatr Surg* 2008, **43**, 1636–1639.

Singham J, Yoshida EM, Scudamore C. Choledochal cysts. Part 3 of 3: Management. *Can J Surg* 2010, **53**, 51–56.

Suzuki M, Shimizu T, Kud T, *et al.* Non breath-hold MRCP in choledochal cyst in children. *J Pediatr Gastroenterol Nutr* 2006, **42**, 539–544.

Tagge EP, Hebra A, Goldberg A, *et al.* Pediatric laparoscopic biliary tract surgery. *Semin Pediatr Surg* 1988, **7**, 202–206.

Tarnasky PR, Palesch YY, Cunningham JT, *et al.* Minimally invasive therapy for choledocolithiasis in children. *Gastrointest Endosc* 1998, **47**, 189–192.

Terui K, Hishiki T, Saito T, *et al.* Pancreas divisum in pancreaticobiliary malfunction in children. *Pediatr Surg Int* 2010, **26**, 419–422.

Terui K, Yoshida H, Kouchi K, *et al.* Endoscopic sphincterotomy is a useful preoperative management for refractory pancreatitis associated with pancreaticobiliary malfunction. *J Pediatr Surg* 2008, **43**, 495–499.

Testoni PA, Mariani A, Curioni S, *et al.* MRCP-secretin test-guided management of idiopathic recurrent pancreatitis: long-term outcomes. *Gastrointest Endosc* 2008, **67**, 1028–1034.

Tipnis NA, Dua KS, Werlin SL. A retrospective assessment of magnetic resonance cholangiopancreatography in children. *J Pediatr Gastroenterol Nutr* 2008, **46**, 59–64.

Todani T, Watanabe Y, Narusue M, *et al.* Congenital bile duct cyst: classification, operative procedures and review of thirty-seven cases including cancer arising from choledocal cyst. *Am J Surg* 1977, **134**, 263–269.

Tringali A, Thomson M, Dumonceau JM, *et al.* Pediatric gastrointestinal endoscopy: European Society for Paediatric Gastrointestinal Endoscopy (ESGE) and European Society of Pediatric Gastroenterology Hepatology and Nutrition (ESPGHAN) guideline executive summary. *Endoscopy* 2017, **49**, 83–91.

Tröbs RB, Hemminghaus M, Cernaianu G, *et al.* Stone-containing periampullary duodenal duplication cyst with aberrant pancreatic duct. *J Pediatr Surg* 2009, **44**, 33–35.

Troendle DM, Fishman DS, Barth BA, *et al.* Therapeutic endoscopic retrograde cholangiopancreatography in pediatric patients with acute recurrent and chronic pancreatitis: data from the INSPPIRE (International Study group of Pediatric Pancreatitis: In search for a cuRE) Study. *Pancreas* 2017, **46**, 764–769.

Varadarajulu S, Wilcox CM, Eloubeidi MA. Impact of EUS in the evaluation of pancreaticobiliary disorders in children. *Gastrointest Endosc* 2005, **62**, 239–244.

Varadarajulu S, Wilcox CM, Hawes RH, *et al.* Technical outcomes and complications of ERCP in children. *Gastrointest Endosc* 2004, **60**, 367–371.

Verting IL, Tabber MM, Taminiau JAJM, *et al.* Is endoscopic retrograde cholangiography valuable and safe in children all ages? *J Pediatr Gastroenterol Nutr* 2009, **48**, 66–71.

Waldhausen JHT. Routine intraoperative cholangiography during laparoscopic cholecistectomy minimized unnecessary endoscopic retrograde cholangiography in children. *J Pediatr Surg* 2001, **36**, 881–884.

Waters GS, Crist DW, Davoudi M, *et al.* Management of choledocholithiasis encountered during laparoscopic cholecystectomy. *Am J Surg* 1996, **62**, 256–258.

38

Endoscopic drainage of pancreatic pseudocysts

Mike Thomson

 KEY POINTS

- EUS is helpful in identifying the optimum site for drainage through the gastric wall and in avoiding gastric vessels.
- A guidewire is inserted, having widened the initial incision with a balloon or a sphincterotome, and then one or more pigtail drainage catheters can be placed through the working channel of the endoscope.
- Specific pancreatic cystotomes are now available requiring a 3.2 mm working channel

- in the endoscope and have the advantage of only requiring one puncture of the cyst through the gastric wall.
- The drainage catheters will drain into the stomach and may extrude spontaneously from the cyst or may be withdrawn after a number of weeks by endoscopy under direct vision when the cyst has collapsed.

Pancreatitis

A number of reports have recently emerged on the utility of endoscopic ultrasosund (EUS) in chronic pancreatitis in childhood. However, the concept in children was utilized as early as 1998, and then later reported specifically for pancreaticobiliary disorders in 2005. This indication is more for diagnostic utility than therapeutic input. EUS-guided fine needle aspiration (EUS-FNA) has been found useful for the diagnosis of idiopathic fibrosing pancreatitis and EUS-guided Trucut needle biopsy may facilitate diagnosis of pathologies such as autoimmune pancreatitis in a relatively minimally invasive fashion. Microlithiasis may be identified as a putative contributor in chronic intermittent pancreatitis in children by EUS (see Chapter 16).

Pancreatic pseudocysts

Pancreatic pseudocysts are secondary to pancreatic damage and may be multietiological: traumatic; post pancreatitis of idiopathic origin; following chemotherapy; or any other cause of acute pancreatitis. They should be differentiated from malignant cysts but this is unusual in childhood and is a distinction necessary predominantly only in adult practice.

Presentation may be with a persistently raised amylase/lipase, with chronic pain, as an abdominal mass, or with consistent nausea/vomiting. Treatment to date has been either conservative, surgical, with the use of (as yet unproven) antisecretory agents such as octreotide or its longer-acting analogues (e.g., lanreotide), or via ERCP. More recently, transgastric cystostomies have been formed by endoscopy [1]. These are

---

Practical Pediatric Gastrointestinal Endoscopy, Third Edition. Edited by George Gershman and Mike Thomson.
© 2021 John Wiley & Sons Ltd. Published 2021 by John Wiley & Sons Ltd.
Companion website: www.wiley.com/go/gershman3e

either guided by endo-ultrasound, which is a safer option avoiding gastric vessels (Figure 38.1), or blind with prior epinephrine injection into the bulge in the gastric wall from the luminal surface and then incision into the injected area. The former is preferable using linear endo-ultrasound ideally but radial endo-ultrasound may at times be sufficient and has been described in children [2–5]. Indeed, EUS has become the accepted imaging and guiding procedure for drainage of pancreatic fluid collections in the past decade. EUS has been shown to be safe and effective and it has been the first-line therapy for uncomplicated pseudocysts.

Where walled-off pancreatic necrosis was originally thought to be a contraindication for endoscopic treatment, multiple case series have now shown that these fluid collections also can be treated endoscopically with low morbidity and mortality [6]. Usually, the cyst can be indirectly identified abutting the lesser or greater curvature and is quite obvious as a mass effect into the gastric lumen hence it is not mandatory to use EUS in obvious cases (Figure 38.2).

The initial incision may be made with an endo-knife (Figure 38.3) and once this is made, a sphincterotome may be inserted and employed to safely expand this incision. Subsequently, either straight ERCP plastic

stents or pig-tailed stents can be inserted into the pseudocyst and left in situ (Figure 38.4). Temporary placement of self-expanding metal stents has been reported [7]. Fluid will then follow the path of least resistance and the presumed communication with the pancreatic duct will close, preventing further accumulation of pancreatic fluid in the cyst. An endoscope may be inserted into the cyst, but this is

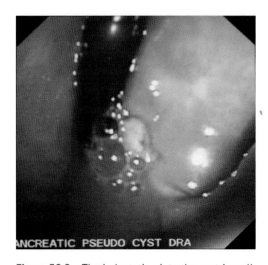

Figure 38.2 The indentation into the gastric wall can be seen easily identifying the position of the pseudocyst.

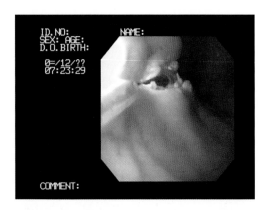

Figure 38.3 After endo-ultrasound has identified the cyst and a site which is free from gastric vessels, an endoknife followed by a sphincterotome (tapertome is best) is used to create a cauterized entry point from the stomach into the cyst. Adrenaline can be injected prior to the incision to further diminish the possibility of hemorrhage during incision.

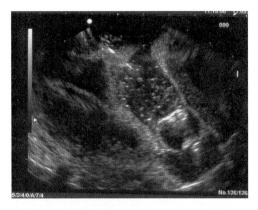

Figure 38.1 Transgastric linear endo-ultrasound needle puncture of a pancreatic pseudocyst. The linear needle can be seen as a straight white line in the upper part of the picture.

not strictly necessary (Figures 38.5 and 38.6). It is hoped that the gastric wall and the cyst will adhese and fibrose, creating a channel so that as the stents become unnecessary as the cyst naturally deflates, the stents are extruded and the fistula closes (Figure 38.7). This is the normal course of events. Patient symptom relief is acute and usually long-lasting. Complications are not common as long as gastric vessels are

avoided initially. A combined approach involving drainage through the papilla and transmural endoscopic drainage can be useful in the larger and more loculated cysts [8].

Efficacy and safety of this procedure in the pediatric population have been described utilizing ultrasound-guided drainage [9]. More recently, sphincterotomes have been devised and employed. These allow puncture, guide-wire insertion, and stent insertion all "through the scope" and prevent the complication of the

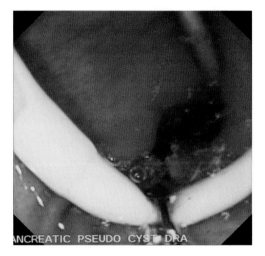

Figure 38.4 Grasping forceps are used to manipulate the stents (pig-tailed [blue] or straight [white]) through the gastrocystostomy that was created.

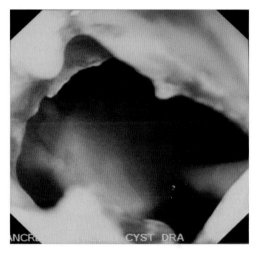

Figure 38.6 The endoscope is withdrawn from the pseudocyst.

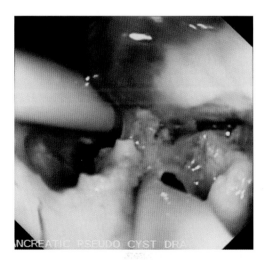

Figure 38.5 The stents are endoscopically observed in the pseudocyst, and membranes between loculations can be punctured as necessary.

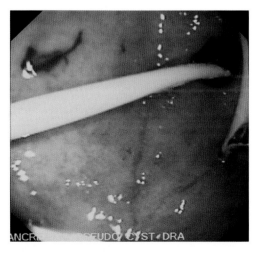

Figure 38.7 The endoscope is withdrawn from the stomach and the gastrocystostomy is left in place.

operator being unable to reinsert a guidewire if the initial endo-knife puncture leads to rapid decompression of the cyst with resultant loss of gastrocyst communication by endoscopy. This is the accessory of choice nowadays.

 • See companion website for videos relating to this chapter topic: www.wiley.com/go/gershman3e

REFERENCES

1 Gumaste VV, Aron J. Pseudocyst management: endoscopic drainage and other emerging techniques. *J Clin Gastroenterol* 2010, **44**(5), 326–331.

2 Theodoros D, Nikolaides P, Petousis G. Ultrasound-guided endoscopic transgastric drainage of a post-traumatic pancreatic pseudocyst in a child. *Afr J Paediatr Surg* 2010, **7**(3), 194–196.

3 Rossini CJ, Moriarty KP, Angelides AG. Hybrid notes: incisionless intragastric stapled cystgastrostomy of a pancreatic pseudocyst. *J Pediatr Surg* 2010, **45**(1), 80–83.

4 Al-Haddad M, El Hajj II, Eloubeidi MA. Endoscopic ultrasound for the evaluation of cystic lesions of the pancreas. *J Pancreas* 2010, **11**(4), 299–309.

5 Park DH, Lee SS, Moon SH, *et al.* Endoscopic ultrasound-guided versus conventional transmural drainage for pancreatic pseudocysts: a prospective randomized trial. *Endoscopy* 2009, **41**(10), 842–848.

6 Galasso D, Voermans RP, Fockens P. Role of endosonography in drainage of fluid collections and other NOTES procedures. *Best Pract Res Clin Gastroenterol* 2009, **23**(5), 781–789.

7 Belle S, Collet P, Post S, Kaehler G. Temporary cystogastrostomy with self-expanding metallic stents for pancreatic necrosis. *Endoscopy* 2010, **42**(6), 493–495.

8 Bhasin DK, Rana SS. Combining transpapillary pancreatic duct stenting with endoscopic transmural drainage for pancreatic fluid collections: two heads are better than one! *J Gastroenterol Hepatol* 2010, **25**(3), 433–434.

9 Jazrawi S, Barth B, Sreenarasimhaiah J. Efficacy of endoscopic ultrasound-guided drainage of pancreatic pseudocysts in a pediatric population. *Dig Dis Sci* 2011, **56**(3), 902–908

39

Duodenal web division by endoscopy

Mike Thomson, Shishu Sharma, Filippo Torroni, and Jonathan Goring

 KEY POINTS

- Preendoscopy MRCP is helpful in identifying the anatomical arrangement between the pancreaticobiliary radicle and the duodenal web or webs.
- Balloon dilation over a guidewire is preferable to incision with an endo-knife or sphincterotome which runs the risk of damaging the

- pancreaticobiliary channels, which may be within the web.
- A number of children have a distal second web and it is therefore important to visualize beyond the first web.
- The procedure may require a repeat if symptoms persist.

Congenital duodenal webs/diaphrams are a rare cause of duodenal obstruction. The incidence is estimated at anywhere from 1 in 10000 to 1 in 40000 patients. Congenital diaphragms are believed to be secondary to incomplete recanalization of the duodenal epithelium during the fourth and fifth weeks of gestation. The most common location of web formation is in the second portion of the duodenum near the ampulla. Patients with congenital webs often present with vomiting, abdominal distension, and failure to thrive. The mainstay of therapy has been surgical intervention with bypass or excision. Modern endoscopic techniques have revolutionized the management of duodenal diaphragms.

Successful endoscopic treatment has been reported and involves two approaches. First, it must be remembered that the pancreaticobiliary tree exit is embryologically inherent in such a congenital defect. Second, this defect

may exist undiagnosed for months and sometimes years as soft food, macerated by the stomach, can pass through even the smallest pinhole defect. In terms of treatment endoscopically, a number of options have been reported and fortunately a major laparotomy can now be avoided in most cases with this approach.

Either membranectomy via balloon dilation (Figure 39.1) or division using a ceramic-tip endo-knife may be successful, but the preferred and more successful (anecdotal) technique involves utilization of a double channel "operating endoscope." This ideal technique involves insertion of a guidewire through the defect (Figure 39.2) which can be very small, then anchoring the web which is of a 'windsock' type towards the scope by passing the balloon beyond the web and inflating it, then retracting the web (Figure 39.3). A ceramic-tip needle-knife can then be used to incise the web

Practical Pediatric Gastrointestinal Endoscopy, Third Edition. Edited by George Gershman and Mike Thomson.
© 2021 John Wiley & Sons Ltd. Published 2021 by John Wiley & Sons Ltd.
Companion website: www.wiley.com/go/gershman3e

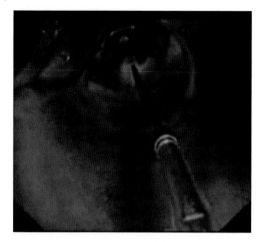

Figure 39.1 Simple balloon dilation of web/ diaphragm can be effective alone but may need repeating to gain adequate luminal patency over time.

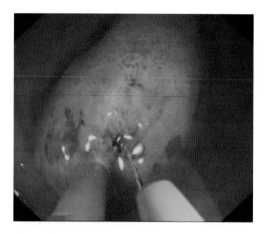

Figure 39.4 Dual-channel endoscope allows deployment of the endoknife to incise the web/ membrane whilst being stabilized by the balloon. Care must be taken to avoid the ampulla of Vater on the medial duodenal wall.

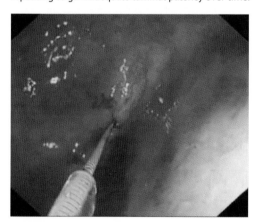

Figure 39.2 Guidewire of endoballoon passing through small apperture in web/diaphragm.

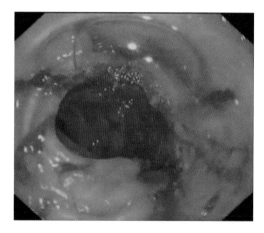

Figure 39.5 Adequate luminal patency achieved.

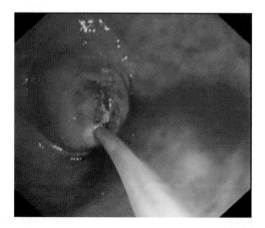

Figure 39.3 Endoballoon has been inflated and gentle traction allows membrane to be drawn towards endoscope for stabilization before incision.

in a direction corresponding to 3–8 o'clock, thereby avoiding the pancreaticobiliary radicles (Figure 39.4); endo-ultrasound can help in identifying these structures if necessary and a preceding MRCP is also useful in doing so. The ceramic tip prevents bursting of the balloon.

Not uncommonly, there may be a second web distal to the first and this one does not usually contain any ampulla-type structures. Full division of the membrane is not usually necessary to allow resolution of obstructive symptoms (Figure 39.5). On-table radiological contrast and imaging can occur at the end of the procedure in order to identify any perforation and an amylase the next day would be ideal to ensure the absence of pancreatitis.

 • See companion website for videos relating to this chapter topic: www.wiley.com/go/gershman3e

 ## FURTHER READING

Asabe K, Oka Y, Hoshino S, *et al.* Modification of the endoscopic management of congenital duodenal stenosis. *Turk J Pediatr* 2008, **50**, 182–185.

Barabino A, Gandullia P, Arrigo S, *et al.* Successful endoscopic treatment of a double duodenal web in an infant. *Gastrointestinal Endosc* 2011, **73**, 401–403.

Beeks A, Gosche J, Giles H, *et al.* Endoscopic dilation and partial resection of a duodenal web in an infant. *J Pediatr Gastroenterol Nutr* 2009, **48**, 378–381.

Goring J, Isoldi S, Sharma S, *et al.* Natural Orifice Endoluminal Technique (NOEL) for the management of congenital duodenal membranes. *J Pediatr Surg* 2020, **55**, 282–285.

Kay GA, Lobe TE, Custer MD, *et al.* Endoscopic laser ablation of obstructing congenital duodenal webs in the newborn: a case report of limited success with criteria for patient selection. *J Pediatr Surg* 1992, **27**, 279–281.

Lee SS, Hwang ST, Jang NG, *et al.* A case of congenital duodenal web causing duodenal stenosis in a Down syndrome child: endoscopic resection with an insulated-tip knife. *Gut Liver* 2011, **5**, 105.

Okamatsu T, Arai K, Yatsuzuka M, *et al.* Endoscopic membranectomy for congenital duodenal stenosis in an infant. *J Pediatr Surg* 1989, **24**, 367–368.

40

Polypectomy

George Gershman, Mike Thomson, and Gabor Veres

 KEY POINTS

- Acquaintance with the principles of electrosurgery and snare loop mechanics is an essential element of safe polypectomy training.
- Good bowel preparation is the key for a safe and successful polypectomy.
- The choice of polypectomy technique is determined by polyp size and type.

- Proper positioning of the scope, gentle opening of the metal loop and coordinated simultaneous advancement of the snare toward the polyp along with tightening of the loop are the key elements of successful polypectomy.

Principles of electrosurgery

The cornerstone of electric cutting and coagulation of living tissue is the heating of the restricted area by radiofrequency (RF) alternating current without stimulation of nerves and muscles. When current alternates up to a million times per second, it does not stimulate muscle and nerve membranes long enough to induce depolarization before the next alternation occurs. Cutting is produced by rapid and strong heating, which creates evaporation of intra- and extracellular fluids.

Coagulation is initiated when the speed and degree of tissue heating are slower and less intense, leading to cellular desiccation. Specific effects of different types of RF currents and heat-related tissue destruction are illustrated in Figures 40.1 and 40.2.

Several factors regulate the degree of tissue heating.

- Voltage (V) is the force required to push current through the tissue. The higher the voltage, the deeper the thermal tissue destruction.
- Tissue resistance (R) or impedance (for alternating current) is the force generated by tissue to resist electrical flow. It is directly proportional to the amount of tissue electrolytes. Resistance increases dramatically during tissue heating and desiccation. Normal tissue resistance is not uniform; it is lowest along blood vessels and highest at the level of the skin.
- Time (T) is an essential factor of energy (E) regulation, which can be expressed as:

$$\mathbf{E}\left(\text{in joules}\right) = \mathbf{P}\left(\text{power in watts}\right) \times \mathbf{T}$$

Practical Pediatric Gastrointestinal Endoscopy, Third Edition. Edited by George Gershman and Mike Thomson.
© 2021 John Wiley & Sons Ltd. Published 2021 by John Wiley & Sons Ltd.
Companion website: www.wiley.com/go/gershman3e

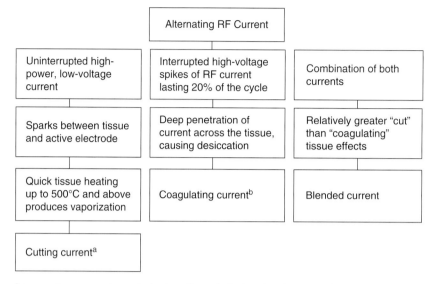

a Low-voltage current penetrates less through desiccation tissue and has limited
  ability to induce deep tissue heating.

b Spikes of high-voltage coagulating current allow a deeper spread through
  desiccated tissue and induce more tissue destruction.

Figure 40.1 Different types of alternating RF currents and specific tissue response.

Tissue heating increases with time, although the process is quite complex.

- Heating produces water loss and increases resistance.
- Increasing resistance shifts the distribution of current from the lowest resistance pathway.
- Fluctuation of resistance affects the power output produced by the generator.
- Some of the released heat is removed from high-temperature areas by blood flow. The cooling effect of blood flow explains why the same energy applied to the tissue generates less destruction if delivered slowly.

Current density is a measure of RF current (I) which flows through a specific cross-section area:

$$\frac{1}{a} = \frac{1}{\pi \tau^2}$$

The amount of heat generated in tissue is directly proportional to the power density (P) expressed as a square value of current density multiplied by resistance:

$$P = \left(\frac{I}{a}\right)^2 \Re = \frac{I^2}{\pi \tau^2} \times \Re$$

This important equation implies that power density has an inverted relationship with the square of the cross-sectional area (πr^2). It means that even a small tightening of the loop produces a profound effect on tissue heating. This can be illustrated by the polypectomy of a 1 cm polyp.

If a snare decreases the diameter of a polyp by half, the cross-sectional area at the level of the loop will be only 0.2 cm². It is four times less than a cross-sectional area at the base of the polyp and about 500 times less than a cross-sectional area of skin under a 10 × 10 cm plate of the return electrode.

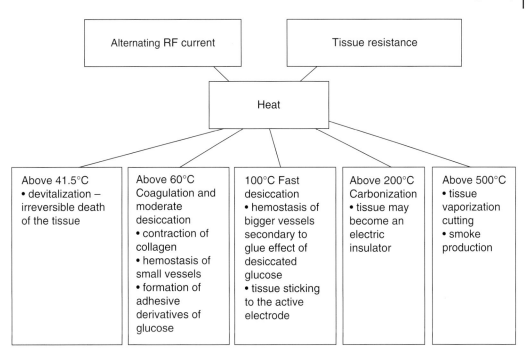

Figure 40.2 Temperature-related tissue destruction always induced by RF current.

If 0.2 A electric current is applied through the snare, it produces a current density of 1 A/cm^2, 0.25 A/cm^2 and 0.002 A/cm^2 at the level of the loop, polyp base, and skin respectively.

The fall of the power density (i.e., power actually delivered to the tissue and generating heat) is even more dramatic: from 1 A/cm^2 × R at the level of the loop, to 0.06 A/cm^2 × R and 0.000004 A/cm^2 × R at the base of the polyp and skin under the return electrode respectively. Narrowing of a cross-sectional area by a closing snare produces the most significant effect on heat production compared with increasing the power setting and time of electric current application. It also allows one to perform a polypectomy at a lower power using a coagulating mode safely.

The law of current density is vital for polypectomy. Narrowing of a cross-sectional area is the most important safety technique, which produces coagulation of the core vessels of the polyps before cutting, restricts the area of max-imal tissue heating around the loop, and limits tissue destruction of the deep bowel wall layers.

Snare loops

Commercially available snares vary by size, configuration of loop, design, mechanical characteristics of handles, and wire thickness. Reusable snares often lose their mechanical properties and can peel and break at the tip. Disposable snares are more durable and pre-dictable. The thickness of the wire loop and handle "attitude" can significantly affect the results of polypectomy. Snares with thick wire loops have two important advantages.

- A decreased risk of snapping a polyp with-out adequate coagulation.
- A large surface contact with tissue resulting in better coagulation.

A standard snare with an opening diameter of 2.5 cm can be used for different size polyps. A special small or "mini" snare (1 cm loop) has been designed for polyps less than 1 cm. It is important for endoscopists to find an "optimal" snare for routine practice in order to avoid any unexpected "surprises" during cutting or coagulation.

The chosen snare should be fully open and then closed to the point when just the tip of the wire loop is outside the outer sheath. Marking of the so-called closing point on the handle of the snare (Figure 40.3) serves two important safety features.

- Protection from premature cutting of a small sessile or pedunculated polyp without adequate coagulation.
- Alerting the endoscopist of a partial polyp's head entrapment or underestimation of the stalk size.

It is very important to check how far the tip of the wire loop is retracted into the outer plastic sheath when the snare is fully closed. A distance of 15 mm provides adequate squeezing pressure (Figure 40.4). If the stalk of a large polyp is not squeezed adequately,

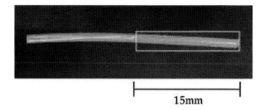

Figure 40.4 Squeezing pressure. A 15 mm retraction of the wire into the plastic sheath provides an optimal narrowing of the polyp base or the stalk for adequate constriction of the blood vessels and generation of an appropriate power density.

this compromises the coagulation of core vessels for two reasons.

- Blood vessels remain open and blood flow continues, producing a cooling effect;
- More importantly, the cross-sectional area is not narrow enough to concentrate the current flow to an appropriate power density to coagulate core vessels.

Closure of a snare loop with excessive pressure can induce premature cutting before coagulation. Both conditions could lead to significant bleeding.

Routine polypectomy

Polypectomy is the most common therapeutic procedure in pediatric GI endoscopy. It can be simple or more complex, depending on the size or location of the polyp and personal experience. No matter how comfortable the endoscopist is with the polypectomy technique, it is always wise to follow a simple rule: safety before action.

Safety routine

A proper assembly and settings check of the electrosurgical unit before each polypectomy should be routine to avoid accidental delivery of excessive power to the tissue. The foot pedal should be conveniently positioned in front of the endoscopist. The polypectomy snare should be

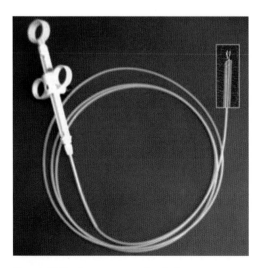

Figure 40.3 Snare preparation before polypectomy: marking of the so-called closing point on the handle of the snare.

checked for smooth opening, thickness of the wire, adequate squeezing pressure, and closing point. It is useful to create a kit of hemostatic accessories such as endo-loops, metal clips, and needle for epinephrine injection.

Preparation and techniques

Good bowel preparation is essential not only for optimal positioning of the snare loop around a polyp stalk or sessile or flat lesion, but also to avoid accidental burning or coagulation of normal mucosa. A large amount of liquid or solid stool increases the chance of missing a small or even a good-sized polyp. An obscure view often leads to excessive use of air and bowel stretching, making it thinner.

Unexpected patient awakening or movements complicate polypectomy, especially during a snare closure, and are avoidable by adequate sedation.

The technique of polypectomy consists of three important elements.

1) Optimal scope navigation.
2) Placement of a wire loop around the polyp.
3) Cold or hot snare polypectomy.

A 6 o'clock position is ideal for polypectomy. The location of a polyp between 4 and 5 or 7 and 8 o'clock is suboptimal. Polypectomy is very difficult and somewhat unsafe if a polyp is located on the upper aspect of a lumen between 9 and 3 o'clock.

An ideal 6 o'clock approach can be established by clockwise or counterclockwise rotation of the shaft and downward deflection of the tip. Careful assessment of the stalk size and location of the polyp is mandatory before polypectomy. Once an optimal position and clear view of the polyp are achieved, the scope is advanced toward the polyp base. An ideal distance from the tip of the scope to the polyp is 1–2cm unless the polyp is hiding beyond a fold. To reveal the polyp, press the mucosal fold down with the tip of the endoscope or a closed snare.

All manipulations with a snare should be performed gradually.

It is good practice to open a snare just enough to embrace the polyp. Full opening of a snare makes the wire loop floppy and less controllable.

An adequately opened and horizontally oriented wire loop above a sessile polyp at 6 o'clock accomplishes snaring just by downward tip deflection. If an opened wire loop creates an angle at the base of the polyp, rotate the shaft of the scope toward the polyp until it is captured. Steer the shaft slightly away from the sessile polyp if it is located between 4 and 5 o'clock or 7 and 8 o'clock and attempts to establish an ideal 6 o'clock position have failed. Advance the snare toward the polyp and open the loop. Once the polyp is inside the loop (Figure 40.5), rotate the scope slowly toward the polyp to align the plane of the snare with the axis of the bowel lumen. Close the snare slowly and move it forward until it reaches the base of the polyp. At this moment, the snare should be completely closed (Figure 40.6).

Occasionally, backward snaring is more effective, especially if the polyp is more than 1.5cm in length. Point a slightly open wire loop down towards the area where a polyp head touches the bowel wall. While the loop is slowly pushing forward, tissue resistance creates a bowing effect and facilitates loop opening. As a result, the loop slides between the

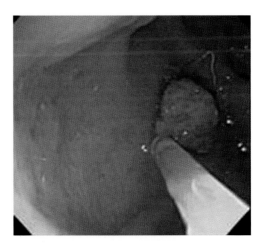

Figure 40.5 The polyp is within the wire loop.

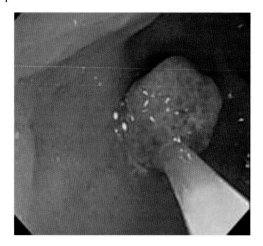

Figure 40.6 The snare is fully closed. Avoid excessive force to prevent amputation of the polyp.

mucosa and the polyp head. An additional clockwise rotation of the tip using both knobs swings a wire loop under the polyp head. Once a snare is positioned properly, it can be closed to complete polypectomy.

If the polyp is facing away from the tip of the scope, advance the snare and open it slowly until the tip of the wire is beyond the polyp's head. Deflect the tip of the scope slightly down to move the wire loop below the polyp. Pull the snare back until the head of the polyp is inside the loop and the wire is just under the polyp head. Close the snare gradually and advance it toward the polyp to prevent sliding of the wire along the stalk.

Advancement of the snare towards the polyp during wire loop closure is a key element in polyp snaring. It secures the polyp within the loop and allows precise navigation of the snare. Capturing a small polyp with a standard snare may be challenging. A slight decompression of the bowel may elevate the polyp above the wire loop and facilitate its capture.

The technique of polypectomy is different when applied to small polyps less than 5 mm, broad-based polyps more than 15 mm, pedunculated polyps more than 20 mm or polyps with a stalk ≥10 mm.

European Society of Gastrointestinal Endoscopy (ESGE) guidelines recommend cold snare polypectomy as the preferred technique for removal of diminutive polyps less than 5 mm. Diminutive colon polyps can also be removed safely by cold biopsy forceps (avoid hot biopsy forceps due to the potential risk of perforation).

Two helpful hints:

- If a polyp is on the edge of a fold, position the tip of the colonoscope within a short distance ('2 cm) from the target, open the forceps cup and orient it perpendicular to the fold, advance the forceps toward the polyp and close it when the polyp is within the cup. Avoid forcefully pushing the forceps up against the mucosa as it will stretch the tissue and result in suboptimal sampling.
- If a small polyp is in between folds, place the forceps with opened cup horizontally to the folds and advance the forceps forward to the point when the polyp is within reach to grasp it.

An alternative technique consists of vertical orientation of the biopsy forceps and positioning the lower biopsy jaw just below the polyp to avoid grasping adjacent mucosa before closing the forceps.

Large sessile polyps are rare in children except patients with Peutz–Jeghers syndrome. Such polyps are usually located in the small intestine, primarily in the jejunum.

Broad-based polyps >15 mm require a piecemeal polypectomy technique. A submucosal injection of epinephrine (1:10 000) solution before polypectomy decreases the risk of deep tissue injury. Injection at the proximal site of the polyp is performed first, followed by injection at the distal edge and lateral sides of the polyp base. Injection of 3–10 cc of the chosen solution in 3–4 sites is usually adequate to create a liquid "cushion" under the polyp. The needle should be oriented tangentially to minimize the risk of transmural injection.

The piecemeal technique consists of removal of the polyp in multiple tangential cuts. This significantly diminishes the risk of full-thickness thermal injury of the intestinal wall and bleeding. Excessive closing pressure should be avoided because it may compromise initiation of cutting, due to lack of electrical arc from the active electrode to the tissue. In addition, decreased wire–tissue contact area increases current density, which may induce excessive desiccation and stop current flow.

En bloc polypectomy of sessile polyps ≤15 mm and pedunculated polyps ≤20 mm with a short stalk is safe if gentle wiggling of the snare with the captured polyp does not produce synchronous movements of the underlying bowel wall (the sign that submucosa and muscularis propria is not trapped within the wire loop).

Polypectomy of pedunculated polyps more than 2 cm is challenging. Attention should be paid to proper positioning of the wire loop at the narrowest portion of the stalk right below the polyp head. Thick blood vessels in the middle of the stalk require slow desiccation for complete coagulation and hemostasis before the final cut. For prevention of bleeding in pedunculated polyps with a head ≥2 cm or stalk ≥1.0 cm, ESGE guidelines recommend injection of dilute adrenaline and/or mechanical hemostasis. It has been shown that the use of endo-loops or endo-clips (Figure 40.7) can be superior to adrenaline injection, and a combination of mechanical prophylaxis with adrenaline injection significantly decreases postpolypectomy bleeding in comparison with injection alone.

It is difficult to avoid direct contact of a large pedunculated polyp with normal mucosa during polypectomy. However, attempts should be made to keep the snared polyp close to the center of the bowel lumen to minimize thermal destruction of adjacent tissue. Careful inspection of a long stalk should precede any manipulations with the snare. The location of the polyp base and position of the long stalk are crucial for an optimal approach to the polyp. To capture the polyp, advance the snare toward the base of the polyp head and open the wire loop slowly until it becomes big enough to embrace the polyp.

Any additional manipulation with the snare should be coordinated with either right or left torque of the shaft toward the 6 o'clock direction. A backward snaring method may be useful. Reserve reduction of polyp size by piecemeal technique for the challenging cases.

A polypectomy can be performed during colonic intubation or the withdrawal phase of a colonoscopy. The decision is made based on polyp size. It is wise to remove a small sessile or pedunculated polyp as soon as it is discovered to eliminate the chance of missing it at a future time. Removal of a large polyp is more convenient after the entire colon has been inspected, except in cases when the position of a polyp is ideal for polypectomy. Careful examination of the colon, especially behind the folds, can be accomplished by circumferential rotation of the tip and the shaft, aspiration of excessive fluid and repeated insertion of the scope for a few segments if the bowel quickly slips away from the tip.

After polypectomy, polyps less than 10 mm can be easily sucked into the biopsy channel and eventually into a filtered polyp suction trap. Water irrigation and proper orientation of a suction nostril at the tip of a scope facilitate the recovery process.

A tripod forceps or Roth net is useful for retrieval of larger polyps (Figure 40.8).

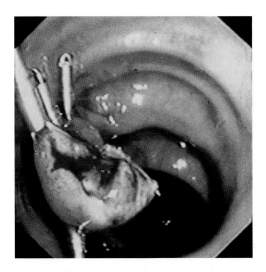

Figure 40.7 Mechanical prophylaxis of bleeding with endo-clips.

(a)

(b)

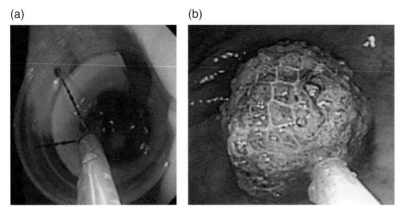

Figure 40.8 (a) Tripod forceps. (b) Roth net.

Nylon polyp retrieval nets or metal baskets can be used for removal of multiple polyps. Grasping of a large polyp using the snare is the most reliable way to bring it to the rectum. Manual assistance to recover a large polyp from the rectum after polypectomy may be necessary.

It is useful to pay attention to the direction in which the polyp falls after polypectomy. The first place to look for a "lost" polyp is in a pool of fluid. If the polyp is not there, flush some water and watch where it flows: backflow indicates that the polyp is distal to the tip of the scope.

Complications

Three types of complications can occur after polypectomy. The most common is bleeding. In contrast to adults, delayed bleeding within two weeks after the procedure is quite rare in children.

Immediate onset of bleeding is more common, although the incidence of this complication is less than 1% in children. This may reflect a smaller size, the number of polyps and the absence of co-morbid conditions such as

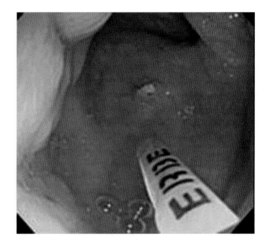

Figure 40.9 Hemostasis with argon plasma coagulation.

hypertension, atherosclerosis, etc. A slow oozing from the polypectomy site is easy to control by injection of epinephrine solution (1:10 000) or bipolar or argon plasma coagulation (Figure 40.9) or application of an endo-clip.

 • See companion website for videos relating to this chapter topic: www.wiley.com/go/gershman3e

FURTHER READING

Cappell MS, Abdullah M. Management of gastrointestinal bleeding induced by gastrointestinal endoscopy. *Gastrointest Endosc Clin North Am* 2000, **29**, 125–167.

Charotini I, Theodoropaulou A, Vardas E, *et al.* Combination of adrenaline injection and detachable snare application as haemostatic preventive measure before polypectomy of large polyps in children. *Dig Dis Sci* 2007, **52**, 338–339.

Cotton PB, Williams C, Hawes RH, *et al. Practical Gastrointestinal Endoscopy. The Fundamentals*, 7th edn. Wiley Blackwell Publishing, Oxford, 2014.

Gershman G, Ament ME. *Practical Pediatric Gastrointestinal Endoscopy*, 2nd edn. Wiley Blackwell Publishing, Oxford, 2012.

Ferlitsch M, Moss A, Hassan C, *et al.* Colorectal polypectomy and endoscopic mucosal resection (EMR): European Society of Gastrointestinal Endoscopy (ESGE) clinical guideline. *Endoscopy* 2017, **49**, 270–297.

Mougenot JF, Vargas J. Colonoscopic polypectomy and endoscopic mucosal resection. In: Winter HS, Murphy MS, Mougenot JF, *et al.* (eds). *Pediatric Gastrointestinal Endoscopy*. BC Decker, Hamilton, 2006, pp. 163–181.

Tappero G, Gaia E, DeFiuli P, *et al.* Cold snare excision of small colorectal polyps. *Gastrointest Endosc* 1992, **38**, 310–313.

Thomson M. Polypectomy. In: Walker WA, Kleinman RE, Goulet OJ, *et al.* (eds). *Pediatric Gastrointestinal Disease. Pathophysiology, Diagnosis and Management*, 6th edn. PMPH, Beijing, 2018, pp. 1874–1875.

Waye JD. New methods of polypectomy. *Gastrointest Endosc Clin North Am* 1997, **7**, 413–422.

Waye JD. Endoscopic mucosal resection of colon polyps. *Gastrointest Endosc Clin North Am* 2001, **11**, 537–548.

41

Endomucosal resection

Mike Thomson and Paul Hurlstone

 KEY POINTS

- Sessile lesions may be elevated to create a tissue plane and minimize perforation risk by injection of a tissue expander mixed with methylene blue and epinephrine.
- A dual-channel "operating endoscope" makes it easier to grasp some of the lesion whilst a polyp snare is manipulated over the anchored piece.

- Piecemeal polypectomy using a snare is ideal.
- Other accessories such as a straight endo-knife, ceramic tip endo-knife or endo-hook may be employed.
- Argon plasma coagulation may be employed to stop any bleeding vessels after resection.
- Any perforation may be closed with endo-clips or over-the-scope clips.

Introduction

Colonoscopic resection methods have traditionally aimed towards biopsy and polypectomy. Endoscopic mucosal resection (EMR) is in its infancy, but it allows early and effective treatment of selected superficial neoplasms and obviates the need for major surgery in these patients. The safety and efficacy of new endoscopic interventional therapeutics in the form of EMR require further evaluation.

It is important to remember that the inflammation–metaplasia–dysplasia–adenocarcinoma sequence is a concept not exclusive to adult patients, and that children and adolescents have a part to play in this evolutionary pathology. The atypia of lesions needs to be carefully evaluated and is made easier with more modern imaging techniques and hardware.

High-magnification chromoscopic colonoscopy

High-magnification colonoscopes enable the magnification of colonic mucosa up to 150 times and also offer higher resolution than older colonoscopes. Their use is maximized in conjunction with chromoscopy and this represents the most common mode of visual enhancement used by endoscopists presently. Using this technique, clear lesion delineation and pit patterns (see Tables 41.1a and 41.1b) can be observed.

Practical Pediatric Gastrointestinal Endoscopy, Third Edition. Edited by George Gershman and Mike Thomson.
© 2021 John Wiley & Sons Ltd. Published 2021 by John Wiley & Sons Ltd.
Companion website: www.wiley.com/go/gershman3e

Table 41.1a Paris classification of endoscopic lesion morphology

Endoscopic appearance	Paris class		Description
Protruded lesions	Ip		Pedunculated polyps
	Ips		Subpedunculated polyps
	Is		Sessile polyps
Flat elevated lesions	IIa		Flat elevation of mucosa
	IIa/IIc		Flat elevation with central depression
Flat lesions	IIb		Flat mucosal change
	IIc		Mucosal depression
	IIc/IIa		Mucosal depression with raised edge

Table 41.1b modified Kudo criteria for the classification of colorectal crypt architecture in vivo using high-magnification chromoscopic colonoscopy (HMCC)

Pit type	Characteristics	Appearance msing HMCC	Pit size (mm)
I	Normal round pits		0.07 +/− 0.02 mm
II	Stella or papillary		0.09 +/− 0.02 mm
IIIs	Tubular/round pits Smaller than pit type I		0.03 +/− 0.01 mm
IIIL	Tubular/large		0.22 +/− 0.09 mm
IV	Sulcus/gyrus		0.93 +/− 0.32 mm
V(a)	Irregular arrangement and sizes of IIIL, IIIs, IV type pit		N/A

The technique involves initial visualization of the colon with conventional video-colonoscopy, looking out for the following mucosal signs, which may be subtle.

- Focal pallor or erythema
- Hemorrhagic spots
- Fold convergence
- Disruption of mucosal vascular net pattern

Table 41.2 Classification of common chromoscopic dyes

Type of dye	Preparation	Application	Advantages	Side effects
Contrast				
Indigo carmine Most commonly used Acetic acid	Standard mucosal toilet	Dye spraying via scope or diffusion catheter		None
Reactive				
Crystal violet Kudo type V pit differentiation Cresyl violet	Mucosal toilet with proteinase solution	Specialized catheter; 2–3 min wait for fixation		Possible long-term toxicity
Absorptive				
Methylene blue	Standard mucosal toilet	Dye spraying via scope or diffusion catheter	Longer staining pattern	Potentially mutagenic

- Mucosal unevenness or discrete mucosal deformity
- Air-induced deformation

Once identified, the suspicious areas are washed down with the appropriate mucosal toilet and the dye applied. Lesions are then sized using an open biopsy forceps whose width is known. Morphological classification is then undertaken by activating the colonoscope's magnification lever and characterizing its appearances.

Pit patterns

Pit patterns have been shown to correlate strongly with their associated histopathological diagnoses and as a result this method of classification is widely used. Types I and II are associated with normal and hyperplastic mucosa. Type III is seen more often in depressed lesions and are associated with carcinomatous change. Type IIIL is associated with adenomas in protuberant lesions. Types IV and V are associated with adenomas with atypical cellularity whereas type V or nonpit patterns are indicative of adenocarcinoma.

A summary of common dyes used in high-magnification chromoscopic colonoscopy (HMCC) is shown in Table 41.2. Indigo carmine (IC) 0.2–1% is the most frequently used agent. It is a contrast enhancer that pools in recesses, aiding the visualization of abnormal mucosa. As there is no actual reaction with the tissues, it washes off easily which makes it unsuitable for prolonged procedures. IC has been shown to be sufficient in the visualization of type I–IV pits but if further visualization is required, crystal violet (CV) can be used to stain the mucosa. This compound is a potentially toxic reactive dye and should only be used sparingly when type V pits are suspected. Methylene blue stains for a longer period of time and is commonly used in ulcerative colitis cancer surveillance.

The introduction of high-frequency "miniprobe" ultrasound has now been reported to have a high overall accuracy when used to determine submucosal invasion Paris class II lesions. However, ultrasound imaging requires further training, has significant expense, and may prolong the procedure.

HMCC in the detection of intraepithelial neoplasia and colitis-associated cancer

Although many pediatric gastroenterologists will see this concept as a theoretical one for their patients, there is no doubt that knowledge of this area is an important corollary of our conception of inflammatory bowel disease (IBD) evolution – this is especially true when counseling adolescents not keen on following treatment regiemes. For instance, azathioprine is now strongly associated with the diminution of colorectal cancer (CRC) risk in long-term IBD. The management and clinical interpretation of dysplasia in the context of chronic ulcerative colitis are radically different from those of sporadic dysplastic lesions in the "normal" population. These patients have an increased risk of interval cancers, especially those with long-standing disease. The morphology of precancerous lesions may be flat and multifocal, making HMCC a useful adjunct in their detection. At the current time, dysplasia is the most reliable biomarker of malignant change, being present in >70% of ulcerative colitis patients with CRC.

The ability to differentiate intraepithelial neoplasia from hyperplastic or inflammatory mucosal change using HMCC in ulcerative colitis offers a sensitive and specific tool. There are, however, indistinct mucosal appearances seen in the presence of acute inflammation which may result in equivocal histological diagnoses. It has therefore been recommended that HMCC targeted biopsies be used only when the disease is quiescent and even then only in clearly demarcated lesions.

Summary of limitations of current imaging technology

- High sensitivity/specificity for the differentiation of nonneoplastic from neoplastic disease but low overall sensitivity for the anticipation of high-grade dysplasia.
- Effective overstaging of submucosal layer 3/T1 neoplasia.
- Operator-dependent error.
- Surface topographical imaging only.
- No ability to image surface/subsurface lymphovascular architecture, except with confocal endomicroscopy which is not widely available to date.

Endoscopic mucosal resection

The benefits or early CRC detection are not exclusively those of increased survival as many patients can be treated curatively using novel resection techniques such as EMR. Such a procedure has a low cost and low associated morbidity and mortality when compared to conventional surgery. As mentioned above, new endoscopic imaging techniques such as chromoscopic colonoscopy and HMCC have highlighted the clinical importance of flat and depressed nonpolypoid colorectal lesions.

Simple snare resection is sufficient for pedunculated lesions. EMR permits the resection of flat and sessile lesions by longitudinal section through the submucosal layer. In the colorectum, EMR may provide curative resection for flat and sessile adenomas in addition to early colorectal cancer. EMR facilitates complete histological analysis of the resected lesion and makes it possible to determine precisely the completeness of excision in both the horizontal and vertical resection planes. This makes it advantageous compared to primary tissue ablative techniques such as argon plasma coagulation and electrocoagulation. Numerous EMR techniques have now been described using transparent caps fitted to the proximal aspect of the endoscope and that using an insulation-tipped cutting knife. With the exception of submucosal posterior rectal tumors, these techniques are reserved for esophageal and gastric resection with the strip biopsy technique used routinely in the colorectum.

Basic EMR technique

The technique of EMR comprises four stages.

1) Diagnosis and localization of the lesion.
2) Evaluation of invasive depth to exclude lesions invading the deep submucosal layer 3 or beyond (i.e., T2 disease) using HMCC or ultrasound techniques.
3) Excision procedure.
4) Postresection evaluation.

Flat and sessile lesions up to 20 mm in diameter can be resected by en bloc or "single pass" resection with larger lesions requiring a piecemeal approach. A needle catheter is then inserted through the side port of the colonoscope with sterile saline injected around the lesion and surrounding mucosa. A cleavage of the submucosa (having the effect of raising the lesion) then permits simple snare resection. A single cannulation can be used for small lesions (<10 mm) diameter with multiple cannulations usually required for lesions of 20 mm or larger. Adrenaline (1/100 000) mixed with saline or a tissue expander as used in IV resuscitation plus a 1:10 dye such as methylene blue is injected into the submucosal plane, allowing for elevation of the lesion and creation of an artificial tissue plane which facilitates resection. Whatever injection medium is used, it is essential to maintain sufficient mucosal lift or detachment throughout the EMR, which minimizes the risk of muscularis propria entrapment and subsequent perforation.

Peripheral margin tattoos can be used prior to saline submucosal injection to delineate the normal mucosal boundaries around the lesion prior to snaring. This is a helpful technique, as at submucosal lift, the lesion can become distorted and indistinct from the surrounding normal mucosa. If the lesion fails to lift (the nonlifting sign of Uno) or has an asymmetrical appearance then the resection should be abandoned as this indicates tethering to the underlying muscularis mucosa. Perforation and risk of noncurative resection can occur in this scenario.

Following successful submucosal lift, a spiked or "barbed" snare is applied over the lesion and slowly closed under gentle suction. This permits the lesion to be retained within the snare boundaries before final resection. Prior to final cutting (usually using a 25 W coagulation current), the snare should be relaxed slightly to allow any entrapped muscularis mucosa to retract. Following resection, the lesion is retrieved using a pronged grasping forcep or Roth net, followed by immediate fixation in 10% formalin solution. Some endoscopists "pin out" the lesion onto a solid cork or polystyrene plate prior to fixation that limits shrinkage of the resection specimen and permits easier and more accurate histopathological sectioning.

Postresection management

Following resection, it is important to reevaluate the cut margin of the mucosa. High rates of adenoma recurrence may occur, despite reported complete excision by the endoscopist. Performing EMR may therefore be considered a hazardous procedure if this is apparent, where remnant adenomatous tissue continues to assume a risk for carcinomatous transformation. Should a further EMR be unsuccessful, argon plasma coagulation (APC) of any remnant tissue, including application to the entire circumference of the cut margin, should be applied. All lesions should have an adjacent submucosal tattoo using Indian ink to facilitate localization at follow-up colonoscopy.

Complications of EMR

The main complications of EMR are hemorrhage, perforation, and stenosis. The immediate and early complications (10% of cases) described in the first 12 hours post resection are principally hemorrhage and rarely perforation. EMR may therefore be a safe and effective endoscopic therapy that may enhance our current strategies aimed at the secondary prevention of colorectal cancer. Accurate in vivo staging is essential at colonoscopy prior to consideration of local endoluminal resection. Flat focal submucosal invasive CRCs which are limited to submucosal layer 1 can be managed by EMR as the risk of lymphovenous invasion and nodal metastasis is low (<5%). For lesions with deeper vertical invasion into submucosal layer 3 or beyond (stage T2), the risk of nodal disease increases to 10–15%. EMR in this group is therefore undesirable due to a higher risk of perforation, noncurative excision and untreated nodal disease. Surgical excision is recommended in this group.

Clinical recommendations and conclusions

Colonic chromoscopy and HMCC have been shown to be useful in discriminating between neoplastic and nonneoplastic Paris 0–II colorectal lesions. The decision to target biopsies or progress to therapeutic intervention using EMR can be guided using this technology and avoid inappropriate biopsy or attempted endoscopic resection of lesions without a malignant potential or those which should be referred for surgical excision.

 • See companion website for videos relating to this chapter topic: www.wiley.com/go/gershman3e

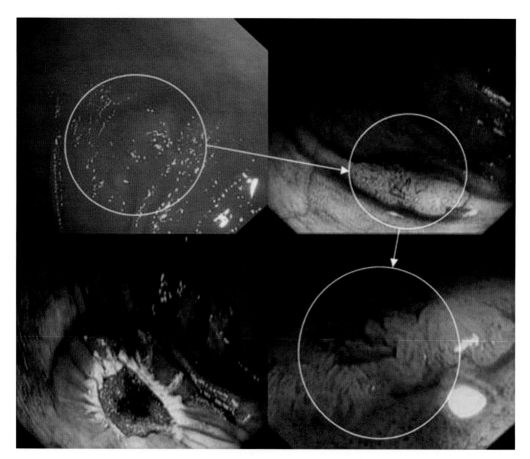

Figure 41.1 (*Top left*) High-definition white light images of a proximal ascending colonic lesion. The lesion highlighted is distinguished by focal erythema and loss of vascular net architecture. (*Top right*) High-definition indigo carmine 0.4% targeted chromoscopy imaging of the lesion. The lesion is now clearly circumscribed and can be classified as a Paris 0–IIa (flat elevated) lesion in the absence of a fixed type 0–IIc component (central depression). (*Bottom right*) High-magnification (100×) imaging shows a normal Kudo type I crypt pattern adjacent to the lesion with a predominant Kudo type IIIL pit pattern at the lesion's apex, i.e., intraepithelial neoplasia positive. Endoscopic excision is indicated. (*Bottom left*) Postendoscopic mucosal resection en bloc resection imaging. The muscularis mucosa can be clearly visualized with no evident neoplastic crypt architecture at the horizontal or vertical resection margins. The lesions has been completely resected (R0 anticipated endoscopically).

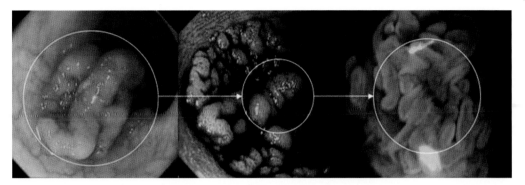

Figure 41.2 (*Left*) Conventional high-definition white light views of a lateral spreading tumor (granular type) positioned at the rectosigmoid junction. (*Middle*) Indigo carmine 0.4% chromoscopy has been applied to the rectosigmoid segment. The peripheral neoplastic pit pattern can now be fully defined and the circumfrential margins of the lesion identified. (*Right*) High-magnification (100×) imaging of the largest nodule (highlighted) shows a Kudo type IV crypt pattern.

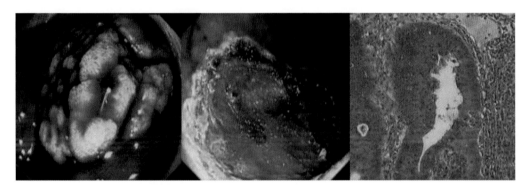

Figure 41.3 **(***Left***)** Endoscopic mucosal resection of the lesion is indicated (neoplastic-noninvasive pit pattern). The lesions has been raised using a submucosal injection of 50% dextrose solution. The lesion has lifted in a symmetrical fashion with no tethering suggestive of submucosal deep invasion. (*Middle*) Postendoscopic mucosal resection appearance shows the muscularis mucosa visible. There are some prominent vessels in the vertical dissection plane which have been prophylactically coagulated using argon plasma. (*Right*) Hematoxylin and eosin stained fixed pathological specimen at high power. Features are of a high-grade villous adenoma without submucosal invasive characteristics. Curative resection was achieved endoscopically in this case.

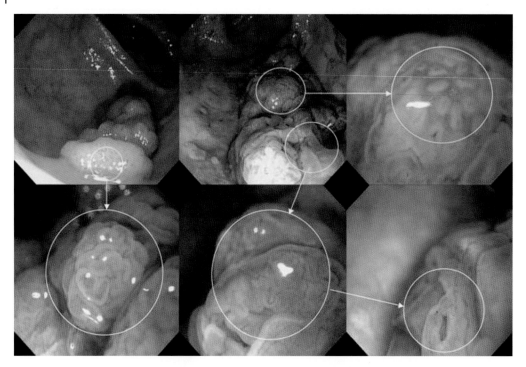

Figure 41.4 (*Top left*) Conventional high-definition white light imaging of a descending colonic Paris class 0–Isp (subpendunculated) lesion. (*Bottom left*) The basal polyp segment highlighted (top left) is shown at 100× magnification using 0.4% indigo carmine chromoscopy. The pit pattern is neoplastic-noninvasive (Kudo type IIIL). (*Top middle*) The lesion is shown at conventional nonmagnified imaging following application of 0.4% indigo carmine chromoscopy. The highlighted areas show the lesion segments undergoing high-magnification (100×) imaging. (*Top right*) High-magnification (100×) imaging of the highlighted segment shows a Kudo type II pit pattern (nonneoplastic noninvasive crypt). (*Bottom middle*) High-magnification (100×) imaging of the highlighted segment shows a tortous vascular net architecture in combination with a IIL crypt pattern (bottom right) highly suggestive of a serrated adenoma component. Postendoscopic mucosal resection showed complete excision (R0) of a "collison" lesion, i.e., villous, tubular, serrated, and hyperplastic component polyp.

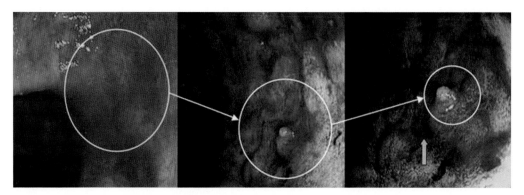

Figure 41.5 (*Left*) Conventional white light views of the distal descending colon in a patient with long-standing ulcerative colitis. There is focal erythema and subtle change in vascular net architecture compared to the surrounding mucosa. (Middle) Methylene blue 0.1% chromoscopy highlights an irregular raised nodule adjacent to a depressed mucosal area. (*Right*) The adjacent mucosal depression is shown highlighted with the blue arrow.

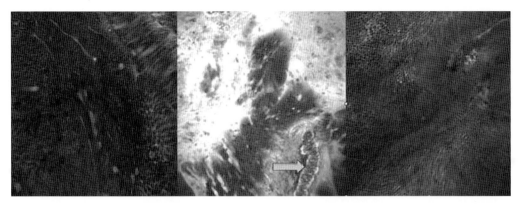

Figure 41.6 (*Left/right*) Confocal laser scanning endomicroscopic imaging using intravenous 10% fluorescein of the adjacent lesional mucosa. At 20 and 80 microns in the z-axis (left figure/right figure respectively), there is clear crypt architectural distortion implying adjacent flat dysplasia. There is mucin depletion, gross loss in regular crypt architecture and ridge lined epithelium present. (*Middle*) The circumscribed lesion has been imaged at 50 microns in the z-axis using confocal endomicroscopy. There is gross extravasation of fluorophore (white-out field) with a central dilated, tortous capillary with red cells "stacked up," i.e., the red cell stack sign of neoplasia. The lesion can be characterized in vivo as a dysplasia-associated lesional mass. Urgent referral for panproctocolectomy should be considered in this clinical scenario.

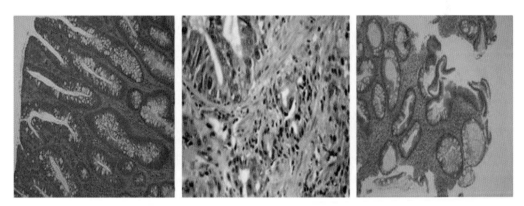

Figure 41.7 (*Left/right*) High-power hematoxylin and eosin staining of the background mucosa shows abnormal crypt architecture compatible with chronic inflammatory bowel disease in addition to dysplastic crypt architecture. (*Middle*) High-power hematoxylin and eosin staining of the circumscribed lesion shows high-grade dysplastic features with an invasive component. Histopathology confirms this lesion to be a dysplasia-associated lesion mass where colectomy should be considered as the management of choice.

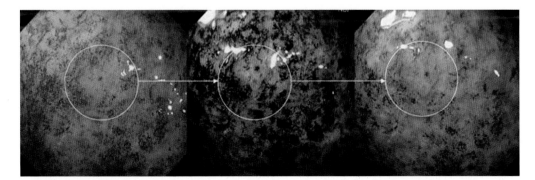

Figure 41.8 (*Left*) High-definition white light imaging of the distal sigmoid colon in a patient with chronic panulcerative colitis. There are florid neovascular changes but also a focus of focal pallor. (*Middle*) Narrow-band imaging of the segment shows the vascular architecture as brown tortuous streaks. The lesion is clearly defined as highlighted. (*Right*) Indigo carmine 0.4% chromoscopy delineated the circumfrential margin of the lesion according to SURFACE guidelines. The lesion was a flat de novo intraepithelial neoplastic lesion (Paris class 0–IIb).

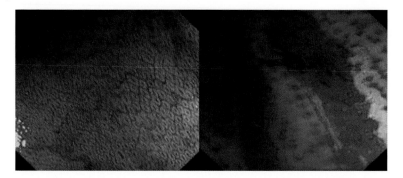

Figure 41.9 (*Left*) High-magnification (100×) chromoscopic colonoscopy (indigo carmine 0.4%) of a "normal" rectal mucosa. Note the regular ordered and "honeycomb" Kudo type Icrypt pattern. (*Right*) High-magnification (100×) chromoscopic colonoscopy (indigo carmine 0.4%) of chronic ulcerative colitis. Note: there is gross fibrotic expansion of the intercrypt spacing, a decrease in overall mucosal crypt density, and prominent linear "tramline" fibrotic ridging characteristic of advanced fibrosis complicating long-standing ulcerative colitis.

42

Endoscopic management of polyposis syndromes

Warren Hyer, Mike Thomson, and Thomas Attard

 KEY POINTS

- Wireless capsule endoscopy with balloon enteroscopy is integral in the management of polyp syndromes.
- Rectal polyp load is the best indicator of the aggressive nature of the phenotype and progression of FAP.
- EGD is not required in FAP until after the age of 20–25 when a side-viewing scope may be employed for surveillance to detect ampullary carcinoma.
- In FAP post colectomy with ileorectal anastomosis (IRA), the rectal stump should be assessed six monthly.

- Endoscopic screening does not usually occur in FAP and juvenile polyposis syndromes until 12–14 years of age.
- In hamartoma syndromes, endoscopic assessment is usually done at younger ages and would be driven by clinical requirement, e.g., in juvenile polyposis of infancy (PTEN and BMPR1A gene defects),
- Surveillance of extraintestinal associated pathologies should not be forgotten.

Introduction and classification

Gastrointestinal (GI) polyps usually present in children with rectal bleeding, or abdominal pain with intussusception in the case of small bowel polyposis. Other children are asymptomatic and come to endoscopy as part of a screening or surveillance program for a familial inherited polyposis syndrome.

Gastrointestinal polyps fall into two main categories: hamartomas or adenomas (Table 42.1). The endoscopic management and the role of GI surveillance of each condition are summarized in Table 42.2. Solitary polyps in children are most commonly hamartomas, predominantly

of the juvenile type, and such polyps are benign. Once removed, repeat colonoscopy is not required unless rectal bleeding reoccurs.

Familial adenomatous polyposis

Familial adenomatous polyposis (FAP) is an autosomal dominant inherited condition caused by a gene mutation in the adenomatous polyposis coli gene (APC). Thirty percent of cases of FAP are de novo mutations and will be identified at colonoscopy after assessment for rectal bleeding or at an older age, presenting with colorectal cancer. Many mutations have

Practical Pediatric Gastrointestinal Endoscopy, Third Edition. Edited by George Gershman and Mike Thomson.
© 2021 John Wiley & Sons Ltd. Published 2021 by John Wiley & Sons Ltd.
Companion website: www.wiley.com/go/gershman3e

Table 42.1 Polyps and polyposis syndromes seen in childhood and associated gene mutations

Gene association	
Adenomatous polyps	
Familial adenomatous polyposis	APC gene on chromosome 5q21
Hamartomatous polyposis	
Solitary juvenile polyp	No gene association
Juvenile polyposis syndrome	SMAD4 or BMPR1A
PTEN – hamartoma syndrome, e.g., Bannayan Riley–Ruvalcaba syndrome Cowden syndrome	PTEN 10q23.3

Table 42.2 Endoscopic surveillance and screening strategies for polyposis syndromes in children and adolescents

Polyposis syndrome	Endoscopic surveillance strategy	Aim of endoscopic surveillance
Familial adenomatous polyposis syndrome	In at-risk children, commence pancolonoscopy age 12–14 years (or earlier if symptomatic). Assess polyp burden, especially rectal polyposis. Repeat surveillance of colon 1–3 yearly. Routine polypectomy not required. Dye spray to improve visualization of adenomas <1 mm if required. Gastroscopy not required before age 20	Refer without delay for colectomy when >500 polyps or polyps >10 mm at colonoscopy. If fewer polyps identified, repeat colonoscopy every 1–3 years and refer for colectomy at a convenient time in later adolescence according to social and educational needs
Juvenile polyposis syndrome	In at-risk children, commence pancolonoscopy age 12–14 or earlier if presenting with rectal bleeding. Remove polyps >1 cm in size. Repeat colonoscopy every 3–5 years, earlier if bleeding returns. Gastroscopy not routinely required until >age 20 years	Remove large polyps >1 cm to prevent blood loss or hypoalbuminemia
Peutz–Jeghers syndrome	In at-risk children, surveillance gastroscopy, colonoscopy and wireless video capsule endoscopy no later than age 8 years. Repeat every three years	Remove small bowel polyps >15 mm in size by polypectomy either by double balloon enteroscopy, laparoscopy or laparotomy to avoid complications of intussusception of small bowel
Solitary juvenile polyp	Once the juvenile polyp has been removed, no repeat colonoscopy is required, unless there is further bleeding	If >5 juvenile polyps identified, then manage as juvenile polyposis syndrome

been identified and correlations have been reported between gene mutation locus and clinical manifestations. Mutations clustered around codon 1250–1464 are associated with a more severe phenotype of FAP, whereas mutations at either extreme end of the gene are associated with a more attenuated appearance and later presentation. Patients may manifest extracolonic features at presentation including bony lesions, such as osteomas, exostosis, supernumerary teeth, or desmoid tumors, congenital hypertrophy of the retinal pigment epithelium, and tumors of the brain or hepatoblastoma.

Genetic screening for at-risk children with an affected parent is usually performed at age 12–14 years if the family-specific gene mutation is known. This genetic testing or colonoscopy should be performed earlier if there are symptoms consistent with colonic polyposis such as rectal bleeding or mucus passage. Pancolonoscopy should be performed in those children predicted to be affected by FAP confirmed at gene testing. The endoscopist should concentrate in the rectum, identifying adenomas >2 mm in size (measured with biopsy forceps), and then inspect the rest of the colon to identify and quantify size and number of adenomas. If no adenomas are visualized, then there is value in using dye spray to identify microadenomas to confirm the phenotype of FAP. Once adenomas have been found, there is no value in routine polypectomy. Instead, the colonoscopy should be repeated every 1–3 years depending on the polyp burden until the adolescent is referred for colectomy.

Colectomy is key to preventing colorectal cancer (CRC) which is ubiquitous in these patients by age 20–50 depending on polyp burden. Patients should be referred for colectomy depending on the appearance of the colon. Those with >500 adenomas, or adenomas measuring >1 cm, should undergo colectomy sooner rather than delay (Figure 42.1). Those with fewer adenomas can undergo repeat colonoscopy every 1–3 years and be referred at a time that suits the social and educational path of the adolescent. Families should be registered with a regional or national polyposis registry so they are recalled for their colonoscopies.

Colectomy will either be by subtotal with an ileorectal anastomosis (IRA) or restorative proctocolectomy with ileal pouch anal anastomosis (IPAA). The choice of procedure will be directed by the surgeon taking into account the colonic and rectal polyp burden, genotype, and

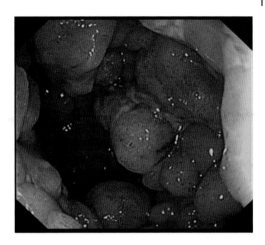

Figure 42.1 Colonoscopic appearance of multiple adenomas >1 cm meriting referral for colectomy

risk of desmoid disease. Post colectomy by IRA, the rectal remnant must be inspected six monthly by flexible sigmoidoscopy to identify and remove any adenomas >5 mm that develop to prevent subsequent rectal cancer. Those would undergo an IPAA and also require annual endoscopic assessment of the pouch

Although upper GI pathology occurs in patients with FAP including gastric adenomas, benign polyps, and duodenal ampullary dysplasia, routine gastroscopy is rarely required until over the age of 20 years. Duodenal disease develops in later years, requiring side-viewing gastroscopy after the age of 25 years.

There is no role for chemoprevention medication to delay or avoid colectomy in patients with FAP.

Juvenile polyposis syndrome

Juvenile polyposis syndrome (JPS) is an autosomal dominant heritable predisposition for colorectal and gastric polyps. The majority of affected individuals harbor mutations in the SMAD4 gene on chromosome 18q21 or BMPR1A gene on chromosome 10q23.2. The syndrome is defined by the presence of multiple (>5) juvenile polyps in the colon, juvenile

(a) (b)

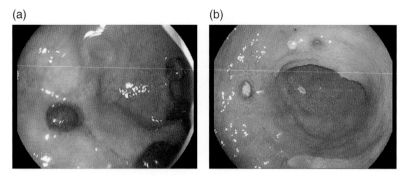

Figure 42.2 (a) Multiple pedunculated polyps in a 6-year-old Caucasian female with JPS presenting with bleeding. (b) Post polypectomy.

polyps in the stomach or any juvenile polyps in the context of a positive family history of JPS. Individuals harboring SMAD4 mutation may, in general, exhibit a more aggressive disease phenotype along with overlap with arterio-venous malformations in hereditary hemor-rhagic telangiectasia (HHT).

Colonoscopic *screening* usually starts by age 12–14 years in at-risk individuals identified by family history, with or without mutation. The goal is to identify juvenile polyps and establish the diagnosis based on the parameters above. *Surveillance* colonoscopy is repeated annually until polyp free, then repeated every 1–5 years, dependent on polyp burden and recurrent symptoms. The goal is to remove polyps with larger lesions submitted for histological changes including atypia and limiting polyp burden that may correlate with bleeding and obstruction risk.

The logistic preparation for these procedures is critical. Colonoscopy in JPS frequently entails multiple, including right-sided, polypectomy. Whenever possible, these procedures should be performed by an experienced team, under gen-eral anesthesia, with good or excellent preoper-ative preparation. Provision should be made for the broadest range of hemostatic techniques and devices (including endo-clips) to be availa-ble. Postoperative bleeding, although uncom-mon, and perforation resulting in peritonitis are significantly more likely than in routine, non-therapeutic procedures; patients and families

need to be counseled to watch for symptoms or signs of adverse outcomes with a clear plan of action to address any concerns.

Relatively large (>2 cm) colonic polyps are characteristic of JPS and can be taken out safely (Figure 42.2). Some polyps are multi-lobular or clustered onto a common stalk. The technique for polypectomy in these instances should include snaring toward the upper quarter of the stalk. Allow best positioning of the polyp ahead of cautery in order to elimi-nate (or maximize) the opportunity for arc occurrence, and leave redundant stalk to be clipped in the case of excessive bleeding post polypectomy. Sometimes, larger or clustered polyps without easy access to the stalk require piecemeal polypectomy. Whenever possible, polyps or fragments of polyps removed during these procedures should be recovered and submitted for histology, although the risk of reintubation of the colon post polypectomy is presumed to be higher and needs to be fac-tored against the loss of histopathological sampling.

Juvenile polyposis of infancy (JPI) reflects a significantly more severe phenotype of juve-nile polyposis that has been associated with contiguous deletions of the BMPR1A and PTEN genes. Given the rarity of this syndrome, management guidelines are unclear but regu-lar, close, multivisceral surveillance, including upper and lower endoscopy from an early age, appears justified.

(a) (b)

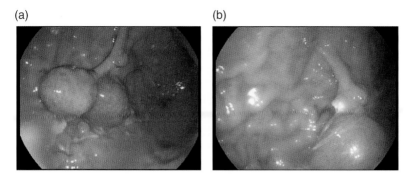

Figure 42.3 (a) Multiple large gastric polyps in the stomach of a 15 year old with Peutz–Jeghers syndrome presenting with profound anemia. (b) Partial resection.

Peutz–Jeghers syndrome

Peutz–Jeghers syndrome (PJS) is a heritable predisposition to polyps and malignancy in several epithelial lined viscera, most notably the gastrointestinal tract. Affected children develop typical mucocutaneous and lip pigmentation. Most affected individuals harbor mutation in the STK11(LKB1) gene on chromosome 19p13. Pediatric PJS is largely defined by polyps in the small bowel resulting in obstruction, larger lesions throughout the intestine relating to blood loss, and colonic polyps harboring a remote risk of dysplasia. Small bowel intestinal obstruction following intussusception often results in surgery and resection, setting the trajectory, in some patients, toward short bowel syndrome.

Gastrointestinal *screening* of at-risk individuals commences no later than 8 years of age while gastrointestinal *surveillance*, usually repeated annually to every three years, is geared toward limiting small bowel polyp burden through a "clean-sweep" approach as well as monitoring for dysplastic changes in larger colonic polyps (Figure 42.3).

Although in many cases it is logistically challenging, the combination of gastroscopy, colonoscopy, routine wireless capsule endoscopy (WCE) +/− double balloon enteroscopy (DBE)

with polypectomy offers a rational approach geared toward abrogating the natural history of PJS. In practical terms, tandem or simultaneous WCE, upper and lower endoscopy will limit repeat preprocedure preparation and hospital visits. Polypectomy in PJS may be associated with a higher risk of perforation whilst the muscularis mucosa may invaginate into the stalk of larger PJS polyps.

In practice, the challenge is to determine, on an individual basis, an early enough age at screening in order to diminish the risk of intussusception and obstruction then surgery leading to adhesions, in turn impacting the success of future surveillance DBE. The counterbalancing factors of limiting iatrogenic harm and unnecessary psychosocioeconomic stress on the patient and family should be carefully factored in. The complexity of medical decision making, the logistic demands, and the technical expertise required to manage this subpopulation of polyposis patients are perhaps the strongest argument fir referral to centers with established pediatric polyposis programs.

 • See companion website for videos relating to this chapter topic: www.wiley.com/go/gershman3e

43

Transnasal gastrointestinal endoscopy

Sara Koo, Kristina Leinwand, Simon Panter, and Joel A. Friedlander

---

 KEY POINTS

- Bronchoscopes may be used in adolescents to determine esophageal pathology by TNE.
- Adequate preparation with local nasal and oropharyngeal analgesia is important.
- The adolescent may be seated in a semi-recumbant postion in a special chair whilst being distracted by videos or a 3D virtual headset.

- The specifically designed TNE scopes may be tolerated by the older adolescent and then gastric and duodenal pathology may be examined.
- Occasional epistaxis is the only observed adverse event.

Introduction

Transnasal gastrointestinal endoscopy (TNE) was first reported in 1994 by Shaker *et al.* as T-EGD with the advent of ultrathin (UT) endoscopes [1]. Since then, use in adult has been increasing worldwide by both gastroenterologists (esophagogastroduodenoscopy [EGD] and esophagoscopy) and otolaryngologists (esophagoscopy) [2,3]. Implementation has occurred mainly in Far Eastern countries such as Japan, but also in Western countries though uptake has been lower (mostly in France and Canada). It is now reported that TNE makes up 9% of hospital practice in Japan compared to 1% in endoscopy units worldwide [4–8]. Pediatric use is limited to a single report in 2016 by Friedlander *et al.* corresponding to 21 cases in children aged 8–17 [9]. The technique was well tolerated. Per unpublished reports from the same center, TNE usage has increased to as

many as 100–140/year (4–5% of practice) in children aged 5–21 years of age.

Ultrathin endoscopes used for adult TNE/EGD and pediatric oral EGD are much narrower, 4.9–5.9 mm (depending on manufacturer and tip maneuverability/optic capability), in comparison to a minimum of 8.6 mm for conventional gastroscopes (Table 43.1) [3,10]. It is important to note that as a result of the narrower scope, the instrument and suction channel are much smaller (2.0–2.4 mm), limiting the flow rate when suctioning and restricting its therapeutic use. However, in recent years several devices have been made to accommodate such channels. These devices include grasping forceps (i.e., Olympus, Boston Scientific), APC probes (i.e., ERBE), and nets (i.e., US Endoscopy). Owing to the smaller channel, the biopsy forceps have a diameter of 1.8 mm, resulting in smaller samples being obtained. Despite this, a large study involving

---

Practical Pediatric Gastrointestinal Endoscopy, Third Edition. Edited by George Gershman and Mike Thomson.
© 2021 John Wiley & Sons Ltd. Published 2021 by John Wiley & Sons Ltd.
Companion website: www.wiley.com/go/gershman3e

Table 43.1 Currently available ultrathin endoscopes

	Olympus GIF-XP260NS	Olympus GIF-XP290N	Olympus BF-XP160/190	Olympus BF-MP160F/P190	Fujinon EG-530NW	Fujinon EG-580NW2	Fujinon EG-530NP	Vision Sciences TNE-5000
Field of view	120°	140°	90°/110°	120°/110°	120°	140°	120°	120°
Distal end outer diameter	5.4 mm	5.4 mm	2.8 mm/3.1 mm	4.0 mm/4.2 mm	5.9 mm	5.8 mm	4.9 mm	4.7 mm/ 5.4 mm/ 5.8 mm
Working length	1100 mm	1100 mm	600 mm	600 mm	1100 mm	1100 mm	1100 mm	650 mm
Instrument channel	2.0 mm	2.2 mm	1.2 mm	2.0 mm	2.0 mm	2.4 mm	2.0 mm	No instrument channel/ 1.5 mm/ 2.1 mm
Angulation	Up 210°Down 90°Right 100°Left 100°	Up 210°Down 90°Right 100°Left 100°	Up 180°/210°Down 130°/130° Rotary 120°	Up 180°/210°Down 130°/130° Rotary 120°	Up 210°Down 90°Right 100°Left 100°	Up 210°Down 90°Right 100°Left 100°	Up 210°Down 120°	Up 140°Down 215°

over 1000 samples obtained using UT scopes showed that its biopsy specimens are comparable in diagnostic yield to samples obtained using conventional gastroscopes and biopsy forceps [11]. There have been more recent studies in pediatrics and adults also demonstrating adequacy of samples in specific conditions such as eosinophilic esophagitis and Barrett's esophagus [9,11–13]. The deeper areas of tissues such as lamina propria seemed to vary between standard biopsies and the smaller samples [12]. There have been other small cohort studies suggesting tissue samples may not be adequate, but larger studies seem to contradict this [11,14].

The pediatric TNE study did not use adult UT endoscopes as they cannot be passed through most children's narrow nasal passages [9]. The Aerodigestive Program, a multidisciplinary airway and digestive disorder clinic responsible for the study, used pulmonary bronchoscopes (2.8–4.0 mm outer diameter) that had channels of 1.2 mm or 2 mm respectively. They used the associated forceps designed for the channels. This study demonstrated that TNE in younger children with movie goggles distraction was also possible with adequate samples obtained [9]. However, in this study TNE was unable to access the duodenum due to the shorter length of the bronchoscope.

Available adult UT endoscopes and pediatric bronchoscopes used in the pediatric studies are listed in Table 43.1 and range in outer diameter (OD) from 2.8 to 4.2 mm with channels of 1.2–2 mm with two-way tip deflection.

The main advantage that TNE offers is the ability to carry out endoscopy without the use of sedation, which carries risks, complications, high cost, and added time for the patient and caregivers. In one adult study, sedation-related cardiopulmonary risk in all forms of endoscopy was 0.6%, while pediatric studies also demonstrate similar events [15–17]. Additionally, in pediatrics there is a further potential risk of anesthesia for the developing brain [18]. Endoscopy in children commonly involves general anesthesia compared to the more common procedural sedation used in adults. The concerns regarding general anesthesia in children continue to be addressed in the literature [18,19].

Additionally, the route of insertion results in less pharyngeal stimulation and gag reflex than unsedated oral endoscopy as the endoscope does not touch the tongue, thereby making it more comfortable for patients [20].

At present, there are no guidelines stipulating indications or contraindications for TNE over and above those for standard oral endoscopy. However, there are relative contraindications for adult or pediatric patients with significant coagulopathy or recurrent and significant epistaxis (especially if related to hereditary haemorrhagic telangiectasia [HHT] – a contraindication for TNE); standard EGD (sEGD) is usually carried out over TNE [3].

Preendoscopy preparation

In pediatrics, preparation for TNE is of the utmost importance because success depends on a cooperative child. The authors recommend a precounseling visit and preparatory video viewing by the family discussing TNE and demonstrating the technique. This could be done by phone or in person per provider preference. Anxiety is not a contraindication as unpublished data demonstrate that children with treated anxiety commonly do well. If a child were to become nervous or would not tolerate the procedure due to a panic attack/anxiety flare, a previsit with a counselor who specializes in anxiety commonly will enable the child to undergo unsedated TNE easily and without complication. For the average child undergoing their first TNE, a child-life expert or a physician with expertise in child distraction and coping is recommended to review techniques with the child.

The above group also reported success with the use of video goggles of various forms. This same group notes that children may also be

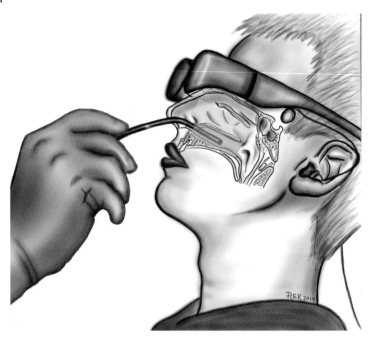

Figure 43.1 (a) Suggested sitting method: TNE insertion pathway below the inferior turbinate (green). Alternate sitting method: TNE insertion pathway above the inferior turbinate, below the middle turbinate (yellow). This area is suggested if swelling or partial nasal obstruction is present at the level of the inferior turbinate. Alternatively, consider a smaller outer diameter endoscope.

able to cope with the technique without goggles, similar to adults, in certain cases. Demonstration of the technique in pediatrics can be seen at www.pediatricendoscopy.com. Following a precounseling visit and consent with the family, the procedure can begin (Figure 43.1).

Nasal preparation is aimed at providing nasal and pharyngeal anesthesia, and improving ease of endoscope insertion via turbinate shrinkage with topical decongestants. In a randomized study, 55.8% patients who underwent unsedated TNE found that the most painful area during endoscope insertion was the nasal cavity, emphasizing the need for adequate preparation [21]. A more recent study reported this to be less than 20% [6]. Various methods of nasal preparation have been described, including pledgetting the nasal cavity with cotton tip and gauze coated in lidocaine, aerosolized spray containing local anesthesia and decongestant (e.g., 5% lidocaine and 0.5% phenylephrine

hydrochloride), a combination of these, or none [10]. Most centers performing TNE would advocate the use of aerosolized spray with topical pharyngeal anesthesia and decongestant. The pediatric group performing TNE currently uses 4% aerosolized lidocaine after blowing the nose, using three sprays to each nostril and one spray orally (total dose 0.3–0.4 mL) per patient. Nasal decongestion was not found helpful nor reported by the pediatric group. The best route for nasal traverse is seen in Figure 43.2, avoiding the inferior turbinate, and then central insertion into the esophagus is as for standard endoscopy (Figure 43.3).

Views and image quality

There were concerns about the quality of images obtained from the first-generation UT scopes, but the more recent models have a brighter light source and improved objective

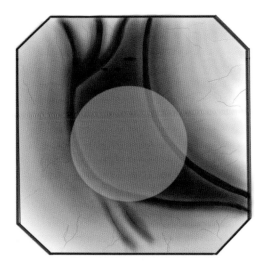

Figure 43.2 Suggested optimal area to pass the transnasal endoscope after insertion. The position is lateral and inferior to the inferior turbinate.

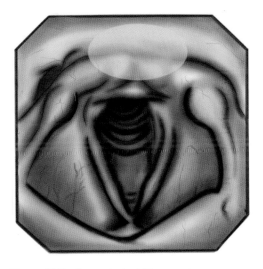

Figure 43.3 Suggested midline area to pass transnasal endoscope from the pharyngeal location to the esophagus. This area is directly superior to the arytenoid cartilages.

optical system, thereby improving views. A randomized control trial involving one experienced endoscopist comparing TNE (Fujinon EG-530N) and conventional gastroscopes found no difference in views obtained in the esophagus, stomach, and duodenum [22]. As expected, the view proximal to the esophagus including the hypopharynx and cricopharyngeal area was better with TNE [22]. The authors also found no difficulty with pyloric intubation with TNE [22]. Crews *et al.* also evaluated the quality of views obtained from TNE (TNE-5000, Vision Sciences) and conventional gastroscopes and found no statistical difference between the quality of videos created with either [23].

Paediatric TNE using bronchoscopes had varying image quality based on generation of scope (video graphics array [VGA] vs high definition [HD]) and usage of air insufflation. UT bronchoscopes are designed without continuous air flow, which if used creates more gagging in the esophagus. When air insufflation is used intermittently, the viewing was optimal barring operator technique, but with air let out the tissues would collapse. The newest UT bronchscopes used for GI TNE have similar HD optics to standard gastroscopes.

Duration

A UK randomized trial compared TNE and sEGD and found that mean preparation time was longer in TNE (5.5 min vs 4.6 min, p < 0.001) [24]. In terms of procedure time, some studies reported that the duration of unsedated TNE was significantly longer compared to sEGD, but one did not [21,22,25]. However, in reality the difference between the two was around a minute; one study reported that the duration for TNE and sEGD was 8.4 ± 3.2 min and 7.7 ± 3.4 min (p = 0.02) respectively [22]. In this same study, patients were observed for an hour post procedure, but 80% of patients from both groups would be happy with a shorter duration of observation post procedure (20 minutes). More importantly, the recovery time for TNE was significantly shorter than sEGD (5.0 min vs 10.0 min, p <0.001) [24].

In the single-center report by Friedlander *et al.*, the average time of TNE was 8.6 minutes with total office time of 60–90 minutes [9]. From newer unpublished data, this center reports average duration of a first-time TNE of 60 minutes in office and 45 minutes for follow-up TNE, and average TNE time has decreased to under six minutes for esophagoscopy/gastroscopy compared to EGD.

Success rates

The success rates for adult unsedated TNE are high. One metaanalysis reports this at 94% (95% confidence interval [CI] 91.6–95.8) in comparison to 97.8% in unsedated UT transoral EGD, but when TNE was compared to unsedated sEGD it performed slightly poorer (RD −2.0%, CI −4.0 to −1.0) [26]. When UT scopes of <5.9 mm was used, similar success rates to sEGD were obtained [26]. Unsuccessful attempts have been attributed to nasal pain, narrow nasal passages or altered anatomy [27].

Success rates in pediatric TNE are also high. As of this publication, the reporting group using TNE has performed 264 TNE that had not been stopped once started. There were six children who came in for TNE but due to motion or anxiety were not able to sit still to start the procedure (97.8% success rate if those children were included).

Patient comfort and preference

A metaanalysis reported that when patients were offered a choice of TNE or sEGD for future endoscopies, a significant proportion of patients opted for unsedated TNE (RD 63%, CI 49–76), and 85.2% of patients were willing to undergo unsedated TNE again in the future [26]. Patients who have undergone unsedated TNE found it more comfortable compared to unsedated EGD (comfort score TNE: 7 ± 2.3 vs EGD: 5.4 ± 2.78, p <0.001) [22]. In the same study, the number of patients who reported gagging was significantly lower in the TNE group (77% vs 26%, p <0.001) [22].

The single-center pediatric study reports that of families of children between 8 and 17 years who had undergone previous EGD, 100% would undergo TNE again while 74% of children would undergo TNE again [9]; 84% of families and 53% of children preferred TNE to sEGD [9].

Complications and safety profile

Esophagogastroduodenoscopy is associated with cardiopulmonary stress with increased heart rate and systolic blood pressure [22,28]. TNE, on the other hand, does not have this effect, and patients undergoing TNE are noted to have a consistent heart rate and systolic blood pressure [22,29]. Furthermore, it is not associated with episodes of desaturation [21,22].

A recent metaanalysis evaluated adverse events associated with TNE; epistaxis was the only event consistently note, comprising 2% of all cases [26]. These are largely self-limiting events [21]. In patients with chronic liver disease or liver cirrhosis, TNE has been found to be safe, with a low rate of self-limiting epistaxis (4–6%) [30,31]. There was only one case of reported esophageal perforation [32]. Reports of presyncopal episodes associated with TNE have also been published (two out of 95 patients in one study) [33].

Using unpublished data from the pediatric TNE center doing esophagoscopy rather than EGD, 5.2% of subjects undergo an episode of spit up or emesis that is brief and limited, 2.6% had nasal irritation without epistaxis, 0.9% presynscope, 0.5% anxiety attack, and 0.4% nausea.

Therapeutic use

The main common therapeutic use would be insertion of nasoenteric tubes. TNE-assisted insertion (either via guidewire assistance or pull-through method with biopsy forceps) was shown to be safe and comparable to fluoroscopic insertion [34,35]. It was found to be safe in critically unwell patients [35]. Overall, the therapeutic use of a TNE scope is limited.

Future considerations

Training in TNE may be a limiting factor as to why its use is not as widespread as one might expect. Further consideration of formalized training for TNE for independent and trainee endoscopists should be undertaken. Some literature exists documenting self-training in operators who are experienced endoscopists [36].

The pediatric center reporting unsedated TNE has implemented a training program for TNE endosocopists. They have reported use of 3D printed models and a curriculum. To date, they have completed a single fellow training and are in the process with two other attending gastroenterologists. Multiple other centers have visited for basic, but not hands-on training due to medical legal US licensing and malpractice issues.

An additional facet with TNE is its potential use in the clinic setting, much like laryngoscopy by ENT specialists. This is currently performed in Japan and was done by the pediatric center in their study [6,9]. Most endoscopy services are set up to be done in procedural units. Perhaps with further training, implementation of TNE, and improvement of endoscopic technology for diagnostic adult and pediatric TNE, bringing diagnostic TNE into the clinic setting may be a possibility.

Such technology has significant potential to transform the practice of pediatric gastroenterology from a method to avoid endoscopy due to risks to a highly valuable tool to make more informed decisions about therapies. With such a tool, careful thought should be given to who truly needs an endoscopy to prevent overuse. Although TNE is safe, effective, and well tolerated, it still carries a cost, discomfort, and potential risk.

Conclusion

In pediatrics, transnasal esophagoscopy using bronchoscopes has been reported to be safe and effective. In both adults and pediatrics, it is well tolerated and is preferred by most patients. With currently available technology, pediatric transnasal EGD is limited to subjects who can tolerate the longer and wider adult UT scopes. As it can be used without sedation, TNE reduces the potential of sedation-related risks. However, due to its smaller diameter and lack of anesthesia, its therapeutic use is limited. With improvement in technology, the quality of UT scope views and imaging is continuing to improve, making TNE an attractive alternative for adult and pediatric patients undergoing upper gastrointestinal tract examination.

 • See companion website for videos relating to this chapter topic: www.wiley.com/go/gershman3e

REFERENCES

1 Shaker R. Unsedated trans-nasal pharyngoesophagogastroduodenoscopy (T-EGD): technique. *Gastrointest Endosc* 1994, **40**, 346–348.

2 Amin MR, Postma GN, Setzen M, *et al.* Transnasal esophagoscopy: a position statement from the American Bronchoesophagological Association (ABEA). *Otolaryngol Head Neck Surg* 2008, **138**, 411–414.

3 Rodriguez SA, Banerjee S, Desilets D, *et al.* Ultrathin endoscopes. *Gastrointest Endosc* 2010, **71**, 893–898.

4 Aviv JE. Transnasal esophagoscopy: state of the art. *Otolaryngol Head Neck Surg* 2006, **135**, 616–619.

5 Aviv JE, Takoudes TG, Ma G, *et al.* Office-based esophagoscopy: a preliminary report. *Otolaryngol Head Neck Surg* 2001, **125**, 170–175.

6 Tanuma T, Morita Y, Doyama H. Current status of transnasal endoscopy worldwide using ultrathin videoscope for upper gastrointestinal tract. *Dig Endosc* 2016, **28**, 25–31.

7 Dumortier J, Napoleon B, Hedelius F, *et al.* Unsedated transnasal EGD in daily practice: results with 1100 consecutive patients. *Gastrointest Endosc* 2003, **57**, 198–204.

8 Cho S, Arya N, Swan K, *et al.* Unsedated transnasal endoscopy: a Canadian experience in daily practice. *Can J Gastroenterol* 2008, **22**, 243–246.

9 Friedlander JA, DeBoer EM, Soden JS, *et al.* Unsedated transnasal esophagoscopy for monitoring therapy in pediatric eosinophilic esophagitis. *Gastrointest Endosc* 2016, **83**, 299–306 e1.

10 Parker C, Alexandridis E, Plevris J, *et al.* Transnasal endoscopy: no gagging no panic! *Frontline Gastroenterol* 2016, **7**, 246–256.

11 Walter T, Chesnay AL, Dumortier J, *et al.* Biopsy specimens obtained with small–caliber endoscopes have comparable diagnostic performances than those obtained with conventional endoscopes: a prospective study on 1335 specimens. *J Clin Gastroenterol* 2010, **44**, 12–17.

12 Philpott H, Nandurkar S, Royce SG, *et al.* Ultrathin unsedated transnasal gastroscopy in monitoring eosinophilic esophagitis. *J Gastroenterol Hepatol* 2016, **31**, 590–594.

13 Saeian K, Staff DM, Vasilopoulos S, *et al.* Unsedated transnasal endoscopy accurately detects Barrett's metaplasia and dysplasia. *Gastrointest Endosc* 2002, **56**, 472–478.

14 Halum SL, Postma GN, Bates DD, *et al.* Incongruence between histologic and endoscopic diagnoses of Barrett's esophagus using transnasal esophagoscopy. *Laryngoscope* 2006, **116**, 303–306.

15 Sharma VK, Nguyen CC, Crowell MD, *et al.* A national study of cardiopulmonary unplanned events after GI endoscopy. *Gastrointest Endosc* 2007, **66**, 27–34.

16 Thakkar K, El-Serag HB, Mattek N, *et al.* Complications of pediatric EGD: a 4-year experience in PEDS-CORI. *Gastrointest Endosc* 2007, **65**, 213–221.

17 Gilger MA, Gold BD. Pediatric endoscopy: new information from the PEDS-CORI project. *Curr Gastroenterol Rep* 2005, **7**, 234–239.

18 Aker J, Block RI, Biddle C. Anesthesia and the developing brain. *AANA J* 2015, **83**, 139–147.

19 Miller TL, Park R, Sun LS. Report on the Fifth PANDA Symposium on "Anesthesia and Neurodevelopment in Children". *J Neurosurg Anesthesiol* 2016, **28**, 350–355.

20 Preiss C, Charton JP, Schumacher B, *et al.* A randomized trial of unsedated transnasal small-caliber esophagogastroduodenoscopy (EGD) versus peroral small-caliber EGD versus conventional EGD. *Endoscopy* 2003, **35**, 641–646.

21 Watanabe H, Watanabe N, Ogura R, *et al.* A randomized prospective trial comparing unsedated endoscopy via transnasal and transoral routes using 5.5-mm video endoscopy. *Dig Dis Sci* 2009, **54**, 2155–2160.

22 Alexandridis E, Inglis S, McAvoy NC, *et al.* Randomised clinical study: comparison of acceptability, patient tolerance, cardiac stress and endoscopic views in transnasal and transoral endoscopy under local anaesthetic. *Aliment Pharmacol Ther* 2014, **40**, 467–476.

23 Crews NR, Gorospe EC, Johnson ML, *et al.* Comparative quality assessment of esophageal examination with transnasal and sedated endoscopy. *Endosc Int Open* 2017, **5**, E340–E344.

24 Despott EH, Baulf M, Bromley J, *et al.* OC-059 Scent: final report of the first UK prospective, randomised, head-to-head trial

of transnasal vs oral upper gastrointestinal endoscopy. *Gut* 2010, **59**, A24.

25 Uchiyama K, Ishikawa T, Sakamoto N, *et al.* Analysis of cardiopulmonary stress during endoscopy: is unsedated transnasal esophagogastroduodenoscopy appropriate for elderly patients? *Can J Gastroenterol Hepatol* 2014, **28**, 31–34.

26 Sami SS, Subramanian V, Ortiz-Fernandez-Sordo J, *et al.* Performance characteristics of unsedated ultrathin video endoscopy in the assessment of the upper GI tract: systematic review and meta-analysis. *Gastrointest Endosc* 2015, **82**, 782–792.

27 Birkner B, Fritz N, Schatke W, *et al.* A prospective randomized comparison of unsedated ultrathin versus standard esophagogastroduodenoscopy in routine outpatient gastroenterology practice: does it work better through the nose? *Endoscopy* 2003, **35**, 647–651.

28 Yuki M, Amano Y, Komazawa Y, *et al.* Unsedated transnasal small-caliber esophagogastroduodenoscopy in elderly and bedridden patients. *World J Gastroenterol* 2009, **15**, 5586–5591.

29 Ai ZL, Lan CH, Fan LL, *et al.* Unsedated transnasal upper gastrointestinal endoscopy has favorable diagnostic effectiveness, cardiopulmonary safety, and patient satisfaction compared with conventional or sedated endoscopy. *Surg Endosc* 2012, **26**, 3565–3572.

30 de Faria AA, Dias CAF, Dias Moetzsohn L, *et al.* Feasibility of transnasal endoscopy in screening for esophageal and gastric varices in patients with chronic liver disease. *Endosc Int Open* 2017, **5**, E646–E651.

31 Choe WH, Kim JH, Ko SY, *et al.* Comparison of transnasal small–caliber vs. peroral conventional esophagogastroduodenoscopy for evaluating varices in unsedated cirrhotic patients. *Endoscopy* 2011, **43**, 649–656.

32 Zaman A, Hahn M, Hapke R, *et al.* A randomized trial of peroral versus transnasal unsedated endoscopy using an ultrathin videoendoscope. *Gastrointest Endosc* 1999, **49**, 279–284.

33 Shariff MK, Bird-Lieberman EL, O'Donovan M, *et al.* Randomized crossover study comparing efficacy of transnasal endoscopy with that of standard endoscopy to detect Barrett's esophagus. *Gastrointest Endosc* 2012, **75**, 954–961.

34 Qin H, Lu XY, Zhao Q, *et al.* Evaluation of a new method for placing nasojejunal feeding tubes. *World J Gastroenterol* 2012, **18**, 5295–5299.

35 Zhihui T, Wenkui Y, Weiqin L, *et al.* A randomised clinical trial of transnasal endoscopy versus fluoroscopy for the placement of nasojejunal feeding tubes in patients with severe acute pancreatitis. *Postgrad Med J* 2009, **85**, 59–63.

36 Maffei M, Dumortier J, Dumonceau JM. Self-training in unsedated transnasal EGD by endoscopists competent in standard peroral EGD: prospective assessment of the learning curve. *Gastrointest Endosc* 2008, **67**, 410–418.

44

Endoscopic bariatric approaches

Mike Thomson and Matjaz Homan

 KEY POINTS

- Bariatric balloons afford temporary weight loss but generally are associated with initial nausea and when removed, the weight loss reverses.
- The endo-sleeve is promising but perihepatic abscesses have been recorded very occasionally so this technology remains under review.

- Pseudopolyps are reported in the duodenal bulb due to the anchor of the sleeve.
- Multiple gastric plications may be used but are not a widespread approach.

Introduction

Over the last 40 years the prevalence of obesity in the pediatric population in developed countries has risen substantially. The high prevalence of obesity in children early in life causes a high incidence of serious health complications, such as diabetes mellitus, hypertension, and nonalcoholic fatty liver disease. In addition to having medical co-morbidities, obese children can also have significant psychosocial problems. Unfortunately, a significant percentage of children with obesity will become obese adults. The combination of medical co-morbidities and psychosocial problems significantly lowers the quality of life so optimal therapeutic modalities should be initiated early in life.

Treatment of obesity and its associated metabolic diseases requires a multidisciplinary approach, with adequate nutrition intervention, lifestyle modification, and physical exercise. However, only a small percentage of

adolescents is able to be compliant with the diet and exercise in the long term. Furthermore, data available for the safety and efficacy of medications that have been studied for the treatment of obesity in children are limited. More enduring weight loss has been achieved with surgical interventions than with diet, physical activity or medications. In morbidly obese adults, Roux-en-Y gastric bypass, sleeve gastrectomy, and laparoscopic banding are well-established methods of losing weight. Due to significant improvement of obesity and obesity-related diseases, the surgical approach is becoming more popular in adolescents as well.

The surgical method most frequently used is Roux-en-Y gastric bypass. However, bariatric surgery is not an optimal method to treat obese children due to several reasons: irreversibility of the procedure, possible important side effects, uncertainty about long-term outcomes, and ethical considerations related to adolescents

Practical Pediatric Gastrointestinal Endoscopy, Third Edition. Edited by George Gershman and Mike Thomson.
© 2021 John Wiley & Sons Ltd. Published 2021 by John Wiley & Sons Ltd.
Companion website: www.wiley.com/go/gershman3e

agreeing to bariatric surgery procedures. As an alternative, a less invasive approach to treat morbidly obese adolescents is a nonsurgical endoluminal intervention performed by flexible endoscopy. Endoscopic bariatric techniques (EBTs) are safer and more cost-effective than current surgical approaches. In the field of metabolic obesity disease in adults, several different endoscopic approaches have been described, such as endoscopic gastroplasty, intragastric balloon, endoscopically placed tube which allows aspiration therapy, endoluminal malabsorptive bariatric procedures, and gastric electrical stimulation. Occupying gastric volume, restricting gastric capacity, and reducing absorption of ingested food are the underlying mechanisms for losing weight in the EBTs.

The rest of the chapter will focus only on those EBTs that have been studied and described in children.

Intragastric balloons

The insertion of intragastric balloons involves a standard upper GI endoscopy and a catheter inserted alongside the endoscope, within which is a tethered balloon. Once in position, the balloon overboard is withdrawn, allowing the balloon to be inflated with fluid containing methylene blue. At this point, 500 mL of fluid is injected and then the balloon is ejected from the catheter into the stomach. The balloon is left for six months and then removed using an endoscopic technique involving a hook grasping forcep and a needle to puncture the balloon, thereby aspirating the fluid and contracting the balloon; once all the fluid is withdrawn then the balloon can be extracted orally.

Our experience is that the median weight loss is around 10% body weight but that weight is put on again after the six months of balloon placement. However, the procedure may allow the individual to know what weight loss feels like and this may motivate them towards their goal (Figure 44.1).

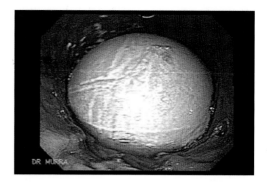

Figure 44.1 Intragastric balloon.

Duodenojejunal bypass liner

The duodenojejunal bypass liner (DJBL) (EndoBarrier gastrointestinal liner, GI Dynamics, Lexington, MA) is an endoscopically placed and removable intestinal liner. The DJBL causes mechanical nonabsorption of nutrients in the proximal part of the small intestine and resembles the most popular bariatric surgical method – Roux-Y-gastric bypass.

The device is composed of a self-expanding nickel-titanium anchor attached to a 61 cm long polymer sleeve (Figure 44.2). In the original form and during delivery, the anchor and sleeve are in a collapsed form packed in a

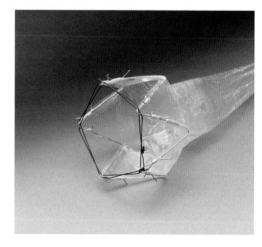

Figure 44.2 Anchor attached to long polymer impermeable sleeve. *Source:* Photo courtesy of GI Dynamics, Inc.

protective white capsule (see Figure 44.2). Three days before the procedure, therapy with proton pump inhibitors (PPI) should be started. In addition, before the procedure antibiotic prophylaxis is indicated.

The endoscopic placement is usually performed in the theater with the patient under general anesthesia. Two pediatric gastroenterologists are required to perform the procedure. The first performs the endoscopy and the second assists with DJBL accessories to position and deploy the device (Figure 44.3). A guidewire is advanced deep into the duodenum with fluoroscopic guidance. The device enclosed in a capsule is advanced over the guidewire (Figure 44.4). The sleeve is then deployed in the proximal intestine (Figure 44.5). When the sleeve is fully extended with the help of the ball, contrast medium and air, and the anchor is located in the duodenal bulb distal to the pylorus, the self-expandable anchor is deployed from the capsule. The position of the device is visualized through the tip of the endoscope kept in stomach during the entire procedure. The position of the crowns (anchor) is carefully inspected again at the end of the placement to correct the crossing or malposition of the crowns with the endoscope (Figure 44.6).

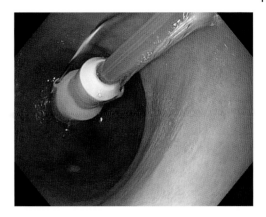

Figure 44.4 The device introduced over the guidewire.

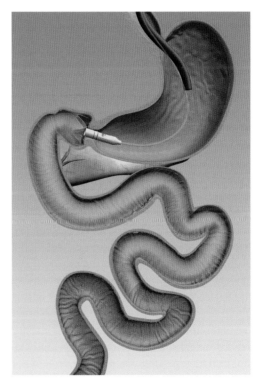

Figure 44.5 The releasing of the device. *Source:* Photo courtesy of GI Dynamics, Inc.

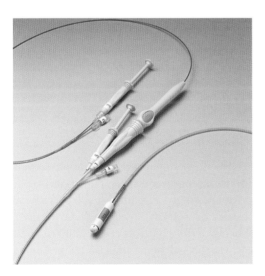

Figure 44.3 The delivery device of the sleeve. *Source:* Photo courtesy of GI Dynamics, Inc.

Placement of the DJBL takes on average half an hour.

Usually painkillers and antiemetics are prescribed for the first few days to prevent vomiting and anchor migration. For the same reason, a liquid diet during the first two weeks after

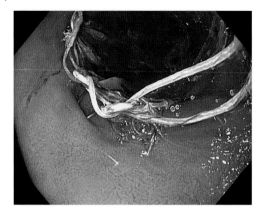

Figure 44.6 The anchor attached to the duodenal mucosa.

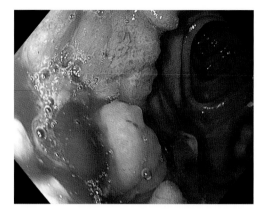

Figure 44.7 Pseudopolyps at the site of anchor attachment.

placement is advised. The device is usually left in place for 12 months. The patient should be kept on regular PPI treatment one year after the procedure to prevent duodenal ulcers and bleeding, and should be advised to avoid any contact sports to prevent possible device migration. Patients are also advised to drink a lot of liquids, chew food well and eat slowly, and avoid raw fruits and vegetables in their diet to prevent mechanical sleeve obstruction.

Device removal is performed under general anesthesia, using a retrieval device. A special foreign body hood is placed at the tip of the endoscope. The tip of the endoscope with the hood is positioned in the duodenal bulb. One of the drawstrings located at the crown of the device is pulled into the hood, thus collapsing the device crowns into the hood. After ensuring fluoroscopically that secure position of all the barbs inside the hood is achieved, the DJBL can be pulled out of the duodenum into the stomach lumen. After complete removal of the device, the endoscopy should be repeated to inspect the site where anchor was attached to the duodenal mucosa for possible bleeding. Usually pseudopolyps can be seen in the duodenal bulb (Figure 44.7). PPI therapy is discontinued two weeks after device removal. The liner can be reimplanted into the same patient after a period of a few months.

In adults, placement of the DJBL device was first described in 2008 by Rodriguez-Grunert

et al., and has been used successfully since as a treatment for morbid obesity with co-morbidities. The American Society for Gastrointestinal Endoscopy recently published a metaanalysis of the DJBL in adults. Out of 135 citations, 11 full-length manuscripts have met strict inclusion criteria. Three trials enrolling 105 patients treated for 12 months indicated that the DJBL achieved 35.3% of excess weight loss (%EWL) (95% confidence interval [CI] 24.6–46.1). In four randomized controlled trials that compared DJBL and control groups of patients after 12–24 weeks of treatment, the mean %EWL difference between the groups was 9.4% (95% CI 8.26–10.65). When the authors looked at the impact on obesity-related co-morbidities, such as glycosylated hemoglobin (HbA1c), they reported significant improvements of -0.7 (95% CI -1.76 to 0.2; p $= 0.16$), -1.7 (95% CI -2.5 to -0.86; p <0.001), and -1.5 (95% CI -2.2 to -0.78; p <0.001) after 12, 24, and 52 weeks of DJBL implantation, respectively.

In a safety analysis, 271 patients with DJBL placement were included. Reported serious adverse events were linear migration (4.9%), gastrointestinal bleeding (3.86%), sleeve obstruction (3.4%), liver abscess (0.13%), cholangitis (0.13%), acute cholecystitis (0.13%), and esophageal perforation (0.13%). Among other adverse events, pain was described in 58.7%, and nausea and vomiting in 39.4% of cases. Early removal of the device because of adverse events was reported in 18.4% of patients. In general, the safety profile of the DJBL was established as acceptable but there was one exception in a US multicenter trial in which a higher than anticipated rate of hepatic abscess was reported and enrolment of new patients was temporarily halted.

For the first time in children, our research group evaluated the efficacy and safety of DJBL and its effects on weight loss, metabolic and cardiovascular parameters. The device was successfully implanted in 14 morbidly obese adolescents out of 17 who underwent the procedure (10 females, mean age 17.7 years, range 15.0–19.2; average body weight 124.3 kg, range 93.2–158.8). Inclusion criteria were BMI ≥35 kg/m² with obesity complications such as hypertension, prediabetes or type 2 diabetes. The BMI (kg/m²) was measured at 0, 3, 6, 9, and 12 months and was shown to have decreased at all time frames (42.3 [range 36.7–48.8], 38.0 [range 34.1–44.5], 37.7 [range 33.3–44.8], 37.5 [range 33.1–45.5], and 36.7 [range 32.4–45.9], respectively). In addition, glucose metabolism significantly improved: mean HOMA-IR level at the beginning of the study was 5.6 (± 2,2) and decreased at six and 12 months after implantation (3.8 ± 1.6 and 2.7 ± 0.9, respectively). The most frequent adverse events were of gastrointestinal origin and were reported mostly in the first two weeks after implantation: nausea in six out of 14 cases, abdominal pain in eight out of 14 children, and diarrhea in two out of 14 adolescents which is comparable with adult data. With the exception of one case of acute cholecystitis that presented three months after liner placement, there were no severe procedure- or postprocedure-related complications similarly to those that are described in adults. Adolescents were followed up for 12 months. Significant weight loss was detected in most adolescent subjects, and glucose metabolism improved in all. The study is still ongoing.

Conclusion

Obesity is a global epidemic and is associated with multiple co-morbidities. It has a great impact on health and quality of life that starts as early as childhood and is even greater later in life. Therefore, it is of great importance to successfully treat obesity early in life to prevent future complications. Diet, lifestyle modification, and medicinal drugs have only minimal efficacy on losing weight. Invasive options, primarily bariatric surgery, have been shown to be more effective, but are rarely utilized in children. EBTs may be a better option for children. Use of space-occupying intragastric balloons offers reversible weight management that has proven to be more effective than diet and lifestyle changes. The new technique of DJBL, resembling the Roux-Y-gastric bypass, is even more effective and regarded as safer than bariatric surgical methods, but more data on use in the pediatric population are needed.

The new endoscopic therapy for obesity will evolve in future, but it is of major importance that only those children who meet strict indications are considered for the endoscopic procedure.

 • See companion website for videos relating to this chapter topic: www.wiley.com/go/gershman3e

 FURTHER READING

Abu Dayyeh BK, Kumar N, Edmundowicz SA, *et al.* ASGE Bariatric Endoscopy Task Force systematic review and meta-analysis assessing the ASGE PIVI thresholds for adopting endoscopic bariatric therapies. *Gastrointest Endosc* 2015, **82**, 425–438.

Ells LJ, Hancock C, Copley VR, *et al.* Prevalence of severe childhood obesity in

England: 2006-2013. *Arch Dis Child* 2015, **100**, 631–636.

Fried M, Yumuk V, Oppert JM, *et al.* Interdisciplinary European guidelines on metabolic and bariatric surgery. *Obes Facts* 2013, **6**, 449–468.

Homan M, Battelino T, Kotnik P, Orel R. Duodenal-jejunal bypass liner- primary experience in morbidly obese adolescents, safety and efficacy. *J Pediatr Gastroenterol Nutr* 2016, **62**, 273.

Kotnik P, Homan M, Orel R, Battelino T. Efficacy and safety of duodenal-jejunal bypass liner in morbidly obese adolescents – 1 year experience. *Hormone Res Paediatr* 2016, **86**, 61.

Nobili V, Vajro P, Dezsofi A, *et al.* Indications and limitations of bariatric intervention in severely obese children and adolescents with and without nonalcoholic steatohepatitis: ESPGHAN Hepatology Committee position statement. *J Pediatr Gastroenterol Nutr* 2015, **60**, 550–561.

Rodriguez-Grunert L, Galvao Neto MP, Alamo M, Ramos AC, Baez PB, Tarnoff M. First human experience with endoscopically delivered and retrieved duodenal-jejunal bypass sleeve. *Surg Obes Relat Dis* 2008, **4**, 55–59.

45

Over-the-scope clip and full-thickness resection device

Mike Thomson

KEY POINTS

- Over-the-scope clips (OTSC) have recently been used successfully in adult, and to a lesser extent pediatric, therapeutic endoscopy.
- The OTSC is constrained in pediatric practice by its size and for upper GI applications should be used by trained expert pediatric endoscopists in children weighing more than 15–20 kg.
- GI bleeding lesions, perforations and fistulae closure (including PEG tracts) are indications for its use.

- OTSC may be used with care for colonoscopic indications such as anastomotic bleeding sites.
- The same device with slight modifications can be used as a full-thickness resection device (FTRD) in order to obtain full thickness transmural biopsy specimens, e.g., in Hirschsprung's disease.

There is relatively recent, but accumulating evidence, showing that the OTSC device can be used in the successful closure of moderate perforations which are too large for endo-clips. The OTSC has also been used for hemostasis, for instance in point bleeding lesions. It may also be applied to perform full-thickness biopsies of the lower GI tract. Specific accessories are available for each indication.

The device is front-loaded onto the endoscope and is controlled by an extraendoscopic channel which is attached to the outside of the scope. The central grasping forceps are deployed to stabilize the tissue of choice and then suction is applied until vision is obliterated – similar to variceal banding; this is generally applied for five seconds and then the jaws of the capture clip are released. They have shape memory to oppose each other like jaws and are released to return to

their original closed position when the handle is turned outside the patient (Figure 45.1). They have been used successfully in a few children to date for perforation closure and recently in our center to stop a point GI bleeding area successfully. A similar case is shown in Figure 45.2.

Various sizes are available and the 12 mm version is appropriate for most children. For perforation the jaws have sharp teeth but the hemostatic clips have more rounded teeth (Figure 45.3). An adaptation of this technique shows promise for obtaining full-thickness biopsies for conditions such as Hirschsprung's disease using a transanal approach (Figure 45.4).

- See companion website for videos relating to this chapter topic: www.wiley.com/go/gershman3e

Practical Pediatric Gastrointestinal Endoscopy, Third Edition. Edited by George Gershman and Mike Thomson.
© 2021 John Wiley & Sons Ltd. Published 2021 by John Wiley & Sons Ltd.
Companion website: www.wiley.com/go/gershman3e

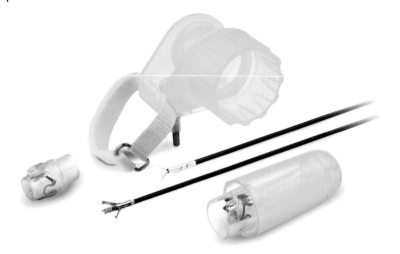

Figure 45.1 The full device components.

(a)   (b)

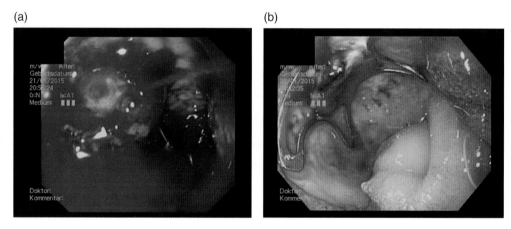

Figure 45.2 Treatment of a point bleeder – before (a) and two days afterwards (b).

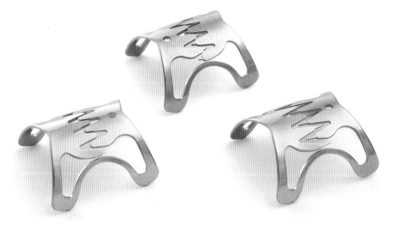

Figure 45.3 Hemostatic clips.

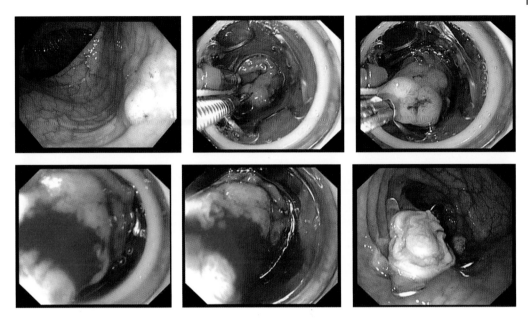

Figure 45.4 Full-thickness resection.

 FURTHER READING

Okada Y, Yokoyama K, Yano T, *et al.* A boy with duodenocolic fistula mimicking functional gastrointestinal disorder. *Clin J Gastroenterol* 2019, **12**, 566–570.

Tran P, Carroll J, Barth BA, Channabasappa N, Troendle DM. Over the scope clips for treatment of acute nonvariceal gastrointestinal bleeding in children are safe and effective. *J Pediatr Gastroenterol Nutr* 2018, **67**, 458–463.

Wedi E, Fischer A, Hochberger J, Jung C, Orkut S, Richter-Schrag HJ. Multicenter evaluation of first–line endoscopic treatment with the OTSC in acute non-variceal upper gastrointestinal bleeding and comparison with the Rockall cohort: the FLETRock study. *Surg Endosc* 2018, **32**, 307–314.

Wedi E, Gonzalez S, Menke D, Kruse E, Matthes K, Hochberger J. One hundred and one over-the-scope-clip applications for severe gastrointestinal bleeding, leaks and fistulas. *World J Gastroenterol* 2016, **22**, 1844–1853.

Weiland T, Rohrer S, Schmidt A, *et al.* Efficacy of the OTSC System in the treatment of GI bleeding and wall defects: a PMCF meta-analysis. *Minim Invasive Ther Allied Technol* 2020, **29**, 121–139.

46

Endoscopic treatment of gastrointestinal bezoars

Andreia Nita and Mike Thomson

 KEY POINTS

- Most bezoars in the stomach and proximal duodenum are radiolucent and endoscopic management and retrieval is possible in most cases.
- It is important to know the composition of the bezoar before its attempted removal.
- Apart from trichobezoars, other bezoars are amenable to enzymatic dissolution or chemical degradation by endoscopy.

- Trichobezoars can be fragmented using various endoscopic devices including polypectomy snares, hook knives, and argon plasma coagulation, with subsequent retrieval of fragmented pieces using rat-toothed forceps, Roth nets, and polyp snares.

Bezoars are classified according to their composition into trichobezoar (hair) (Figure 46.1), lactobezoar (milk), pharmacobezoar (medicines/chemicals), and phytobezoar (vegetable matter) (Figure 46.2). While most bezoars can be treated by enzymatic dissolution (with proteolytic enzymes or Coca-Cola™), a trichobezoar may be a greater challenge for the endoscopist.

The gold standard for diagnosis of bezoars is endoscopy, while the treatment is either endoscopic or surgical. Surgery was the treatment of choice in the past, but endoscopy is gaining ground, being reported as the preferred treatment in 66–77% of bezoars [1,2]. Endoscopic removal is less invasive and more cost-effective, provided that the shape and dimensions of the trichobezoar enable endoscopic retrieval. Sometimes, endoscopic treatment is not successful because of the extension of the trichobezoar tail into the small bowel, the size of the bezoar or its embedding into gastric mucosa.

The endoscopic intervention usually consists of two steps: fragmentation and removal of fragmented parts. The whole procedure can involve many passages over 3–4 hours (Figure 46.3).

The trichobezoar can be fragmented using various endoscopic devices including polypectomy snare, hook knife, and argon plasma coagulation, and then retrieval of fragmented pieces may be carried out with rat-toothed forceps and polyp snares (Figure 46.4).

Endoscopic attempts to remove gastric trichobezoars have been reported [3–8]. Starting from the first attempt in 1989 with Nd:YAG laser and extracorporeal shockwave lithotripsy for fragmentation in multiple endoscopic sessions, and keeping up with technological progress, other methods have been tried

Practical Pediatric Gastrointestinal Endoscopy, Third Edition. Edited by George Gershman and Mike Thomson.
© 2021 John Wiley & Sons Ltd. Published 2021 by John Wiley & Sons Ltd.
Companion website: www.wiley.com/go/gershman3e

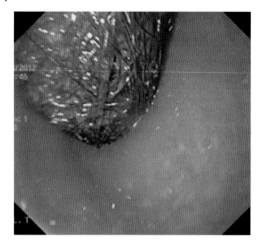

Figure 46.1 Trichobezoar.

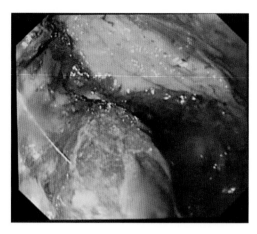

Figure 46.3 Trichobezoar endoscopic intervention usually consists of two steps: fragmentation and removal of fragmented parts.

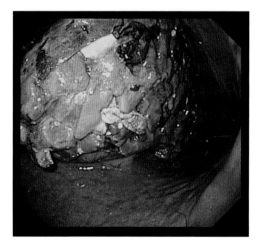

Figure 46.2 Phytobezoar.

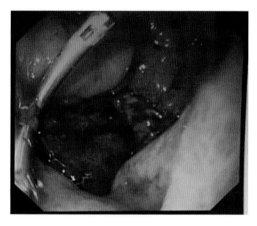

Figure 46.4 The trichobezoar can be fragmented using various endoscopic devices including polypectomy snare, hook knife, and argon plasma coagulation, and then retrieval of fragmented pieces may be carried out with Roth nets, rat-toothed forceps, and polyp snares.

such as the use of a double channel endoscope and overtube, removing the trichobezoar as a single unit. As a new alternative for trichobezoar fragmentation, electrocautery can be used (argon plasma coagulation and polypectomy snare).

A combined method using laparoscopy-assisted fragmentation (laparoscopic scissors used through a 1 cm gastric incision) and endoscopic retrieval of fragments has been reported recently [9]. It is important to know that the constituents of the bezoar are organic and not chemical so that application of electrocautery does not produce a chemical reaction with the potential for caustic effects topically on the GI mucosa.

REFERENCES

1 Park SE, Ahn JY, Jung HY, *et al*. Clinical outcomes associated with treatment modalities for gastrointestinal bezoars. *Gut Liver* 2014, **8**, 400–407.

2 Lee SJ, Cheon GJ, Oh WS, *et al*. Clinical characteristics of gastric bezoars. *Korean J Helicobacter Up Gastrointest Res* 2010, **10**, 49–54.

3 Van Gossum A, Delhaye M, Cremer M. Failure of nonsurgical procedures to treat gastric trichobezoar. *Endoscopy* 1989, **21**, 113.

4 Soehendra N. Endoscopic removal of a trichobezoar. *Endoscopy* 1989, **21**, 201.

5 Saeed ZA, Ramirez FC, Hepps KS, *et al*. A method for the endoscopic retrieval of trichobezoars. *Gastrointest Endosc* 1993, **39**, 698–700.

6 Konuma H, Fu K, Morimoto T, *et al*. Endoscopic retrieval of a gastric trichobezoar. *World J Gastrointest Endosc* 2011, **3**, 20–22.

7 Aybar A, Safta AM. Endoscopic removal of a gastric trichobezoar in a pediatric patient. *Gastrointest Endosc* 2011, **74**, 435–437.

8 Benatta MA. Endoscopic retrieval of gastric trichobezoar after fragmentation with electrocautery using polypectomy snare and argon plasma coagulation in a pediatrci patient. *Gastroenterol Rep (Oxf)* 2016, **4**, 251–253.

9 Kanetaka K, Azuma T, Ito S, *et al*. Two-channel method for retrieval of gastric trichobezoar: report of a case. *J Pediatr Surg* 2003, **38**, e7.

47

Natural orifice transendoluminal surgery

Mike Thomson

 KEY POINTS

- Natural orifice transendoluminal surgery (NOTES) involves performing procedures previously only occurring with standard laparoscopy or laparotomy, i.e., with an extraluminal component and application.
- Animal models of organ resection have been followed by proof of concept in adult humans but not as yet in children.

- Certain constraints exist such as lack of a triangulation capability, infection, and development of specific accessories.
- To a certain extent, it is a technology still looking for an application in children as small port and single port laparoscopy is safe and well established but this may change once the constraints mentioned above are dealt with in the coming years.

Kalloo first entered the peritoneal cavity via a gastrotomy in 2004 with an endoscope. A proposed paradigm shift from laparoscopy/laparotomy was anticipated by some, similar to that which had occurred on shifting from open surgery to minimally invasive surgery. This has not transpired as quickly or as widely as was hoped, for a number of reasons.

To a degree, certainly in children, this is an area that is still looking for an application which may make it superior to single-port laparoscopy approaches. One might class some of the endoscopic therapeutic procedures detailed in this textbook as technically fulfilling the definition of natural orifice transendoluminal surgery (NOTES), for example transoral endoscopic fundoplication, peroral endoscopic myotomy (POEM), duodenal web division, etc. However, to truly be identified as a NOTES

procedure, it really should operate in the extraluminal compartment, that is, the peritoneum.

Potential benefits are obvious as these procedures have a scarless result, may cause less catabolic stress to the patient and less postoperative discomfort and may consequently be associated with a shorter hospital stay.

Conversely, challenges remain significant to all those working in this rapidly changing field and include sepsis; lack of a triangulation approach for instruments when only one endoscope is employed – although with dual-orifice approaches with two endoscopes from different angles, this is mitigated; an evolving but still relatively young/early instrumental toolbox for transendoscopic work (needle placers and endo-scissors, etc. are constantly evolving, however); and closure of the port of entry – again, development of devices such as

Practical Pediatric Gastrointestinal Endoscopy, Third Edition. Edited by George Gershman and Mike Thomson.
© 2021 John Wiley & Sons Ltd. Published 2021 by John Wiley & Sons Ltd.
Companion website: www.wiley.com/go/gershman3e

the over-the-scope clip (OTSC), endo-clips which are rotatable and allow multiple open/close maneuvers, endo-loops, etc. have almost solved this problem. Hemorrhage may be more easily contained with the advent of approaches such as Hemospray® but standard techniques such as argon plasma cautery, uni- or bipolar cautery or hot biopsy forceps and endo-clips can also usefully be employed.

Challenges that set the child apart from the adult include different anatomy such as a more horizontal stomach, an intraabdominal bladder and proportionately larger viscera such as liver and spleen, so these factors may limit the working space available to the pediatric transluminal endoscopist. CO_2 insufflation is now standard for endoscopy in many units and hypercarbia does not seem to be an issue with endoscopy or laparoscopy using this gas.

Animal models for proof of concept are published with a number of ports of entry including oral, anal, vaginal, and combinations thereof. Procedures that have occurred in animal models include gastrojejunostomy; cholecystectomy; hysterectomy; direct visual liver biopsy; splenectomy; appendicectomy; and fallopian tube ligation.

Published work in adult humans with transgastric, transcolonic or transvaginal entry points includes appendectomy; cholecystectomy; hysterectomy; enteroenterostomy; lesion biopsy, etc.

In reality, there will increasingly be a blurring in the demarcations between the endoscopist and laparoscopist and indeed, a closer working relationship already exists in many centers with dual approaches, such as percutaneous laparoscopic-assisted jejunostomy placement. The development of a specific specialist with both of these skills is well under way in larger centers. A successful model is likely to include a multidisciplinary combined effort involving endoscopists, laparoscopists, and radiologists providing real-time imaging such as that which now occurs in MRI-guided neurosurgery and the future application of robotics.

There has been concern that NOTES would be prematurely adopted and applied to children but there now exists a sufficient body of adult work which may suggest that targeted application of this technology is ready for the pediatric field. It goes without saying that close scrutiny of safety and efficacy will be paramount in the evolution in our speciality in order that these technologies find the right home, in the right hands, and thereby avoid discreditation by more traditional practitioners.

 • See companion website for videos relating to this chapter topic: www.wiley.com/go/gershman3e

Index

Practical Pediatric Gastrointestinal Endoscopy, Third Edition. Edited by George Gershman and Mike Thomson.
© 2021 John Wiley & Sons Ltd. Published 2021 by John Wiley & Sons Ltd.
Companion website: www.wiley.com/go/gershman3e